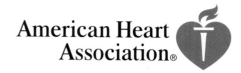

American Heart Association®

Fighting Heart Disease and Stroke

ACLS—The Reference Textbook

ACLS for Experienced Providers

Editor
Richard O. Cummins, MD, MPH, MSc
  ECC Senior Science Editor

Associate Editors
John M. Field, MD
  ACLS Science Editor
Mary Fran Hazinski, RN, MSN
  ECC Senior Science Editor

Illustrator
Anne Jorunn Svalastog

Special Contributors

Thomas A. Barnes, EdD, RRT
Robert A. Berg, MD
Paul Berlin, MS, EMT-P
Fred W. Chapman, PhD*
Alidene Doherty, RN, CCRN
Harald Eikeland*
Helge Fossan, MSc*
Henry Halperin, MD, MA
Robert S. Hoffman, MD
Judd E. Hollander, MD
William Kaye, MD
Richard E. Kerber, MD
Karl B. Kern, MD

Walter Kloeck, MD, BCh
Rashmi U. Kothari, MD
Peter J. Kudenchuk, MD
Murray Lorance, NREMT
Thomas G. Martin, MD, MPH
David G. C. McCann, MD
Steven G. Miller, MD
William H. Montgomery, MD
Graham Nichol, MD, MPH
Robert Niskanen, MSEE*
Robert O'Connor, MD, MPH
Joseph P. Ornato, MD
Mary Ann Peberdy, MD

Anthony Scalzo, MD
Steven M. Schexnayder, MD
Gregory Sinibaldi
Edward Stapleton, EMT-P
Ronald E. Stickney*
David Szpilman, MD
Robert Walker*
Ron M. Walls, MD
Roger D. White, MD
Arno Zaritsky, MD
Carolyn M. Zelop, MD

*Indicates persons asked by the editor to contribute expert review and commentary.
 At the time of their reviews they were employed by companies with products related to resuscitation.

ISBN 0-87493-424-9

i

Special Acknowledgments

Successful organizations achieve their success by employing people who come to work each day, do their job, and do it well. Over time a few individuals begin to stand out in special ways. For the American Heart Association two such people are Mary Ann McNeely, Director, ECC Product Development, and F. G. Stoddard, ECC Editor in Chief.

Mary Ann possesses a special goal-oriented blend of leadership, maturity, professionalism, and wisdom. Without her presence, perseverance, and patience this textbook would not exist. She has provided support and friendship that have been invaluable.

F.G. is also a special blend. He is that once-in-a-lifetime person we all hope to meet and know. To actually work alongside him on a project like this textbook is a special privilege. A true renaissance man, he combines a level of skill, creativity, insight, erudition, and professionalism before which I can only stand in awe. Best of all he has been my friend. Thank you, F.G.

Acknowledgments

David Barnes contributed the creative eye of an artist to his coordination of design and production; Julie Noe, Jackie Haigney, and Sarah Johnson exercised superb copyediting skills; Kara Robinson meticulously reviewed and proofread all page galleys; Colleen Halverson, Jerry Potts, and Jo Haag provided precise scientific review.

Statements of Possible Conflicts of Interest

During the preparation of this textbook Mary Fran Hazinski, RN, Richard Cummins, MD, and John Field, MD, served as part-time compensated consultants to the American Heart Association. Dr. Cummins has reported receiving financial support for noncategorical research projects from the Laerdal Foundation for Acute Medicine and from Medtronic Physio-Control Corporation. Ms. Hazinski has reported receiving equipment and expense support from Medtronic Physio-Control Corporation for one research project.

For information about contributors' potential conflicts of interest visit **www.americanheart.org/cpr** and click the link "CPR Science" to read the conflict of interest statements.

Contents

Chapter 4
Special Resuscitation Situations
Part 1: Hypothermia

Chapter 4
Part 2: Submersion

Chapter 4
Part 3: Severe, Life-Threatening Asthma

Chapter 4
Part 4: Anaphylaxis

Introduction to ACLS for Experienced Providers

ACLS for Experienced Providers: The Premise

The idea for ACLS for Experienced Providers (ACLS-EP) emerged while trying to answer two simple questions:

■ If you know the cause of a cardiac arrest, how will that knowledge change your approach to the attempted resuscitation?

■ If you encounter the potential victim of cardiac arrest 10 minutes *before* the cardiac arrest and you know the cause, will you be able to prevent the cardiac arrest?

The ACLS *Algorithm Approach*—attach a defibrillator/monitor; identify the rhythm; follow the algorithm for the rhythm—is effective for the treatment of many victims of cardiac arrest. This approach has been referred to as the "find-a-rhythm/pick-a-drug" approach. During some cardiovascular emergencies, however, the ACLS provider will need more resuscitation information and skills.

In the ACLS Course providers learn a systematic method—the Primary and Secondary Survey—that is appropriate for every resuscitation attempt. Experienced providers can expand this Primary and Secondary Survey into what is termed the *5 Quadrads Approach*. This approach can be applied to patients in cardiac arrest and to unstable patients at risk for development of a cardiopulmonary arrest.

Critical Concepts: The 5 Quadrads

Cardiac Arrest

1. Primary ABCD Survey

3. Secondary ABCD Survey

Periarrest

3. Oxygen–IV–Monitor–Fluids

4. Temperature–Heart Rate–Blood Pressure–Respirations

5. Tank volume–Tank resistance–Pump–Rate

The 5 Quadrads Approach to ACLS for Experienced Providers

The 5 quadrads are 5 sets of 4 items that cover *assessment* actions and *management* actions that apply to almost any emergency setting. Clinicians can apply the memory aid for

■ Patients in full cardiac arrest

■ Patients in full cardiac arrest who are not responding to therapy

■ Patients "on their way" to a cardiac arrest: patients who—if rescuers fail to identify specific problems and start appropriate treatments—will progress to full cardiac arrest

■ Patients who have responded to resuscitative efforts and are in the postresuscitation period

■ Any major clinical challenge or decision-making point

Important Points

■ The first 2 quadrads, the Primary and Secondary ABCD Surveys, apply to people in full cardiac arrest. These 2 quadrads can also be used to highlight fundamental assessment and actions for all patients. When rescuers evaluate airway, breathing, and circulation and perform the Secondary ABCD Survey, they may be able to correct problems and prevent deterioration to cardiac arrest.

The 3rd, 4th, and 5th quadrads apply in general to people experiencing a cardiopulmonary emergency but who have not yet developed cardiac arrest.

■ Experienced clinicians need to tailor the use of the 5 quadrads to the clinical situation. For example, cervical spine immobilization needs to be added to the Primary and Secondary ABCD Surveys when dealing with patients suffering from cardiac arrest associated with trauma, drowning, electric shock, or hypothermia. Modifications are also necessary when dealing with hypothermic cardiac arrest and cardiac arrest associated with pregnancy.

■ Some redundancy exists among the 5 quadrads. For example, the pulse and breathing checks in the Primary ABCD

Survey may identify problems with heart rate, blood pressure, and respirations that are components of the 4th quadrad (temperature–heart rate–blood pressure–respirations). Also, the support provided in the "C: Cardiovascular" step in the Secondary ABCD Survey can include elements of the "oxygen–IV–monitor–fluids" components in the 3rd quadrad. As a memory aid the "5 Quadrads" is not perfect, but it may be helpful.

Applying the 5 Quadrads

Cardiac Arrest Patients

Quadrad 1. Primary ABCD Survey

This easily remembered series of assessments and treatments covers basic CPR and defibrillation:

- **Airway:** Unresponsive (assessment); open airway (treatment).

- **Breathing:** Check breathing (assessment); if not breathing or if breathing is inadequate, provide 2 ventilations (treatment). If you cannot provide 2 ventilations (assessment), then correct a possible obstructed airway (treatment).

- **Circulation:** Check for pulse (assessment); if no pulse, provide chest compressions (treatment).

- **Defibrillation**: Check rhythm for presence of ventricular fibrillation/ventricular tachycardia (assessment); if VF or VT is present, provide direct-current shocks (treatment).

Quadrad 2. Secondary ABCD Survey

This series of assessments and treatments addresses advanced airways and pharmacologic treatment of arrhythmias. The experienced ACLS team leader also begins to think about the cause of the emergency, differential diagnoses, and alternative approaches to treatment.

- **Airway:** Determine if initial airway techniques and ventilations are adequate (assessment); if inadequate, establish advanced airway (treatment).

- **Breathing:** Check effectiveness of advanced airway and breathing support, including tube placement, oxygenation, and ventilation (assessment); provide positive-pressure ventilations through tracheal tube or other advanced airway device (treatment).

- **Circulation:** Check heart rate and attach monitor leads to determine the rhythm (assessment); establish IV access to administer fluids and medications (treatment); administer rhythm-appropriate medications (treatment).

- **Differential diagnoses:** This critical part of the treatment of a cardiopulmonary emergency requires the experienced provider to *think*. Most other steps involve dichotomous yes/no decision making. But at this time the rescuer should pause

Using the Primary and Secondary ABCD Surveys: Key Principles

Here are key principles to keep in mind when using the Primary and Secondary ABCD Surveys:

- The survey sequence addresses problems in their order of importance, using the alphabet as a helpful memory aid.

- Whenever the surveys identify a problem, *go no further* with the survey until the identified problem is resolved. For example, if you are unable to make the chest rise with ventilation ("B" of the Secondary Survey), you must solve that problem before you start an IV and administer medications.

- The survey assessments and treatments can be followed only as far as personnel and equipment resources allow. A single rescuer, for example, would be limited to basic CPR and automated defibrillation until other help arrived.

The "5 Quadrads Approach" provides an organized reminder to help the clinician recall elements of patient **assessment** *and patient* **management.**

---

to think carefully and try to identify the cause of the cardiac arrest. As various causes are considered, think of the treatment for each cause.

The differential diagnoses become of paramount importance when dealing with *asystolic* and *pulseless electrical activity* cardiac arrest. The Critical Concepts box explains how the "D" in the Secondary ABCD Survey can be expanded by using the *6 H's and 6 T's,* a memory aid for the most common and potentially reversible causes of *asystolic* and *pulseless electrical activity* cardiac arrest. The accompanying table also shows how the steps of *assessment* and *treatment* are linked with each differential diagnosis.

- When additional personnel arrive, the survey sequence tells them exactly where to enter the resuscitative effort. To illustrate, personnel arriving to assist a lone rescuer doing CPR ("ABC" of the Primary Survey) would assume responsibility for defibrillation, advanced airway management, IV access, and medications—and in that order.

- If a sufficient number of skilled personnel are available, they can proceed with the survey steps simultaneously. But the surveys supply a useful review to make sure someone has responsibility for every task.

- The Secondary Survey ends with *"D: Differential Diagnosis,"* a reminder to stop and *think*. This "D" directs rescuers, especially the team leader, to think about *why* the arrest occurred in the first place and *why* the person remains in arrest or remains unstable.

Periarrest Patients

Quadrad 3. Oxygen–IV–Monitor–Fluids

Experienced ACLS providers learn *oxygen–IV–monitor–fluids* as a single term. These assessment and treatment actions are required in virtually every cardiopulmonary emergency and should be provided for every patient. Making these actions a core part of the 5 quadrads fosters a routine that will help prevent delays or omission of these actions.

Quadrad 4. Temperature–Heart Rate–Blood Pressure–Respirations

The vital signs are probably one of the most neglected areas in training for cardiopulmonary emergencies. Nevertheless the vital signs provide critical information needed to manage these patients and evaluate their response to therapy.

Quadrad 5. Tank volume–Tank resistance–Pump–Rate

These terms summarize the concept of the 5th or *cardiovascular quadrad*. The cardiovascular quadrad directs experienced ACLS providers to consider whether patients with shock, hypotension, and

---

Critical Concepts:
"D" in the Secondary ABCD Survey: Developing Expanded Differential Diagnoses

"The 6 H's and the 6 T's"

The following table uses the memory aid of the "6 H's and 6 T's" to provide an expanded list of possible causes of asystolic or PEA cardiac arrest. Such a reminder list comes into play during the "D" part of the Secondary ABCD Survey, the *Differential Diagnoses*. The table also lists the critical assessments and treatments associated with each potential cause. The emphasis is on *reversible, treatable conditions.*

The 6 H's: Causes	Assessments	Treatments
Hypovolemia ■ Occult bleeding ■ Anaphylaxis ■ Pregnancy with gravid uterus	■ History, exam ■ Hematocrit ■ β-HCG test	■ Administer volume ■ Administer blood if needed ■ If the victim has a large uterus, turn the victim to the left side (see *ACLS-EP* Chapter 4, Part 6)
Hypoxia ■ Inadequate oxygenation	■ Breath sounds ■ Tube placement? ■ Arterial blood gas	■ Oxygen ■ Ventilation ■ Good CPR technique
Hydrogen ion ■ Acidosis ■ DKA ■ Drug overdoses ■ Renal failure	■ Clinical setting ■ Arterial blood gas ■ Lab tests	■ See *ACLS-EP* Chapter 5 ■ Maintain good CPR technique ■ Optimize perfusion ■ Establish effective oxygenation and ventilation ■ Tricyclic antidepressant overdose: bicarbonate ■ Other toxicologies: see *ACLS-EP* Chapter 3
Hypo-/hyperelectrolytes ■ Potassium, sodium, magnesium, calcium ■ History, exam	■ Risk factors	■ Treat specific electrolyte balance: see *ACLS-EP* Chapter 5 ■ Hyperkalemia: give calcium, bicarbonate, insulin, glucose
Hypo-/hyperglycemia ■ Low glucose = insulin reactions ■ DKA ■ Nonketotic, hyperosmolar coma	■ History, exam ■ Lab tests	■ See *ACLS-EP* Chapter 5 ■ Fluids ■ Potassium ■ Hyperglycemia: insulin ■ Hypoglycemia: 50% glucose
Hypo-/hyperthermia ■ Profound hypothermia ■ Heat stroke	■ Touch ■ Core body temperature	■ Hypothermia: see *ACLS-EP* Chapter 4, Part 1 ■ Hypothermia: Active/passive, external/internal rewarming ■ Hyperthermia: surface cooling

The 6 T's: Causes	Assessments	Treatments
Tablets (drug overdoses) ■ TCA, phenothiazines ■ β-Blockers, calcium channel blockers ■ Cocaine, digoxin, aspirin, acetaminophen	■ Risk factors ■ History, toxidrome	■ Specific antidotes and more comprehensive list of therapies: see *ACLS-EP* Chapter 3 ■ Possible volume therapy (titrate carefully) and vasopressors for hypotension ■ TCA overdose: bicarbonate ■ Calcium channel blocker or β-blocker overdose: glucagon, calcium ■ Cocaine overdose: benzodiazepines; do not give β-blockers ■ Prolonged CPR may be justified ■ Cardiopulmonary bypass
Trauma ■ Massive trauma ■ Electrocution, lightning strike ■ Submersion	■ History ■ Clinical setting ■ Physical exam	■ See *ACLS-EP* Chapter 4, Parts 2 "Submersion", 5 "Trauma" and 7 "Electric Shock and Lightning" ■ Rescuer safety ■ Reverse triage (give priority to patients in cardiac arrest) ■ Early tracheal intubation ■ In blunt trauma, survival after prehospital cardiac arrest is unlikely ■ In some situations (eg, small child submerged in icy water), prolonged resuscitation may be justified
Tamponade, cardiac ■ Trauma ■ Renal failure ■ Chest compressions ■ Carcinoma ■ Central line perforations	■ Risk factors ■ History ■ Prearrest picture ■ Distended neck veins ■ Echo	■ Administer volume ■ Pericardiocentesis ■ Thoracotomy
Tension pneumothorax ■ Asthma ■ Trauma ■ COPD, blebs ■ Ventilators + positive pressures	■ Risk factors ■ Lung sounds diminished ■ Tracheal deviation ■ Neck vein distention	■ Needle decompression ■ Chest tube
Thrombosis, heart ■ Acute MI ■ Other acute coronary syndromes	■ Prearrest symptoms ■ ECG ■ Serum markers	■ See Volume 1, Chapter 17, and *ACLS-EP* Chapter 2 ■ MONA (Morphine, Oxygen, Nitroglycerin, Aspirin), vasopressors ■ Emergent PTCA ■ Empiric tPA ■ Balloon pump, CABG
Thrombosis, lungs ■ Pulmonary embolus	■ Risk factors ■ History ■ Echo or V/Q	■ Administer volume ■ Dopamine ■ Heparin ■ Thrombolytics

β-HCG, human chorionic gonadotropin, beta subunit; CABG, coronary artery bypass graft; COPD, chronic obstructive pulmonary disease; DKA, diabetic ketoacidosis; PTCA, percutaneous transluminal coronary angioplasty; TCA, tricyclic antidepressant; tPA, tissue plasminogen activator; V/Q, ventilation/perfusion scan.

acute pulmonary edema have a clinical problem dominated by

■ Inadequate or excessive vascular volume (Tank volume)

■ Excessive or inadequate peripheral vascular resistance (Tank resistance)

■ Poor cardiac function as a pump (Pump)

■ Inadequate blood pressure and perfusion due to hemodynamically significant tachycardias or bradycardias (Rate)

The next section provides more detail on this topic.

The 5th (Cardiovascular) Quadrad

"Tank volume–Tank resistance–Pump–Rate" as an Aid to Diagnosis and Treatment

The *cardiovascular quadrad* is a conceptual aid to use when faced with a variety of prearrest cardiovascular emergencies and cardiac arrest unresponsive to the Primary and Secondary Surveys. The starting point for the Algorithm for Acute Pulmonary Edema, Hypotension, Shock (see *ECC Handbook*, page 21, Figure 11, and Chapter 5 in this volume) is *clinical signs of shock, hypoperfusion, congestive heart failure, acute pulmonary edema.* Just below that box is the question *"What is the most likely problem?"* This question asks the clinician to try to classify the patient's condition (if possible) into one or more categories of altered cardiovascular physiology:

■ **Intravascular volume.** The intravascular volume may be too low (*hypovolemia*) or too high. This problem can be simplified by characterizing the cardiovascular system as a hydraulic tank of a certain *size* (see below) with a certain *content* or *volume* (Tank volume).

■ **Peripheral vascular resistance.** Altered peripheral vascular resistance plays a major role in pathologic conditions like shock and acute cardiac failure. The peripheral vascular resistance (Tank resistance) affects the *size* or *capacity* of the "tank" that contains the intravascular volume and how much

work the pump must do to perfuse the lungs and the system.

■ **Pump.** The cardiovascular quadrad, in essence a *hydraulic* model, includes the heart as a variable-capacity pump that drives the flow of the intravascular volume.

■ **Rate.** Each beat of the heart or *pump* injects a certain volume into this hydraulic system. The number of times per minute that the pump beats affects the rate and volume of blood flow.

Using the Cardiovascular Quadrad

As a memory aid the 5th quadrad asks whether a patient with low blood pressure, shock, vascular congestion, or pulmonary edema has a problem with 1 or more of the 4 determinants of cardiac output:

■ Tank volume problem? (intravascular volume, fluid status): fluid loss, bleeding, gastrointestinal losses

■ Tank resistance problem? (peripheral vascular resistance, vasomotor tone): vasodilation, vasoconstriction, redistribution of blood flow and cardiac output

■ Pump problem? (contractility): either primary or secondary cardiac dysfunction

■ Rate problem? (the electrical system): either too fast or too slow

Rules for Multiple or Overlapping Problems

Once the rescuer identifies the patient's problem, the rescuer can select the appropriate therapy. The following priority of actions is recommended: First, correct *Rate* problems if present.

■ Second, correct any *Tank volume* problems with fluid or transfusions or diuresis. Always correct Tank volume problems before treating Tank resistance problems. Vasopressors will reduce tank size by increasing peripheral vascular resistance, and vasodilators will increase the tank size by reducing peripheral vascular resistance.

■ Third, treat *Pump* problems with pressors, inotropes, or both.

Each patient requires individualized treatment. But 3 rules will help you avoid major errors:

1. Do not use fluids or vasopressors when the hypotension is caused by tachycardia or bradycardia (treat rate problems first).

2. Do not use vasopressors alone to treat hypotension caused by hypovolemia (eg, shock due to gastrointestinal bleeding). Treat Tank volume problems before treating with vasopressors.

3. Do not use fluids when the tank is full and the problem is the pump. Pump problems can include acute myocardial infarction, congestive heart failure, or cardiomyopathy with acute pulmonary edema. Treat pump problems with vasopressor or inotropic agents rather than fluids.

Vasodilators may be needed to treat inadequate cardiac output with poor myocardial function. Ensure that intravascular volume is adequate before administering vasodilators, and be ready to administer additional volume if needed during vasodilator therapy.

Summary: The 5 Quadrads

Quadrad 1. Primary ABCD Survey

Airway:

■ If unresponsive, open airway.

Breathing:

■ If not breathing adequately, provide positive-pressure ventilations.

Circulation:

■ If no signs of circulation, perform chest compressions.

Defibrillation:

■ Identify and shock VF/pulseless VT, attempt defibrillation.

Quadrad 2. Secondary ABCD Survey

Airway:

- Determine the effectiveness of the primary ventilation and airway techniques.
- Remove any airway obstruction.
- Achieve airway control and protection with advanced airway techniques if indicated.

Breathing:

- Confirm placement and function of advanced airway device, verify with exhaled CO_2 device.
- Provide positive-pressure ventilations through advanced airway device.
- Support oxygenation, verify with oxygen saturation measurement.
- Treat any condition that interferes with effective oxygenation and ventilation (eg, tension pneumothorax).

- Support ventilation that produces bilateral chest wall movement.

Circulation:

- Continue chest compressions.
- Establish IV access, administer volume if needed.
- Attach monitor leads.
- Identify rhythm and rate.
- Measure blood pressure.
- Administer medications appropriate for rhythm, rate, and blood pressure.

Differential diagnosis:

- Identify and treat reversible causes of cardiovascular emergencies.
- Employ memory aids such as the 6 H's and 6 T's.

Quadrad 3. Oxygen–IV–Monitor–Fluids

- Administer oxygen.

- Establish IV access and administer IV fluids as needed.
- Monitor heart rate and rhythm.

Quadrad 4. Temperature–Heart Rate–Blood Pressure–Respirations

- Evaluate vital signs.
- Treat any reversible problems identified (eg, hypothermia, bradycardia, hypotension, inadequate breathing).

Quadrad 5. The Cardiovascular Quadrad: Tank volume–Tank resistance–Pump–Rate

- Identify and support problems with
  - Heart rate
  - Intravascular volume (Tank volume)
  - Vascular resistance (Tank resistance)
  - Pump

The ACLS 5 Quadrads Approach for Experienced Providers

Memory Aid: The ACLS *5 Quadrads Approach* for experienced providers gives a comprehensive checklist for immediate assessment and management of patients with a variety of cardiovascular emergencies, such as trauma, drug overdoses, environmental emergencies, and critical medical conditions.

Survey Step	Assess	Manage
Quadrad 1. Primary ABCD Survey		
■ **A**irway	■ Open?	■ Head tilt–chin lift; jaw thrust
(C-spine)	■ Suspicious mechanism?	■ Chin lift, jaw thrust, NO head tilt; immobilize head, neck and torso; backboard
■ **B**reathing	■ Pulse/signs of circulation?	■ Give 2 breaths; follow obstructed airway protocols if needed
■ **C**irculation	■ Moving air?	■ Chest compressions; continue CPR until AED is available
■ **D**efibrillation	■ Attach AED; paddles; monitor	■ Deliver shock(s) for VF/pulseless VT
Quadrad 2: Secondary ABCD Survey		
■ **A**irway (C-spine)	■ Adequate? ■ Signs of airway protective mechanisms (cough/gag)? ■ Signs of obstruction (noisy breathing) or pooled secretions?	■ Remove obstructions; suction — Insert oropharyngeal airway; nasal trumpet — Determine if advanced airway is needed: tracheal tube/LMA/combitube; nasotracheal intubation; surgical airways

Survey Step	Assess	Manage
■ **B**reathing (Oxygen)	■ Cords visualized? tube in trachea and confirmed by primary (5-point auscultation) and secondary confirmation techniques (exhaled CO_2 or esophageal detector device)? ■ Chest x-ray: pneumothorax? flail chest? open chest? ■ Cyanosis? moving air? Order ABG; attach O_2 saturation monitor	■ Support of airway and ventilation: see Volume 1 Chapter 8. ■ Provide oxygen by nasal cannula, face mask, Venturi mask, nonrebreathing mask at 15 L/min; with airway devices use high FiO_2 + hyperventilation + PEEP — Verify placement of advanced airway — Perform needle decompression; insert chest tube; cover/release sucking wounds as needed — Obtain mechanical ventilator
■ **C**irculation (IV-monitor-fluids)	■ Heart rate? attach monitor; assess rhythm — Is blood pressure adequate or too high? ■ Send blood for type and cross-match, lab tests (A-A-A-A-B-B-Tox*)	■ Establish IV access; administer volume as needed — Give rhythm-appropriate medications — For trauma, hemorrhage: order blood type and cross; stop visible hemorrhage; obtain serial hematocrits — If victim is pregnant with large uterus, place on left side (45°)
■ **D**ifferential **D**iagnosis **(THINK!)**	■ Assess using the "D-(CP)-D-E-E-E-F-F-F-G-G" system ■ Consider differential diagnoses by "H's and T's" mnemonic	■ Begin management of identified diagnoses
■ **D**isability-**D**-(CP)-**D**	■ Mental status? pupil response? ■ GCS score: best eye, vocal, motor response ■ For altered mental state, see Coma Protocol (right column) and reassess	■ Coma Protocol (CP): give 50 mL of $D_{50}W$; give thiamine 100 mg IV; give Narcan 2 mg IV $D_{50}W$ ■ Assess response
■ **E**xpose-**E**xamine-**E**xtremities	■ Completely expose the patient; perform quick visual check for gross injuries, signs of pregnancy, skin lesions, skin temperature, medic alert ■ Check pulse in extremities	■ Stabilize obvious injuries — Intervene if needed to restore pulse to compromised extremities — Treat other wounds
■ **F**ingers-**F**oley-**F**lip	■ Rectal, vaginal exam; check for injuries of pelvis, perineum, and genitalia, then insert Foley catheter ■ "Flip" (log-roll) patient to check back areas	■ Foley to straight drainage; send for urine specimen for analysis, including toxicology screen; observe rate of urine output

(Continued on next page)

Survey Step	Assess	Manage
■ Gastric tube-"Gunk"	■ Check contraindications to nasal insertion of tubes ■ Observe aspirate for blood, pills, odors	■ Instill "Gunk" (activated charcoal 50 g plus cathartic) down the gastric tube for suspected drug overdoses and appropriate indications
■ History	■ Document expanded history to increase differential diagnoses	■ Delay history until patient is stable ■ Question family, friends, EMS personnel
Quadrad 3. O$_2$–IV–Monitor–Fluids	■ Assess response to 1st treatment; check lab tests, x-rays	■ Continue management of identified diagnoses — Evaluate response
Quadrad 4. Temperature–HR– BP–Respirations	■ Assess excessively low or high temperatures	■ Continue management as indicated — Evaluate response
Quadrad 5. Tank volume–Tank resistance–Pump– Rate	■ Consider problems in these categories	■ Continue management as indicated — Evaluate response

*A-A-A-A-B-B-Tox indicates alcohol, acetylsalicylic acid (aspirin), acetaminophen, amylase, β-human chorionic gonadotropin, bilirubin, and toxicology screen; ABG, arterial blood gas analysis; GCS, Glasgow Coma Scale; PEEP, positive end-expiratory pressure.

Advanced Acute Coronary Syndromes Part 1: Non–ST-Elevation MI and Unstable Angina

Overview of Chapter 2

Volume 1, Chapter 17 presents the assessment and management of patients with acute chest pain suggestive of infarction. Specifically that chapter discusses patients who have ST-segment elevation MI.

This chapter presents other major aspects of ACS. Parts 1 and 2 discuss the assessment and management of patients with acute ischemic chest pain who present with ST-segment depression or nondiagnostic ST-segment or T-wave changes on ECG. Part 3 discusses potential complications of ACS, including cardiogenic shock and acute pulmonary edema. Part 4 describes several conditions that cause life-threatening chest pain, conditions that the ACLS provider must be able to distinguish from ACS.

This advanced material includes the recommendations of the international *ECC Guidelines 2000*.[1] In September 2000 a Joint Task Force on Practice Guidelines from the American College of Cardiology and the American Heart Association (ACC/AHA) published guidelines for the management of patients with unstable angina and non–ST-segment elevation myocardial infarction.[2,3] These guidelines were updated in October 2002.[4,5] To provide the most current information for ACLS providers, these ACC/AHA recommendations are included in this chapter. Although the ACC/AHA guidelines have not yet been subjected to the international ECC and resuscitation review process, the ACLS provider should be familiar with the recommendations. The American Heart Association

helped develop all of these guidelines. To avoid confusion in the following discussion, the source of each recommendation will be labeled as ECC (for AHA ECC international guidelines recommendations)[1] or ACC (for ACC/AHA guidelines).[2,4-6] The definitions of Classes of Recommendations from the Emergency Cardiovascular Care Committee are very similar to those developed by the American College of Cardiology/American Heart Association Task Force.

Part 1: Non–ST-Elevation MI and Acute Angina

Volume 1, Chapter 17 began the walk through the Acute Ischemic Chest Pain Algorithm, presenting Boxes 1 through 12 of the algorithm (see Figure 1). This portion of the algorithm is relevant to patients with ST-segment elevation indicative of infarction.

This first part of Chapter 2 continues the presentation of the Ischemic Chest Pain Algorithm:

■ Figure 2 highlights Boxes 13 through 20 of the algorithm. This part starts with the second of the 3 groups of patients with acute chest pain characterized by the initial ECG. These are the patients with ST depression or dynamic T-wave inversion on their initial 12-lead ECG.

■ Figure 3 highlights Boxes 21 through 25. These are the patients with a normal ECG or with nondiagnostic changes in

the ST segment or T waves. In the setting of acute chest pain, many of these patients will fall into the clinical category of possible "unstable" or "new-onset" angina.

12-Lead ECG: ST Depression or Dynamic T-Wave Inversion

This section discusses the care of patients with ST-segment depression or dynamic T-wave inversion on initial 12-lead ECG. It also presents the management of patients who have nondiagnostic changes on initial ECG but have positive cardiac troponins (cardiac-specific biochemical markers of cardiac necrosis, called troponin T or troponin I). The care of these patients is depicted in Boxes 13 through 20 of the Ischemic Chest Pain Algorithm (Figure 2). Patients with ischemic ST-segment depression or positive troponins constitute a high-risk subgroup, with a mortality competing with anterior Q-wave MI. They have high coronary event rates called MACE (Major Adverse Coronary Events)—death, nonfatal MI, need for urgent revascularization—despite conventional treatment with aspirin and heparin. Some of these patients will develop ST-elevation MI and develop Q-wave MI.

Because of the high risk of coronary events, the ACC/AHA Task Force[4,5] now recommends that patients with ST-segment depression or positive troponins be referred for early invasive strategy (PCI). This

FIGURE 1. ST-segment elevation MI (Boxes 1 through 12).

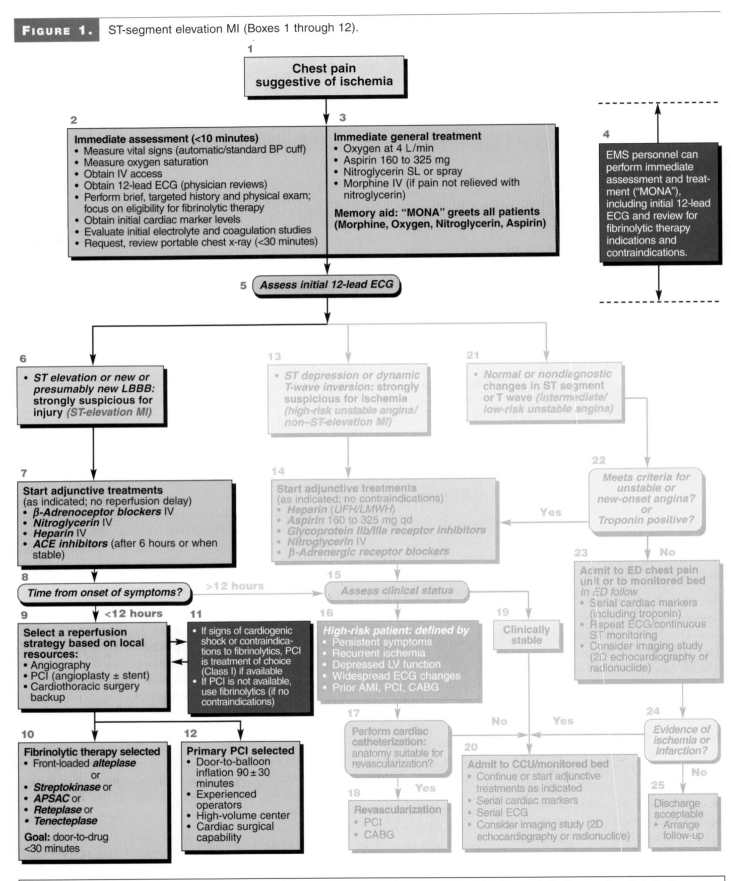

This algorithm provides general guidelines that may not apply to all patients. Carefully consider proper indications and contraindications.

FIGURE 2. Non–ST-elevation MI and high-risk angina.

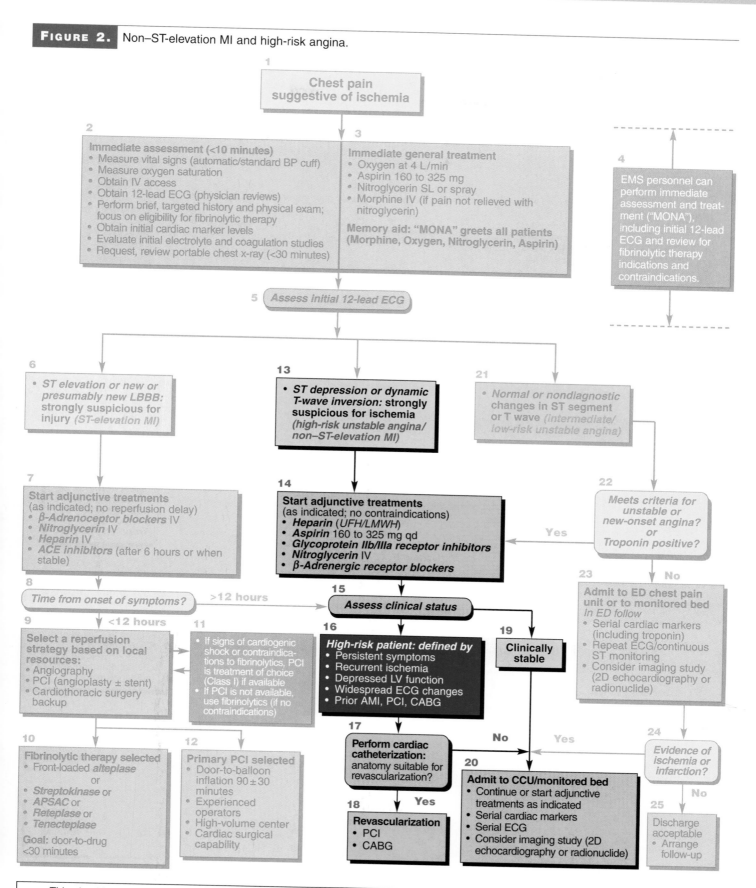

This algorithm provides general guidelines that may not apply to all patients. Carefully consider proper indications and contraindications.

FIGURE 3. Normal or nondiagnostic ECG.

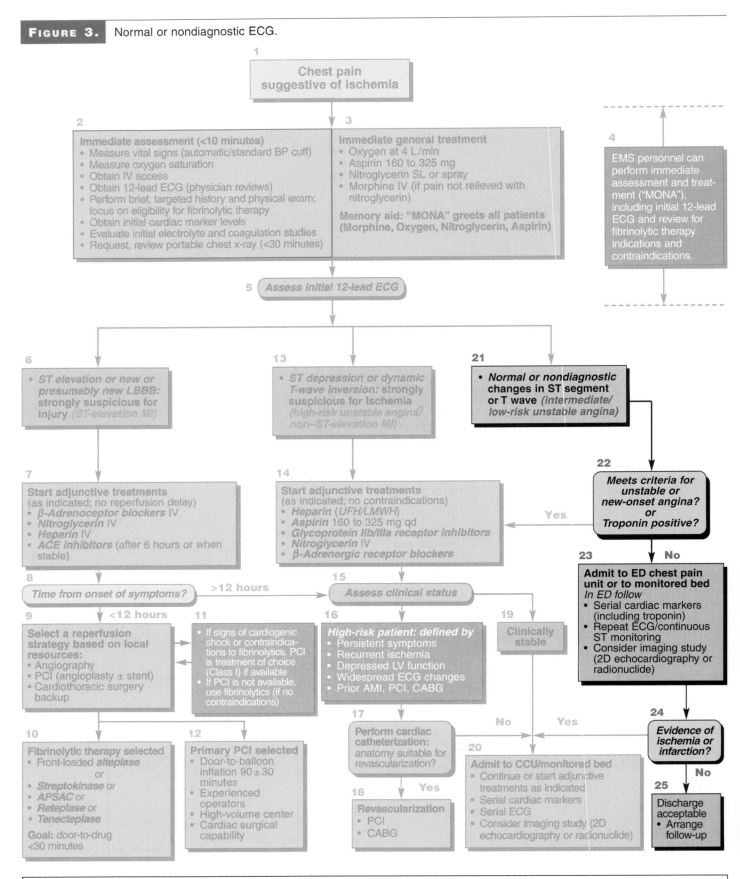

This algorithm provides general guidelines that may not apply to all patients. Carefully consider proper indications and contraindications.

recommendation is consistent with the AHA ECC Ischemic Chest Pain Algorithm, with the presumption that these patients are now known to be high-risk patients (Figure 2, Box 16).

Box 13. ST-Segment Depression or Dynamic T-Wave Inversion: Strongly Suspicious for Ischemia (High-Risk Unstable Angina/ Non–ST-Elevation MI)

The ACLS provider will initially stratify the patient's risk based on ECG. When the patient presents with ST-segment depression or dynamic T-wave changes, the ACLS provider should appreciate that this patient is at high risk for adverse cardiac events. The provider will institute therapy and also check for the presence of positive serial markers indicative of infarction. Initial markers are obtained on patient presentation and repeated once the patient is admitted to the hospital.

- **Positive serial markers (troponin positive).** If troponins are present in the patient with either ST-segment depression or nonspecific ECG changes, the patient has experienced a myocardial infarction, termed *non–ST-elevation MI.*[7]

- **Negative serial markers (troponin negative).** If serial markers are negative in the patient with ST-segment depression, the patient has *unstable angina.*

- Some patients with positive serial markers will develop Q-wave MI.

Candidates for Fibrinolytic Therapy?

Clinical trials have observed no benefit and even harm when fibrinolytic agents are administered to acute coronary syndrome (ACS) patients with ST-segment depression or T-wave inversion on initial 12-lead ECG.[4,5] Fibrinolysis releases thrombin and, paradoxically, increases the tendency toward thrombosis. In a platelet-rich initial clot, thrombin and platelet activation favor thrombogenesis. The TIMI-IIIB study concluded that the addition of a fibrinolytic

drug is not beneficial and may be harmful to patients with non–ST-elevation MI. Four intracranial hemorrhages occurred in the tPA-treated group versus none in the placebo group.[8] The 2002 ACC/AHA guidelines list intravenous fibrinolytic therapy a Class III intervention for patients without acute ST-segment elevation, a true posterior MI, or a presumed new left bundle branch block.[4,5]

Consider Posterior Current of Injury

ST-segment depression in the precordial leads V_1-V_4 may represent reciprocal depression due to a posterior wall MI. The differentiation from ST-segment depression indicative of anterior wall ischemia can be difficult. Posterior wall MI can be due to lesions in the circumflex or right coronary artery and may produce both inferior and posterior-lateral changes of infarction or posterior-lateral changes only. When ST-segment depression in V_1-V_4 is the only ECG manifestation, differential diagnosis can be difficult. The diagnosis of posterior infarction can be made if typical ST-segment elevation is present in posterior leads placed over the back of the heart, eg, V_7-V_9. Echocardiography can also be useful if it demonstrates a regional wall motion abnormality in this area. The diagnosis of posterior MI should be made with some certainty before administering fibrinolytics.

Box 14. Start Adjunctive Treatments

As indicated; no contraindications

- **Heparin** (UFH/LMWH)

- **Aspirin** 160 to 325 mg qd

- **Glycoprotein IIb/IIIa receptor inhibitors**

- **Nitroglycerin** IV

- **β-Adrenergic receptor blockers**

- *Also consider* **clopidogrel** 300 mg PO, then 75 mg PO qd

Note that patients with ST-segment depression on initial ECG are now labeled high-risk in the most recent ACC/AHA guidelines.[4,5] During the first minutes or hours

of therapy, you will also learn if the patient is troponin-positive, indicating that the patient has experienced a non–ST-segment elevation MI. Either of these conditions—ST-segment depression or troponin-positive—labels the patient as high-risk. Either of these conditions will influence the selection of adjunctive drug therapy and suggests the need for early invasive therapy (PCI).[4,5]

The international *ECC Guidelines 2000,* published in August 2000,[1] recommended addition of 2 new agents to the Ischemic Chest Pain Algorithm:

- Low-molecular-weight heparin (LMWH)

- Glycoprotein IIb/IIIa receptor inhibitors

The other adjunctive treatments recommended in *ECC Guidelines 2000* are aspirin, nitroglycerin, and β-adrenergic receptor blockers.

The more recent recommendations published by the American College of Cardiology and the American Heart Association, in September 2000,[2,3] and updated in October 2002,[4,5] added the agent clopidogrel. Clopidogrel was always indicated if the patient was aspirin intolerant; now it is used in specific instances *in addition* to aspirin.

Once you begin these therapies, you should continue to evaluate the patient for the presence of clinical indicators of high risk for MACE (see below).

Heparin (Unfractionated or Low-Molecular-Weight)

Heparin, an indirect inhibitor of thrombin, has been widely used as an adjunctive therapy for fibrin-specific lytics and, in combination with aspirin, for the treatment of unstable angina. The major advantages of low-molecular-weight heparin (LMWH) are ease of subcutaneous administration and absence of need for laboratory monitoring. The substitution of enoxaparin for unfractionated heparin in high-risk patients undergoing PCI is currently under continuing evaluation. The SYNERGY trial is randomizing approximately 8000 patients with high-risk unstable angina to receive either enoxaparin or unfractionated heparin. In addition, point of care testing for Factor Xa inhibition has recently become available for use in the catheterization suite. The effectiveness of enoxaparin can now be estimated at the time of PCI.

Recommended:

- **ECC (no class given)[1]:** Treat patients with ST-segment depression or T-wave inversion and ischemic-type chest pain with aspirin and heparin. For patients identified as high-risk for clinical deterioration (see following sections), give:

  — Aspirin and glycoprotein IIb/IIIa inhibitors *and* unfractionated heparin **or**

  — Low-molecular-weight heparin (efficacy of combination with glycoprotein IIb/IIIa inhibitors not yet established at time of international *ECC Guidelines 2000*).

- **ACC Class I[4]:** Parenteral anticoagulation with intravenous unfractionated heparin (UFH) or with subcutaneous LMWH should be added to antiplatelet therapy with ASA or a thienopyridine (clopidogrel or ticlopidine).

- **ACC Class IIa[4]:** Enoxaparin (LMWH) is preferred over unfractionated heparin in patients with ST depression or dynamic T-wave inversion in the absence of

  — Renal failure

  — Plans for coronary artery bypass graft surgery (CABG) within 24 hours

Precautions, Contraindications:

- Bleeding effects increase at higher aPTT for intravenous unfractionated heparin

- Precautions for LMWH are hypersensitivity. Use enoxaparin with caution— if at all—in patients with heparin-induced thrombocytopenia

Aspirin

Although a time-dependent effect of aspirin is not supported by evidence, aspirin should be given as soon as possible to all patients with suspected ACS unless the patient has aspirin allergy, sensitivity, or active bleeding disorders. A dose of 160 to 325 mg

causes rapid and near-total inhibition of thromboxane A_2 production, so it reduces platelet aggregation. It can reduce death and vascular events. In high-risk patients it can reduce nonfatal MI and vascular death, and it is effective in patients with unstable angina. Aspirin is often administered as four 81-mg tablets. Enteric-coated formulations are not used. An aspirin suppository is given if oral administration is not effective (eg, with nausea, vomiting).

Recommended:

- **ECC (no class given):** In the absence of contraindications, administer aspirin 160 to 325 mg PO to all patients with an ACS or ischemic-type chest pain. *Note:* You should give aspirin as soon as possible to all patients presenting with chest pain suggestive of ischemia.

- **ACC Class I[4]:** Antiplatelet therapy should be initiated promptly. ASA should be administered as soon as possible after presentation and continued indefinitely.

Cautions, Contraindications:

- Contraindicated in patients with active peptic ulcer disease, a history consistent with aspirin hypersensitivity, or bleeding disorders

Glycoprotein IIb/IIIa Receptor Inhibitors

After plaque rupture in the coronary artery, tissue factor in the lipid-rich core is exposed and forms complexes with or triggers other coagulation factors. Platelet adhesion, activation, and aggregation may result in formation of an arterial thrombus and are pivotal in the pathogenesis of ACS. The integrin glycoprotein IIb/IIIa (GP IIb/IIIa) receptor is the final common pathway to platelet aggregation, leading to binding of circulating adhesive macromolecules. Administration of a GP IIb/IIIa receptor antagonist (inhibitor) is one way of reducing acute ischemic complications after plaque fissure or rupture.

Recommended:

- **ECC Class IIa[1]:** The guidelines 2000 recommend the use of glycoprotein IIb/

IIIa receptor inhibitors for all patients with non–ST-elevation MI or high-risk unstable angina. GP IIb/IIIa inhibitors have incremental benefit in addition to conventional therapy with UFH and aspirin (Class IIa).

- **ACC 2000-2002 Recommendations:** Note that the ACC 2000 recommendations advocated the use of GP IIb/IIIa inhibitors when cardiac catheterization is planned.[2,3] The 2002 recommendations advocate the use of GP IIb/IIIa inhibitors for high-risk patients as Class I if PCI is planned and as Class IIa even if no PCI is planned.[4,5] Note that patients with ST-segment depression or positive troponins qualify as having high-risk features, so the GP IIb/IIIa inhibitors are advocated.

  — **ACC Class I:** In the absence of contraindications, administer a platelet glycoprotein IIb/IIIa inhibitor (eptifibatide, tirofiban, or abciximab) if cardiac catheterization and a PCI are planned (Box 17).

  — **ACC Class IIa:** In the absence of contraindications, administer a platelet glycoprotein IIb/IIIa inhibitor (eptifibatide or tirofiban but *not* abciximab), in addition to ASA and LMWH or UFH, to patients with continuing ischemia, an elevated troponin, or with other high-risk features if an *invasive management strategy* (cardiac catheterization and PCI) is not planned.

  — **ACC Class IIb:** For Box 14 patients who are *not* defined as high risk by continuing ischemia or other high-risk features and who will *not* be treated with PCI, consider eptifibatide or tirofiban but not abciximab. Note that this recommendation refers to patients with nondiagnostic ECG who remain troponin negative with no evidence of continuing ischemia (Boxes 23 and 25).

Precautions, Contraindications:

- Active internal bleeding or bleeding disorder in past 30 days (thrombocytopenia, platelets <150 000)

- History of intracranial hemorrhage, neoplasm, arteriovenous malformation, aneurysm, or stroke within 30 days, major surgical procedure or trauma within 1 month

- Aortic dissection, pericarditis, and severe hypertension

- Hypersensitivity

Nitroglycerin IV Infusion

Nitroglycerin reduces myocardial oxygen demand while enhancing myocardial oxygen delivery. Nitroglycerin, an endothelium-independent vasodilator, has both peripheral and coronary vascular effects that contribute to increased oxygen delivery and reduced oxygen demand. By dilating the capacitance vessels (ie, the venous beds), it increases venous pooling to decrease myocardial preload and myocardial oxygen consumption. More modest effects on the arterial circulation decrease afterload, contributing to further reduction in myocardial oxygen consumption and increased oxygen delivery.[3,4]

Recommended:

- **ECC (no class indicated)[1]:** Nitroglycerin is indicated for the initial management of pain and ischemia with ACS without hypotension (SBP <90 mm Hg) except in patients with RV infarction. Evidence does not support the routine administration of nitroglycerin in patients with uncomplicated AMI. Give IV nitroglycerin for the following:

  - If pain is not controlled with up to 3 sublingual nitroglycerin tablets, 3 metered spray doses, or nitroglycerin paste

  - If pain recurs after initial abatement

  - If blood pressure is elevated after giving β-blockers

  - If signs of congestive heart failure develop

- **ACC Class I[2-5]:** Nitroglycerin, sublingual tablet or spray, followed by intravenous administration, for the immediate relief of ischemia and associated symptoms.

Contraindications:

- Hypotension (systolic blood pressure <90 mm Hg)

- Right ventricular infarction

- Viagra use within previous 24 hours

Precautions:

- Use with caution if SBP <100 mm Hg

- Inferior ECG changes (possible RV infarction)

β-Adrenoceptor Blocking Agents (β-Blockers)

β-Blockers block sympathetic nervous system stimulation of heart rate and contractility, resulting in vasodilation and reduced ventricular afterload. They can reduce infarct size, decrease postinfarction ischemia, and reduce incidence of ventricular ectopy and fibrillation.

Recommended:

- **ECC (no class indicated)[1]:** Start β-blocker therapy within 12 hours of onset of infarction; β-blockers are usually administered in the ED unless contraindications are present. β-Blockers are also indicated for recurrent or continuing ischemia.

- **ACC Class I[2-5]:** In the absence of contraindications, start β-blocker therapy in all patients with ST depression or dynamic T-wave inversion (non–ST-elevation MI and unstable angina).

- **ACC Class IIa[2-5]:** In the absence of contraindications, give β-blockers to ischemic chest pain patients with a nondiagnostic ECG who develop

  - Continuing or recurrent ischemic pain

  - Tachyarrhythmias (eg, atrial fibrillation with a rapid ventricular response)

Precautions, Contraindications:

The following are absolute contraindications to β-blocker therapy:

- Severe LV failure and pulmonary edema

- Bradycardia (heart rate <60 bpm)

- Hypotension (SBP <100 mm Hg)

- Signs of poor peripheral perfusion

- Second- or third-degree heart block

Clopidogrel

Clopidogrel is a thienopyridine, or an adenosine diphosphate (ADP) antagonist, that is used for antiplatelet therapy. It is at least as effective as ASA. It is indicated in patients who are unable to tolerate ASA. Note that full effect will not develop for several days.

Recommended:

- **ACC Class I[4]:** In the absence of contraindications, administer clopidogrel (300 mg PO, followed by 75 mg PO qd for 1 to 9 months) as soon as possible to all patients with ST depression or dynamic T-wave inversion (non–ST-elevation MI and unstable angina) if

  - An in-hospital conservative approach is planned *or*

  - Cardiac catheterization and PCI are planned and the risk for bleeding is not high

Box 15. Assess Clinical Status ("Risk Stratification")

Box 15 directs the clinician to assess clinical status. This step translates as *clinical* "risk stratification," based on the patient's clinical appearance and likelihood of further deterioration. Do not make this step more complicated than it should be. Patients with ST-segment depression or positive troponins are already at high risk for adverse cardiac events. These patients are not candidates for fibrinolytic therapy because no benefit results and there is a risk of potential harm. These patients may have any of the following:

- ST-segment depression ≥0.5 mm or dynamic T-wave inversion pain.

- Transient ST-segment elevation ≥0.5 mm for <20 minutes. Note: This transient

ST-segment elevation for <20 minutes is treated the same as ST-segment *depression* in the ACC/AHA recommendations. To group this transient elevation with ST-segment depression, cardiologists use the term "ST-segment *deviation* ≥0.5 mm."

■ Nonspecific or nondiagnostic ST or T-wave changes with release of cardiac markers (specifically troponin I or T)

See Part 2 of this chapter for more specific recommendations for clinical risk stratification.

Early Conservative vs Early Invasive Strategies

By 2002 treatment strategies have been developed using evidence-based trials and clinical bedside risk-stratification of patients.[4,5]

■ The *early invasive strategy* recommends *routinely* taking patients with unstable angina or non–ST-elevation MI to cardiac catheterization and angiographically directed revascularization when indicated.

■ The *early conservative strategy* recommends initial management of stable patients with antiplatelet, antithrombin, and antianginal therapy. The recurrence of symptoms despite adequate therapy or the finding of high-risk features based on clinical criteria or on stress testing is then an indication for coronary angiography.

Note that the Ischemic Chest Pain Algorithm reflects the early conservative strategy but does indicate the option for the early invasive strategy. The ACC/AHA Task Force on the Management of Patients With Unstable Angina recently concluded that the latest clinical trials comparing early conservative and early invasive strategies showed an improved outcome for patients at intermediate or high risk when assigned to the invasive strategy. For this reason the task force made the early invasive strategy a Class I recommendation in the 2002 update of the guidelines for patients with unstable angina and non–ST-elevation MI at intermediate or high

risk of MACE.[4,5] This class of recommendation is consistent with the algorithm if you note that the patient with ST-segment depression or positive troponins is included in the high-risk categories listed in Box 16.

Box 16. High-Risk Patient

Patients with ST depression, dynamic T-wave inversion, or unstable angina are considered high-risk candidates for an early invasive strategy of cardiac catheterization and PCI.

Consensus panels[2,4,9-14] and clinical trial coordinators[15] have developed a variety of approaches to defining high-risk patients. These approaches often mix historical factors (prior AMI, prior PCI), prior CAD (known stenosis >50%), and demographic factors (male gender, age >65 years).

In the Ischemic Chest Pain Algorithm, *ECC Guidelines 2000* provides a brief list of clinically useful factors for defining high risk. These are contemporaneous "bedside criteria":

■ Persistent symptoms

■ Recurrent ischemia

■ Depressed LV function

■ Widespread ECG changes

■ Prior AMI, PCI, or CABG

In 2002 the ACC/AHA Task Force on the Management of Patients With Unstable Angina published a detailed list of high-risk indicators that now include all patients with ST-depression and positive troponins[4]:

■ Recurrent angina or ischemia at rest or with low-level activities (occurs despite intensive anti-ischemic therapy)

■ Recurrent angina or ischemia with symptoms of CHF, an S_3 gallop, pulmonary edema, worsening rales, or new or worsening mitral regurgitation

■ Elevated troponin T or I

■ New or presumably new ST-segment depression

■ High-risk findings on noninvasive stress testing

■ Depressed LV systolic function (eg, ejection fraction <40% on noninvasive study)

■ Hemodynamic instability

■ Sustained ventricular tachycardia

■ PCI within previous 6 months

■ Prior CABG

According to the 2002 ACC/AHA guidelines, PCI or CABG, when indicated and feasible, would be a Class I recommendation for any patients with any of the above high-risk indications and an unstable coronary syndrome.[4,5] This means that the 2002 ACC/AHA guidelines recommend referral of these high-risk patients to facilities with cardiac catheterization suites and interventional capability.[2,4,16,17] For the more than 80% of US hospitals that are not equipped for cardiac catheterization, the clinician should consider EMS triage or transfer to a medical center that has such capabilities.

Box 17. Perform Cardiac Catheterization: Anatomy Suitable for Revascularization?

Coronary angiography identifies lesions at-risk for occlusion, with a high level of ischemic potential. These are called "target lesions." When technically feasible, angioplasty is performed to dilate these target lesions. In addition, the majority of patients today also receive a metal scaffold, called a stent, to maintain vessel patency. This is possible in most single vessel disease and in some patients with more than one lesion. Coronary artery bypass surgery, if not contraindicated, is performed for patients with multiple target lesions, particularly diabetic patients.

Box 18. Revascularization

When indicated, PCI—either angioplasty alone or angioplasty with stent placement—may reduce the incidence of MACE and decrease the incidence of recurrent ischemia.[9,16,18]

Coronary artery bypass grafting is indicated primarily for patients with stenosis of the left main coronary artery or severe multivessel disease when other therapies have failed.[19] The ACC/AHA indications for urgent CABG surgery in patients with anatomy suitable for surgery are

- Failed angioplasty with persistent pain (Class I)
- Hemodynamic instability (Class I)
- Ischemia refractory to medical therapy plus the patient is not a candidate for catheter-based intervention (Class I)
- Cardiogenic shock (Class IIa)
- Failed PTCA with a small area of myocardium at risk (Class IIb)

Box 19. Clinically Stable

Patients presenting with ischemic chest pain and ST-segment depression or T-wave inversion should not be considered clinically stable unless they are free of pain and virtually asymptomatic. Exercise stress testing should not be performed in patients with high-risk unstable symptoms until they are pain free on medical therapy for 24 to 48 hours. A functional study, eg, adenosine thallium or dobutamine stress echocardiography, may be appropriate in selected patients.

Morphine, intravenous nitroglycerin, and intravenous β-blockers may still be needed. These patients display none of the high-risk criteria (Box 16). With rare exceptions these patients will require hospital admission (Box 20).

Box 20. Admit to CCU/Monitored Bed

- **Continue or start adjunctive treatments as indicated (see Box 14)**
- **Obtain serial cardiac-specific markers**
- **Obtain serial ECGs**
- **Consider imaging study (2D echocardiography or radionuclide)**

Patients can arrive at this point in the Ischemic Chest Pain Algorithm from 4 different subsets:

- **Clinically stable patients with ST-segment depression or dynamic T-wave inversion (Box 19):** This group represents part of the continuum between chronic stable angina and non–ST-elevation MI. Unlike patients with ST-segment elevation, these patients probably do not have total occlusion of the coronary artery. The majority of these patients will not develop Q-wave MI.

- **High-risk patients with ST-segment depression or dynamic T-wave inversion who are not candidates for revascularization (Box 17):** Continue or start all indicated adjunctive therapy, in particular aspirin, nitroglycerin, heparin, β-blockers, or calcium channel blockers. Continue oxygen and analgesia.

- **Patients with an initially nondiagnostic ECG who produce evidence of rest ischemia or infarction (Box 24):** Many patients will probably evolve to have a non–Q-wave infarction. This course is more common in the elderly and in patients with a prior MI. The incidence appears to be increasing because of the greater use of aspirin and β-blockers.

- **Clinically stable patients with ST elevation who are more than 12 hours from the onset of symptoms (Box 8).**

All 4 groups need admission to the Coronary Care Unit or a monitored bed:

- Continue or start adjunctive treatments as indicated (see Box 14). Making these patients pain-free continues to be a major goal. Adjunctive treatments should continue or be started on the basis of specific indications (Box 14).

- Obtain serial cardiac-specific markers and serial ECGs. If serial ECGs reveal development of persistent ST *elevation,* consider fibrinolytic therapy. Consider the indications and contraindications for alternative reperfusion strategies (Boxes 9 and 10).

- Consider obtaining an imaging study (radionuclide or 2D echocardiography). These studies can diagnose abnormalities in wall motion and will help to further "risk stratify" the patient.

12-Lead ECG: Nondiagnostic or Normal

This section discusses Boxes 21 through 25 of the Ischemic Chest Pain Algorithm (Figure 3).

Box 21. Normal or Nondiagnostic ECG: Absence of Diagnostic Changes in ST Segment or T Waves (Intermediate/Low-Risk Unstable Angina)

- For patients who have not yet received aspirin, nitroglycerin, and morphine as indicated, immediately administer these agents, especially if pain continues.

- Control of pain with intravenous morphine and nitroglycerin should be a major goal, as it is for all patients with a suspected acute coronary syndrome.

Box 22. Meets Criteria for Unstable OR New-Onset Angina? OR Troponin I or T Positive?

Box 22 focuses the clinician on an important decision: Does the patient meet criteria for unstable or new-onset angina? This decision has major therapeutic implications.

- Patients who are classified as having unstable or new-onset angina or who are troponin positive, need to be started on intravenous heparin. This requires that you shift the patient's care to Box 14 and pursue the high-risk therapy.

- Other adjunctive treatments, discussed in Box 14, may be indicated.

The Nomenclature of Angina[2,3]

- **Stable angina:** Stable angina is a clinical syndrome usually characterized by a deep, poorly localized chest or arm discomfort. Stable angina is *reproducibly* associated with physical exertion or emotional stress and is *predictably* and promptly (less than 5 minutes) relieved with rest or sublingual nitroglycerin.

Patients learn, through experience, how much physical exertion they can perform before the symptoms of angina begin. They also learn how soon and to what degree rest or nitroglycerin relieves the pain.

- **Unstable angina:** Acute process of myocardial ischemia that is not of sufficient severity and duration to cause myocardial necrosis. Patients with unstable angina typically do not present with ST-segment elevation on ECG and do not release cardiac-specific biomarkers.[2,3] In general, unstable angina is a change in the pattern of predictability of stable angina. There are 3 principal presentations of unstable angina:

    — **Rest angina:** Angina that occurs at rest, usually lasting more than 20 minutes.

    — **New-onset angina:** Chest pain that starts with physical exertion and that produces marked limitation of ordinary physical activity. It occurs on walking 1 to 2 blocks on the level and climbing 1 flight of stairs under normal conditions and at normal pace. Symptom onset is within the past 2 weeks.

    — **Increasing angina:** Previously diagnosed angina that is distinctly more frequent, longer in duration, or lower in threshold. *Threshold* refers to the level of activity (or class of angina) that induces pain.

- **Classes of angina:** Angina can be graded according to the amount of physical activity that causes the pain:

    — **Class I:** Ordinary physical activity does not cause the angina. Pain requires strenuous, rapid, or prolonged exercise.

    — **Class II:** Slight limitation of ordinary activity. Pain occurs on (1) walking or climbing stairs rapidly, walking uphill, climbing stairs after meals, or walking in the wind or cold, or (2) walking more than 2 blocks or climbing more than 1 flight of stairs at normal pace.

    — **Class III:** Marked limitation of ordinary physical activity. Pain occurs after walking 1 or 2 blocks on the level or climbing 1 or 2 flights of stairs at normal pace.

    — **Class IV:** Inability to carry on any physical exertion without discomfort.

New-Onset Angina vs AMI?

What is the distinction between new-onset angina and the pain of a classic AMI? The most frequent presentation of documented AMI is the sudden onset of severe, prolonged (>20 minutes), substernal chest pain or pressure *at rest*.

By definition, angina has a clear relation to physical activity and exertion. But the majority of patients with new-onset angina, a form of unstable angina, have pain at rest. The pain is due to the dynamic nature of the partially occluding thrombus. In these patients endothelial function is also impaired and focal spasm may further reduce coronary flow. Experiments have shown cyclical reduction in coronary flow corresponding to ST-segment changes, both with and without clinical symptoms.

For this reason the distinction between unstable angina and AMI is difficult to make on history alone. *The most urgent clinical obligation is to identify the subset of patients who have associated ST-segment elevation. An ECG is obtained within 10 minutes of presentation and interpreted by the physician most experienced in the risk-stratification of patients with acute coronary syndromes and the risk-benefit application of fibrinolytic therapy. These patients are the urgent reperfusion candidates.*

Troponin I or T Positive?

The identification and refinement of sensitive and cardiac-specific markers indicating myocardial necrosis has significantly altered our understanding of acute coronary syndromes. The release of troponin I or T by patients with ischemic chest pain, even if they have a normal or nondiagnostic ECG, predictably defines a group at risk for adverse outcomes. These patients have non–ST-elevation MI. For this reason

Box 22 directs the clinician to use the adjunctive treatments listed in Box 14 to assess and manage chest pain patients with nondiagnostic ECGs but with acute troponin I or T release.

Box 23. Admit to ED Chest Pain Unit or to Monitored Bed

In the ED follow:

- **Serial cardiac-specific markers (including troponin T and I)**

- **Repeat ECG/continuous ST-segment monitoring**

- **Consider imaging study (2D echocardiography or radionuclide)**

At this point the clinician must make several critical decisions about patients with the following features:

- Ischemic-like chest pain on presentation but now pain-free, either with or without morphine, nitroglycerin, or β-blockers

- A nondiagnostic or normal ECG

- Absence of criteria for unstable angina

- Negative initial cardiac-specific markers

The clinician must be aware of and understand the following critical observations:

- A normal ECG does not rule out an acute coronary syndrome; the sequence of ECG changes that indicate an AMI may start within 1 hour or may take up to 24 hours to develop. For this reason you should obtain a second ECG if the chest pain persists or recurs to any degree. Obtain a second ECG during pain if the pain recurs, preferably before the administration of nitroglycerin, Do not, however, impose a significant delay in nitroglycerin administration solely for an "ECG-during-pain."

- Cardiac-specific markers of MI do not begin to become positive until several hours after damage to myocardial cells occurs. The ACC/AHA guidelines recommend obtaining a *second* set of cardiac markers (troponin I or T and CK-MB) when initial levels are not elevated.

Recommendations vary, even within the ACC/AHA guidelines, on when to obtain the second set of enzymes.[5] The issues, discussed in detail in the ACC/AHA guidelines, relate to the "release-kinetics" of the different biomarkers and laboratory familiarity with particular assay techniques. Neither troponin I and T nor CK-MB achieves accuracy sensitivity until approximately 6 hours after symptom onset. Ideally you should obtain the second set 8 to 12 hours after the onset of chest pain, but 6 hours is acceptable in low-risk chest pain patients.

- Radionuclide imaging and 2D echocardiography can detect abnormalities in wall motion early in MI, even earlier than ECG and serial marker changes.

- Early rest or provocative testing (eg, treadmill stress testing) of these low-risk and some intermediate-risk patients has an acceptable degree of sensitivity and safety for further risk-stratifying these patients. The type of stress test is usually determined by local expertise, preferences, and availability of personnel.

- Patients presenting with chest pain syndromes require continuous risk factor stratification during evaluation. (See Part 2.) In isolation neither the history nor the ECG will identify patients at risk or free of disease. At a point during the evaluation when a noncardiac etiology is identified, patients are treated for this noncardiac diagnosis and discharged from the chest pain evaluation protocol.

- For those patients at low or intermediate risk of coronary artery disease, with unchanged ECGs, no recurrent discomfort, and negative cardiac-specific markers, a stress study to provoke ischemia is indicated:

  — Low-risk patients with a low likelihood of coronary artery disease may be discharged with a stress evaluation scheduled within 72 hours. These patients constitute the minority of patients evaluated for acute chest pain.

  — Intermediate risk patients should undergo stress testing before discharge, and if ischemia is demonstrated, they are admitted for treatment as an "UA/NSTEMI" patient. (See Part 2 of this chapter.)

Objective evaluation can take the form of

- Serial cardiac markers
- Serial or continuous ECGs
- 2D echocardiography or radionuclide cardiac imaging
- Provocative testing

A variety of alternatives are available to replace the expensive practice of "admit to CCU—rule out AMI." These approaches are acceptable provided that you closely monitor the patient. They include

- Hospital admission to an intermediate level "telemetry observation" or "step-down" unit

- Admission to a "chest pain evaluation unit" (often a designated area within the ED), where 2D echocardiography, radionuclide cardiac imaging, or stress testing can be performed or initiated

- Continued evaluation for several hours in a monitored ED bed

Box 24. Evidence of Ischemia or Infarction?

If objective evidence confirms ischemia or infarction during the hours of ED observation and evaluation, you should admit the patient to the Coronary Care Unit or equivalent monitored bed.

In the past physicians weighed evidence to determine whether to admit a patient with chest pain to the hospital. Physicians must abandon this subjective balancing of "pros and cons" when making decisions for chest pain patients. Contemporary decision making can no longer be dependent on implicit clinical judgment (see "Critical Concepts: The Clinical Judgment Fallacy"). It is now dependent on explicit objective information. Multiple changes in practice are occurring:

- **Fewer CCU admissions:** Fewer patients are immediately admitted to rule out AMI than in the past. AMI can now be ruled out over 4 to 8 hours in the ED.

- **Fewer rapid ED discharges:** Fewer patients are discharged quickly from the ED on the basis of the history, physical examination, a normal initial ECG, and normal initial cardiac markers. They now need to stay for 4 to 8 hours for evaluation of at least 1 repeat ECG, at least 1 repeat set of cardiac-specific markers, and the clinical course over several hours.

- **Longer ED stays:** Not only are fewer patients discharged quickly, the ED stay is longer. Patients spend more time in the ED or "chest pain center" waiting for the 2 sets of cardiac markers and serial ECGs, which are obtained several hours apart.

- **More complex ED workups:** Longer stays in the ED allow more evaluations, in particular early provocative testing, to be performed. These evaluations often initiate a series of cardiology outpatient evaluations.

- **More use of intermediate care units, step-down units, and short hospital stays (<24 hours):** Physicians can now more accurately place patients into various risk categories.

Box 25. Discharge Acceptable

- **Arrange follow-up**

Note: Patients to be discharged should have experienced complete relief of pain early after presenting to the ED unless a noncardiac cause of pain has been identified. If the pain was not quickly eliminated soon after ED presentation or if pain recurs during evaluation, then the patient is considered at least intermediate risk.

If objective evidence (minimum of 2 normal ECGs with no ST-segment deviation or significant changes plus 2 sets of normal cardiac markers obtained 6 or more hours apart) excludes myocardial necrosis and stratifies the patient as low-risk for MACE, the patient can be discharged

Critical Concepts:
The "Clinical Judgment"
Fallacy

Recently published consensus guidelines clearly establish that clinicians cannot rule out an acute coronary syndrome in patients with typical ischemic chest pain symptoms on the basis of history, physical examination, risk factor evaluation and "clinical judgment" alone. This principle holds even if the initial 12-lead ECG is normal or nondiagnostic and even if the initial cardiac biomarkers are normal. Since the acute coronary syndromes require the passage of time in order to be definitively diagnosed (or to be ruled out) most of these patients are looking at a 6 to 12 hour period of observation with both a repeat ECG and a repeat set of cardiac biomarkers near the end of that observation period. ED nurses and staff commonly refer to getting "the 6-hour EKG and CPP" (chest pain panel). Physicians, following initial evaluation, may refer to a patient's status as another "6-hour rule-out."

Failure by the responsible clinician to understand and follow these principles has led to many bad outcomes for these patients. Many of them will later prove to have been experiencing an acute coronary syndrome. These bad outcomes can include greater loss of myocardium through untreated infarctions, and even death from related arrhythmias. The current "standard of care" has become for the "reasonably prudent" physician to obtain additional objective evidence that myocardial ischemia or infarction has not occurred, or is not occurring in patients with a "good story" of chest pain. This is no longer a matter left to "clinical judgment."

with specific instructions and follow-up. These actions not only constitute appropriate clinical care but also are prudent risk management for ED physicians.

■ The responsible physician should arrange for timely follow-up of the patient. Document these arrangements in writing in the medical record. If practical, communicate directly (voice-to-voice) with the physician who will take responsibility for the patient's continued evaluation.

■ Ask the patient to sign a statement confirming the patient's understanding and acceptance of the follow-up plans, and place the statement in the medical record. In contemporary emergency medicine practice this statement most conveniently takes the form of a copy of the signed discharge instructions to the patient.

■ Instruct patients to phone 911 and request EMS transport to return to the ED if any of their symptoms recur.

References

1. American Heart Association in collaboration with International Liaison Committee on Resuscitation. Guidelines 2000 for Cardiopulmonary Resuscitation and Emergency Cardiovascular Care: International Consensus on Science, Part 7: The Era Of Reperfusion: Section 1: Acute Coronary Syndromes (Acute Myocardial Infarction). *Circulation.* 2000;102:I172-I203.

2. Braunwald E, Antman EM, Beasley JW, Califf RM, Cheitlin MD, Hochman JS, Jones RH, Kereiakes D, Kupersmith J, Levin TN, Pepine CJ, Schaeffer JW, Smith EE 3rd, Steward DE, Theroux P, Gibbons RJ, Alpert JS, Eagle KA, Faxon DP, Fuster V, Gardner TJ, Gregoratos G, Russell RO, Smith SC Jr. ACC/AHA guidelines for the management of patients with unstable angina and non-ST-segment elevation myocardial infarction: executive summary and recommendations. A report of the American College of Cardiology/American Heart Association task force on practice guidelines (committee on the management of patients with unstable angina). *Circulation.* 2000;102:1193-1209.

3. Braunwald E, Antman EM, Beasley JW, Califf RM, Cheitlin MD, Hochman JS, Jones RH, Kereiakes D, Kupersmith J, Levin TN, Pepine CJ, Schaeffer JW, Smith EE III, Steward DE, Theroux P, Alpert JS, Eagle KA, Faxon DP, Fuster V, Gardner TJ, Gregoratos G, Russell RO, Smith SC Jr. ACC/AHA guidelines for the management of patients with unstable angina and non-ST-segment elevation myocardial infarction. A report of the American College of Cardiology/American Heart Association Task Force on Practice Guidelines (Committee on the Management of Patients With Unstable Angina). *J Am Coll Cardiol.* 2000;36:970-1062.

4. Braunwald E, Antman EM, Beasley JW, Califf RM, Cheitlin MD, Hochman JS, Jones RH, Kereiakes D, Kupersmith J, Levin TN, Pepine CJ, Schaeffer JW, Smith EE 3rd, Steward DE, Theroux P, Gibbons RJ, Alpert JS, Faxon DP, Fuster V, Gregoratos G, Hiratzka LF, Jacobs AK, Smith SC Jr. ACC/AHA guideline update for the management of patients with unstable angina and non-ST-segment elevation myocardial infarction—2002: summary article: a report of the American College of Cardiology/American Heart Association Task Force on Practice Guidelines (Committee on the Management of Patients With Unstable Angina). *Circulation.* 2002;106:1893-1900.

5. Braunwald E, Antman EM, Beasley JW, Califf RM, Cheitlin MD, Hochman JS, Jones RH, Kereiakes D, Kupersmith J, Levin TN, Pepine CJ, Schaeffer JW, Smith EE 3rd, Steward DE, Theroux P, Gibbons RJ, Alpert JS, Faxon DP, Fuster V, Gregoratos G, Hiratzka LF, Jacobs AK, Smith SC Jr. ACC/AHA 2002 guideline update for the management of patients with unstable angina and non-ST-segment elevation myocardial infarction—summary article: a report of the American College of Cardiology/American Heart Association task force on practice guidelines (Committee on the Management of Patients With Unstable Angina). *J Am Coll Cardiol.* 2002;40:1366-1374.

6. Braunwald E, Antman EM, Beasley JW, Califf RM, Cheitlin MD, Hochman JS, Jones RH, Kereiakes D, Kupersmith J, Levin TN, Pepine CJ, Schaeffer JW, Smith EE 3rd, Steward DE, Theroux P, Alpert JS, Eagle KA, Faxon DP, Fuster V, Gardner TJ, Gregoratos G, Russell RO, Smith SC Jr. ACC/AHA guidelines for the management of patients with unstable angina and non-ST-segment elevation myocardial infarction. A report of the American College of Cardiology/American Heart Association Task Force on Practice Guidelines (Committee on the Management of Patients With Unstable Angina). *J Am Coll Cardiol.* 2000;36:970-1062.

7. Alpert JS, Thygesen K, Antman E, Bassand JP. Myocardial infarction redefined—a consensus document of The Joint European Society of Cardiology/American College of Cardiology Committee for the redefinition of myocardial infarction. *J Am Coll Cardiol.* 2000;36:959-969.

8. TIMI-3B Investigators. Effects of tissue plasminogen activator and a comparison of early invasive and conservative strategies in unstable angina and non-Q-wave myocardial infarction. Results of the TIMI IIIB Trial. Thrombolysis in Myocardial Ischemia. *Circulation.* 1994;89:1545-1556.

9. Scanlon PJ, Faxon DP, Audet AM, Carabello B, Dehmer GJ, Eagle KA, Legako RD, Leon DF, Murray JA, Nissen SE, Pepine CJ, Watson RM, Ritchie JL, Gibbons RJ, Cheitlin MD, Gardner TJ, Garson A Jr, Russell RO Jr, Ryan TJ, Smith SC Jr. ACC/AHA guidelines for coronary angiography: executive summary and recommendations. A report of the American College of Cardiology/American Heart Association Task Force on Practice Guidelines (Committee on Coronary Angiography) developed in collaboration with the Society for Cardiac Angiography and Interventions. *Circulation.* 1999;99:2345-2357.

10. Guideline for the management of patients with acute coronary syndromes without persistent ECG ST segment elevation. British Cardiac Society Guidelines and Medical Practice Committee and Royal College of Physicians Clinical Effectiveness and Evaluation Unit. *Heart.* 2001;85:133-142.

11. Clinical policy: critical issues in the evaluation and management of adult patients presenting with suspected acute myocardial infarction or unstable angina. American College of Emergency Physicians. *Ann Emerg Med.* 2000;35:521-525.

12. Doukky R, Calvin JE. Risk stratification in patients with unstable angina and non-ST segment elevation myocardial infarction: evidence-based review. *J Invasive Cardiol.* 2002;14:215-220.

13. Doukky R, Calvin JE. Part II: risk stratification in patients with unstable angina and non-ST segment elevation myocardial infarction: evidence-based review. *J Invasive Cardiol.* 2002;14:254-262.

14. Braunwald E, Jones RH, Mark DB, Brown J, Brown L, Cheitlin MD, Concannon CA, Cowan M, Edwards C, Fuster V, et al. Diagnosing and managing unstable angina. Agency for Health Care Policy and Research. *Circulation.* 1994;90:613-622.

15. TIMI Investigators, Antman EM, Cohen M, Bernink PJ, McCabe CH, Horacek T, Papuchis G, Mautner B, Corbalan R, Radley D, Braunwald E. The TIMI risk score for unstable angina/non-ST elevation MI: A method for prognostication and therapeutic decision making. *JAMA.* 2000;284:835-842.

16. Smith SC Jr, Dove JT, Jacobs AK, Kennedy JW, Kereiakes D, Kern MJ, Kuntz RE, Popma JJ, Schaff HV, Williams DO, Gibbons RJ, Alpert JP, Eagle KA, Faxon DP, Fuster V, Gardner TJ, Gregoratos G, Russell RO. ACC/AHA guidelines for percutaneous coronary intervention (revision of the 1993 PTCA guidelines)—executive summary: a report of the American College of Cardiology/American Heart Association Task Force on Practice Guidelines (Committee to Revise the 1993 Guidelines for Percutaneous Transluminal Coronary Angioplasty) endorsed by the Society for Cardiac Angiography and Interventions. *Circulation.* 2001;103:3019-3041.

17. Pollack CV Jr, Gibler WB. 2000 ACC/AHA guidelines for the management of patients with unstable angina and non-ST-segment elevation myocardial infarction: a practical summary for emergency physicians. *Ann Emerg Med.* 2001;38:229-240.

18. Smith SC Jr, Dove JT, Jacobs AK, Kennedy JW, Kereiakes D, Kern MJ, Kuntz RE, Popma JJ, Schaff HV, Williams DO, Gibbons RJ, Alpert JP, Eagle KA, Faxon DP, Fuster V, Gardner TJ, Gregoratos G, Russell RO. ACC/AHA guidelines of percutaneous coronary interventions (revision of the 1993 PTCA guidelines)—executive summary. A report of the American College of Cardiology/American Heart Association Task Force on Practice Guidelines (Committee to Revise the 1993 Guidelines for Percutaneous Transluminal Coronary Angioplasty). *J Am Coll Cardiol.* 2001;37:2215-2239.

19. Eagle KA, Guyton RA, Davidoff R, Ewy GA, Fonger J, Gardner TJ, Gott JP, Herrmann HC, Marlow RA, Nugent W, O'Connor GT, Orszulak TA, Rieselbach RE, Winters WL, Yusuf S, Gibbons RJ, Alpert JS, Garson A Jr, Gregoratos G, Russell RO, Ryan TJ, Smith SC Jr ACC/AHA guidelines for coronary artery bypass graft surgery: executive summary and recommendations : A report of the American College of Cardiology/American Heart Association Task Force on Practice Guidelines (Committee to revise the 1991 guidelines for coronary artery bypass graft surgery). *Circulation.* 1999;100:1464-1480.

Advanced Acute Coronary Syndromes Part 2: New Concepts From 2000 and Beyond

Overview

Since the last edition of the *ACLS Textbook,* researchers, experts, and experienced clinicians have added important new recommendations to the assessment and management of the patients discussed in this chapter (see Part 1, "Overview"). These patients present with ischemic-type chest pain or ischemic equivalents. They have ST-segment depression, dynamic T-wave inversion, or nondiagnostic changes on their initial ECG. A small percentage will have a normal or unchanged ECG.

Many of these patients eventually will be diagnosed as having a non–ST-segment elevation MI or unstable angina. Morbidity and mortality in these patients with ST-segment depression compete with those rates for patients with ST-segment elevation MI. When you apply these new recommendations to such a large, high-risk subset of AMI patients, a strategy that modestly improves survival can benefit a large number of patients.

Part 2 of this chapter discusses the following new treatment recommendations for these patients:

1. Risk stratification: These patients can have any of several imprecisely defined disorders. Each disorder has a wide range of risks. The patient's level of risk serves as a critical "driver" of management decisions, particularly decisions based on the new recommendations.[1]

2. Early conservative versus early invasive strategies: Recent publications and guidelines have clarified the role of these complementary strategies.

3. Low-molecular-weight heparin: LMWH, specifically *enoxaparin,* is now considered equivalent and possibly superior to unfractionated heparin (UFH) for all current indications in this patient group.

4. Glycoprotein IIb/IIIa inhibitors: These antiplatelet agents are now recommended for high-risk patients in this group with a few exceptions.

5. Clopidogrel: This antiplatelet agent is also now recommended for high-risk patients in this group with a few exceptions.

Note: The clinical trials supporting these new recommendations enrolled subjects who were already receiving 1 or more antiplatelet or antithrombin agents. For this reason you should consider each new recommendation to be "conditionally effective." This caveat means the new agents are recommended most often on the condition that they are added to the antiplatelet or antithrombotic agents used in the various clinical trials.

1. Risk Stratification
ST-Segment Depression and T-Wave Inversion

High-Risk Patients

Data from the early fibrinolytic trials suggested that ST-segment depression is a high-risk indicator for major adverse coronary events (MACE)—death, nonfatal MI, or need for urgent surgical revascularization. In some studies[2] morbidity and mortality for patients with ST-segment depression MI rival the rates for patients with anterior Q-wave and ST-segment elevation MI.

Significantly, fibrinolytic therapy not only fails to help these patients but may be harmful. In addition, despite conventional therapy with aspirin and heparin, the rate of MACE in these patients is high.

The "Number-Needed-to-Treat" Statistic

The number-needed-to-treat statistic, which is being used more frequently in clinical trials, allows investigators to easily comprehend and convey the clinical impact of adding new therapies. Researchers have observed that when most new interventions for acute coronary syndromes are extended to high-risk patients, the number needed to treat to prevent 1 adverse clinical outcome was much less than in lower–risk patients.

There is a strong rationale for treating only the patients most likely to benefit and excluding the patients most likely to be harmed. Such straightforward reasoning accounts for the current widespread acceptance of risk stratification.

Defining Risk Strata 1: ACC/AHA Committee on Unstable Angina

By 2000 there was clear understanding that risk stratification not only pointed clinicians in the proper therapeutic direction but also predicted outcomes and survival. Soon after presentation clinicians should "risk stratify" patients with chest pain who do not have significant ST-segment elevation on their initial ECG (treatment strategies for patients who do not have significant ST-segment elevation are depicted in Boxes 13 and 21 of the Ischemic Chest Pain Algorithm in Volume 1, Chapter 17 and in Part 1 of this chapter).

Many different sets of criteria have been used to risk stratify patients with chest pain. The most widely recognized and clinically used approach is the one initially proposed and later refined by Braunwald and his colleagues on the ACC/AHA Task Force on the Management of Patients With Unstable Angina.[1,3-9] This approach is based on a combination of historical, clinical, laboratory, and ECG variables.

Table 1 is a modified version of what has been a work in progress by Braunwald and colleagues over several publications.[6,7,9] Part I starts with adults with chest pain but no ST-segment elevation MI. Their ECGs can display a variety of other changes. Using the data gathered, clinicians can place these patients in 1 of 3 "likelihood" categories (high, intermediate, and low) for "ischemic etiology." Ischemic etiology is a composite group that includes unstable angina and non–ST-segment elevation MI (UA/NSTEMI).

The next step in this process is to consider the short-term risk of death or nonfatal MI in patients determined to have a high or intermediate risk of UA/NSTEMI. Part II of the table addresses this question.

This detailed (and consequently complex) approach ends with criteria for high-risk patients (Table 1, Part II). Note that these criteria are similar to the criteria listed in Box 16 of the Ischemic Chest Pain Algorithm.

TABLE 1. Likelihood of Ischemic Etiology and Risk of Death or Nonfatal MI Over the Short Term in Patients With Chest Pain Who Present Without ST-Segment Elevation (note that patients with ST-segment elevation are already characterized as having ischemic etiology)

Part I. Chest Pain Patients Without ST-Segment Elevation: Likelihood of Ischemic Etiology			
	A. High likelihood There is high likelihood that chest pain is of ischemic etiology if patient has *any* of the findings in the column below:	**B. Intermediate likelihood** There is intermediate likelihood that chest pain is of ischemic etiology if patient has NO findings in column A and *any* of the findings in the column below:	**C. Low likelihood** There is low likelihood that chest pain is of ischemic etiology if patient has NO findings in column A or B. Patients may have any of the findings in the column below:
History	■ Chief symptom is chest or left arm pain or discomfort *plus* — Current pain reproduces pain of prior documented angina — Known CAD, including MI	■ Chief symptom is chest or left arm pain or discomfort ■ Age >70 years ■ Male gender ■ Diabetes mellitus	■ Probable ischemic symptoms ■ Recent cocaine use
Physical exam	■ Transient mitral regurgitation ■ Hypotension ■ Diaphoresis ■ Pulmonary edema or rales	■ Extracardiac vascular disease	■ Chest discomfort is reproduced by palpation
ECG*	■ New or presumably new transient ST deviation (≥0.5 mm*) *or* ■ T-wave inversion (≥2 mm) with symptoms	■ Fixed Q waves ■ Abnormal ST segments *or* ■ T waves that are not new	■ Normal ECG *or* ■ T-wave flattening *or* ■ T-wave inversion in leads with dominant R waves
Cardiac markers	■ Elevated cardiac troponin I or T ■ Elevated CK-MB	*Any finding in column B above PLUS* ■ Normal	■ Normal
High (A) or Intermediate (B) Likelihood of Ischemia			

Part II. Risk of Death or Nonfatal MI Over the Short Term in Patients With Chest Pain With High or Intermediate Likelihood of Ischemia (Columns A and B in Part I)

	High risk: Risk is high if patient has *any* of the following findings:	**Intermediate risk:** Risk is intermediate if patient has *any* of the following findings:	**Low risk:** Risk is low if patient has NO high- or intermediate-risk features; patient may have any of the following:
History	■ Accelerating tempo of ischemic symptoms over prior 48 hours ■ Prolonged, continuing (>20 min) rest pain	■ Prior MI *or* ■ Peripheral-vascular disease *or* ■ Cerebrovascular disease *or* ■ CABG, prior aspirin use *or* ■ Prolonged (>20 min) rest angina is now resolved (moderate to high likelihood of CAD) ■ Rest angina (<20 min) or relieved by rest or sublingual nitrates	■ New-onset angina (Class III or IV) in past 2 weeks ■ No prolonged rest pain (moderate to high likelihood of CAD)
Physical exam	■ Pulmonary edema secondary to ischemia ■ New or worse mitral regurgitation murmur ■ Hypotension, bradycardia, tachycardia ■ S_3 gallop or new or worsening rales ■ Age >75 years	■ Age >70 years	
ECG*	■ Transient ST-segment deviation (≥0.5 mm*) with rest angina ■ New or presumably new bundle branch block ■ Sustained VT	■ T-wave inversion ≥2 mm ■ Pathologic Q waves or T waves that are not new	■ Normal or unchanged ECG during an episode of chest discomfort
Cardiac markers	■ Elevated cardiac troponin I or T ■ Elevated CK-MB	Any of the above findings PLUS ■ Normal	■ Normal

*NOTE: When the international *ECC Guidelines 2000* were written, ST-segment depression of ≥1 mm was established as a significant predictor of adverse myocardial events (MACE). In recent years new evidence has confirmed that ST-segment depression of ≥0.5 mm is also a significant predictor of risk. Whereas formerly only patients with ≥1 mm ST-segment depression entered the UA/NSTEMI treatment and evaluation pathway, now patients with ≥0.5 mm get treated. This lower threshold is now used in the ACC/AHA recommendations and will be used in this chapter, although it has not yet been subjected to the ECC Evidence Evaluation process.

Modified from Braunwald et al.[1,4-7,9]

Defining Risk Strata 2: The TIMI Risk Score

The researchers who derived the important TIMI risk score[10] used data from the TIMI-11B and ESSENCE trials, for unstable angina/non–ST-elevation MI[10,11] and from the In-TIME trial for ST-elevation MI.[12]

The TIMI risk score comprises 7 independent prognostic variables (see Table 2). These variables were significantly associated with the occurrence, within 14 days, of at least 1 of the primary end points: death, new or recurrent MI, or need for urgent revascularization.

Derived by complex multivariate logistic regression, the score includes variables that seem counterintuitive. Aspirin use within the previous 7 days, for example, would not seem to be an indicator of a bad outcome. But aspirin use was, in fact, found to be one of the most powerful predictors.[10]

It is possible that aspirin use identified a subgroup of patients at higher risk or on active but failed therapy for coronary artery disease.

The creators of the TIMI risk score confirmed its validity with 3 groups of patients. Further validation studies in 4 clinical trials demonstrated a significant interaction between the TIMI risk score and treatment.[13-16] These findings confirm the value of the TIMI risk score as a guide to therapeutic decisions.

The TIMI risk score has immense clinical appeal. By classifying patients into 1 of 3 risk strata (see Table 3), it serves as the dominant clinical guide for predicting morbidity and mortality in patients with acute coronary syndromes. It also enables clinicians to direct therapy towards only those patients at higher risk of adverse cardiac events and thus to avoid unnecessary

therapy and the potential for adverse consequences in patients who are at lower risk for adverse cardiac events.

The TIMI risk score has become the primary driver for therapeutic recommendations (see Figure at the end of Part 2). A TIMI Risk score calculator that incorporates the 2002 updated ACC/AHA guidelines is available for download into handheld organizers (eg, Palm Pilot or PDAs) at **www.timi.org/files/palmsoftware/ TIMI%20Risk%20Calculator.htm** and at the ACC website for clinical statements: **www.acc.org/clinical/statements.htm.**

Defining Risk Strata 3: Indicators for Early Invasive Strategies

Risk stratification helps the clinician identify patients with non–ST-segment elevation MI and unstable angina who should be referred immediately for cardiac catheterization. Catheterization then allows the

clinician to determine whether patients are appropriate candidates for revascularization with PCI or CABG (Box 18 of the Ischemic Chest Pain Algorithm, Figure 2 in Part 1 of this chapter).

In 2002 the ACC and AHA published an updated list of Class I, high-risk indicators for an early invasive strategy.[1] *ECC Guidelines 2000* defines high-risk patients using similar criteria (persistent symptoms, recurrent symptoms, depressed LV function, widespread ECG changes, or prior AMI or PCI or CABG).[17] The major difference between the two lists now is that the recent ACC/AHA recommendations include new ST-segment depression and positive troponins in the list of high-risk indicators. These indicators overlap to a considerable degree with the more rigorously validated TIMI risk score.[10]

TABLE 2. TIMI Risk Score for Patients With Unstable Angina and Non–ST-Elevation MI: Predictor Variables[10]

Predictor Variable	Point Value of Variable	Definition
Age ≥65	1	
≥3 risk factors for CAD	1	Risk factors: ■ Family history of CAD ■ Hypertension ■ Hypercholesterolemia ■ Diabetes ■ Current smoker
Aspirin use in last 7 days	1	
Recent, severe symptoms of angina	1	≥2 anginal events in last 24 hours
Elevated cardiac markers	1	CK-MB or cardiac-specific troponin level
ST deviation ≥0.5 mm*	1	ST depression ≥0.5 mm is significant*; transient ST elevation ≥0.5 mm for <20 minutes is treated as ST-segment depression and is high risk; ST elevation ≥1 mm for more than 20 minutes places these patients in the STEMI treatment category.
Prior coronary artery stenosis ≥50%	1	Risk predictor remains valid even if this information is unknown

*NOTE: When the international *ECC Guidelines 2000* were written, ST-segment depression of ≥1 mm was established as a significant predictor of adverse myocardial events (MACE). In recent years new evidence has confirmed that ST-segment depression of ≥0.5 mm is also a significant predictor of risk. Whereas formerly only patients with ≥1 mm ST-segment depression entered the UA/NSTEMI treatment and evaluation pathway, now patients with ≥0.5 mm get treated. This lower threshold is now used in the ACC/AHA recommendations and will be used in this chapter, although it has not yet been subjected to the ECC Evidence Evaluation process.

Table 4 presents these various lists of high-risk features, categorized by when physicians identify them. The 3 sets of indicators appear in columns for easy comparison.

"Take-Home" Message: Risk Stratification

The existence of multiple criteria for risk stratification may confuse rather than clarify the risk of death and major cardiovascular events in various patient groups. The essential take-home message for ACLS providers is that risk stratification is a compass that points clinicians in a general direction with options for different therapeutic pathways. The process allows the most effective care for patients with ischemic pain who end up, by whatever route, defined as high risk. In addition, risk stratification maximizes benefits in high-risk groups by identifying those patients most likely to benefit from a therapy. Risk stratification also avoids subjecting patients to unnecessary therapy with the associated risk of therapeutic complications.

2. Early Invasive vs Early Conservative Strategy for High-Risk Patients

Early Invasive Strategy

Many medical centers have adopted the *early invasive strategy* as the default or dominant strategy for patients with suspected UA/NSTEMI. With this strategy all patients with suspected UA/NSTEMI and without obvious contraindications to coronary revascularization undergo coronary angiography with angiographically directed revascularization (ie, PCI or CABG).[1]

Patients can get to this early invasive strategy by 1 of 3 pathways:

- High-risk criteria (see Table 4) are present during the patient's first evaluation.

- High-risk criteria develop after initial presentation.

TABLE 3. TIMI Risk Score for Patients With Unstable Angina and Non–ST-Elevation MI: Risk Status[10]

Calculated TIMI Risk Score	Risk of ≥1 Primary End Point* in ≤14 Days	Risk Status
0 or 1	5%	Low
2	8%	Low
3	13%	Intermediate
4	20%	Intermediate
5	26%	High
6 or 7	41%	High

*Primary end points: death, new or recurrent MI, or need for urgent revascularization.

- High-risk criteria develop after provocative testing or risk-oriented evaluation.

Early Conservative Strategy

Aggressive medical therapy for high-risk patients with UA/NSTEMI calls for multiple agents to be given simultaneously or in sequence. It is helpful to group these interventions in some easy-to-remember manner. Clinician-teachers have found the *Triple A's* (antianginal/anti-ischemic, antiplatelet, and antithrombin agents) to be a useful reminder of the therapies they must consider (see Table 5).

Initial distinctions between treatment of non–ST-segment elevation MI and high-risk unstable angina are not significant. Clinicians initiate similar therapy for the two conditions.

Early Invasive vs Early Conservative Strategy: The Evidence

Whether patients with UA/NSTEMI benefit most from a conservative or an initially invasive strategy has been the subject of multiple studies and continuing discussion.[5,7,18-20] The effectiveness of both conservative and

catheterization strategies has increased substantially in recent years. For example, the invasive strategies in studies completed a few years ago did not include stenting or the use of glycoprotein receptor inhibitors. In addition, better PCI equipment and operator skill at high volume centers is now available. Recent risk stratification tools using troponin and ST-segment deviation are only now becoming widely appreciated.

The *integration* of these therapies is more important than the individual agents. The most important strategy is to apply the right therapy to the right patients in a timely manner.

Two trials comparing current invasive and conservative strategies in patients with UA/NSTEMI were recently completed.[21,22] On the basis of these results the ACC/AHA committee updated their recommendations about an early invasive versus an early conservative strategy[1,6]:

- An early invasive strategy is *more beneficial* for high-risk patients with UA/NSTEMI (Class I, level of evidence A). High-risk is defined as having 1 of the indicators listed in column A of Table 4.

TABLE 4. High-Risk Features for Patients Presenting With ST-Segment Depression, Dynamic T-Wave Inversion, or Unstable Angina: Indications for Referral for Angiography and Angiographically Directed PCI or CABG

Identification of High-Risk Feature	A. ACC/AHA Unstable Angina Committee[1,6]	B. *ECC Guidelines 2000*[17]	C. TIMI Risk Score Predictor Variables[10]
On presentation to ED	■ PCI within previous 6 months ■ Prior CABG	■ History of 2 or more risk factors for CAD, including prior AMI, prior angioplasty, or prior CABG (Class IIa)	■ Age ≥65 ■ 3 or more risk factors for CAD ■ Aspirin use in last 7 days ■ Prior coronary artery stenosis >50%
12-Lead ECG (either initial or serial)	■ New or presumably new ST-segment depression ≥0.5 mm* ■ Sustained VT	■ ECG changes of ST depression ≥1 mm* suggestive of cardiac ischemia (Class IIa)	■ ST deviation ≥0.5 mm*
Cardiac biomarkers	■ Elevated cardiac markers (troponin T or I preferred)	■ Elevated cardiac markers	■ Elevated cardiac markers
During initial assessment and treatment	■ Recurrent angina or ischemia at rest (2000 edition listed for >20 minutes) or with low-level activities (occurs despite intensive anti-ischemic therapy)	■ Recurrent (stuttering) breakthroughs of ischemic pain despite morphine, nitroglycerin, and β-blockers (Class I)	■ Recent, severe symptoms of angina
	■ Recurrent angina or ischemia with symptoms of CHF, S_3 gallop, pulmonary edema, worsening rales, or new or worsening mitral regurgitation	■ Unremitting ischemic discomfort despite aggressive use of morphine, nitroglycerin, and β-blockers (Class II)	
	■ Depressed LV systolic function (eg, ejection fraction <40% on noninvasive study)	■ Signs of depressed LV function, shock, and pulmonary congestion (Class I)	
	■ Hemodynamic instability		
During noninvasive provocative (stress) testing	■ High-risk findings on noninvasive stress testing		

*NOTE: When the international *ECC Guidelines 2000* were written, ST-segment depression of ≥1 mm was established as a significant predictor of adverse myocardial events (MACE). In recent years new evidence has confirmed that ST-segment depression of ≥0.5 mm is also a significant predictor of risk. Whereas formerly only patients with ≥1 mm ST-segment depression entered the UA/NSTEMI treatment and evaluation pathway, now patients with ≥0.5 mm get treated. This lower threshold is now used in the ACC/AHA recommendations and will be used in this chapter, although it has not yet been subjected to the ECC Evidence Evaluation process.

- An early invasive strategy and an early conservative strategy are equivalent in hospitalized patients *without* high-risk features or contraindications to revascularization (Class I, level of evidence B).

3. Low-Molecular-Weight Heparins

The Need for Antithrombins

When plaque rupture occurs at the start of an acute coronary syndrome, platelets are activated. The exposure of tissue factors activates the extrinsic coagulation system. The activated platelets begin to transform

TABLE 5. The Triple A's: Pharmacotherapy for Non–ST-Elevation MI (ST-Segment Depression, Dynamic T-Wave Inversion) and Unstable Angina

Antianginal or anti-ischemic agents

- Morphine sulfate
- Oxygen
- β-Adrenergic blockers
- Nitroglycerin

Antiplatelet agents

- Cyclooxygenase inhibitor
  — Aspirin
- Glycoprotein IIb/IIIa inhibitors
  — Abciximab (ReoPro®)
  — Eptifibatide (Integrilin®)
  — Tirofiban (Aggrastat®)
- Adenosine diphosphate inhibitors
  — Clopidogrel (Plavix®)
  — Ticlopidine (Ticlid®)

Antithrombin agents

- Unfractionated heparin
- Low-molecular-weight heparin
  — Dalteparin (Fragmin®)
  — Enoxaparin (Lovenox®)
  — Nadroparin (Fraxiparine®)

prothrombin to thrombin, which in turn begins the conversion of fibrinogen to the fibrin matrix of a thrombus.

Heparin provides indirect inhibition of thrombin, slowing the fibrinogen-to-fibrin conversion. For this reason heparin is classified as an antithrombin agent.

In its unfractionated form, heparin is a heterogeneous mixture of sulfated glycosaminoglycans with chains of various lengths. There are several disadvantages to the use of unfractionated heparin in patients with ACS:

- UFH produces an unpredictable anticoagulant response in individual patients.

- UFH requires intravenous administration.

- UFH requires frequent monitoring of activated partial thromboplastin time (aPTT).

- UFH stimulates platelet activation, causing thrombocytopenia.[23] Heparin-induced thrombocytopenia can cause serious or even fatal complications in a small percentage of patients.

The Evidence

There are 3 new forms of low-molecular-weight heparin available. Each one has been compared with UFH in clinical trials:

- Enoxaparin (Lovenox, Clexane)[20,24]

- Dalteparin (Fragmin)[25,26]

- Nadroparin (Fraxiparine)[27]

The new low-molecular-weight heparins have several advantages over UFH:

- They can be administered subcutaneously so do not require IV administration.

- They do not require periodic aPTT measurements.

Controlled clinical trials have confirmed that LMWHs are equivalent in efficacy to UFH for patients with UA/NSTEMI.[14,28,29] One LMWH, enoxaparin, has been found to be superior to UFH for the treatment of unstable angina.[14,30]

A recent trial confirmed the safety and efficacy of combining a LMWH with a glycoprotein IIb/IIIa inhibitor.[31] The updated (2002) ACC/AHA guidelines for unstable angina cite 2 additional abstracts.[1,6]

Recommendations

- The ACC/AHA guidelines now recommend enoxaparin over UFH for patients with high-risk UA/NSTEMI.[1,6] Updated recommendations in high-risk patients await completion of a large open-label phase 3 trial (SYNERGY).

- For low- and intermediate-risk patients with unstable angina, the guidelines recommend only enoxaparin.

4. Glycoprotein IIb/IIIa Receptor Inhibitors

Glycoprotein IIb/IIIa receptor inhibitors block the final common pathway of platelet aggregation. More than 40 000 patients with an ACS but no ST-segment elevation have now been studied in clinical trials of these inhibitors.[32] These trials have confirmed the following observations:

- These agents have a modest ability to reduce adverse cardiac events such as MI and death.[32]

- These agents reduce the incidence of complications in patients undergoing PCI.[33]

- These agents improve the prognosis for high-risk UA/NSTEMI patients with ST-segment depression, positive cardiac markers, and refractory ischemia.[34,35]

- Short-acting agents such as eptifibatide and tirofiban are useful as "upstream" therapy compared with initial therapy started in the catheterization suite.

- Diabetic patients, already at highest risk for coronary events and procedural complications, seem to experience a particular positive benefit.

Recommendations

Glycoprotein IIb/IIIa inhibitors are recommended for *all* high-risk patients with UA/NSTEMI and no contraindications. But the strength of the ACC/AHA recommendation and the level of evidence vary for different subsets of patients:

- **High-risk patients, planned invasive management:** If an invasive management strategy (cardiac catheterization and PCI) is planned, administer eptifibatide, tirofiban, or abciximab (Class I).

- **High-risk patients, no invasive management:** If an invasive management strategy is *not* planned, administer eptifibatide or tirofiban but not abciximab (Class IIa).

- **Low- or intermediate-risk patients:** If an invasive management strategy is *not* planned, consider eptifibatide or tirofiban but not abciximab (Class IIb).

5. Clopidogrel

Adenosine Diphosphate Inhibitors: Clopidogrel and Ticlopidine

These newly approved agents join aspirin and glycoprotein IIb/IIIa inhibitors as the third antiplatelet therapy available for patients with UA/NSTEMI.

Two randomized, clinical trials of clopidogrel in patients with UA/NSTEMI were published after the international *ECC Guidelines 2000* was published.[36,37] The trials compared clopidogrel with aspirin and with placebo. The benefits of clopidogrel in reducing composite end points (a composite of death, nonfatal MI, or need for urgent revascularization) were modest. The number needed to treat to prevent 1 adverse end point was approximately 50.

Clopidogrel has a more rapid onset of action and better safety profile than ticlopidine. Clopidogrel is now preferred over ticlopidine for ACS.[1,6]

The ACC/AHA recommendations were published in 2002:[1,6]

- Clopidogrel should be given as soon as possible to all patients with high-risk ST-segment depression or dynamic T-wave inversion (non–ST-segment elevation MI and unstable angina) if percutaneous intervention is not immediately planned.

Summary Algorithm for Risk Stratification and Treatment of Patients With UA/NSTEMI

The clinician faces an imposing array of clinical trial data and therapeutic choices. More than any single intervention, a comprehensive strategy that selects patients at highest risk during a defined time period will provide the most benefit. Such a therapeutic strategy should be based on evaluation of clinical variables that are easily available to the bedside clinician at initial evaluation. Early risk stratification is essential to guide therapy.

The Figure is an algorithm that integrates current trial data and management strategies. This algorithm, developed specifically for this text, summarizes the evolving interventions and strategies for patients with UA/NSTEMI, including new ACC/AHA recommendations that were not available when the international *ECC Guidelines 2000* was published. The algorithm is a way of presenting clinical information. It is intended for educational purposes and to integrate current information into a clinical framework. This algorithm does not represent "official" evidence-based consensus recommendations from the AHA ECC Committee and Subcommittees.

FIGURE. Risk Stratification and Treatment Strategies for Patients With Unstable Angina or Non–ST-segment Elevation MI

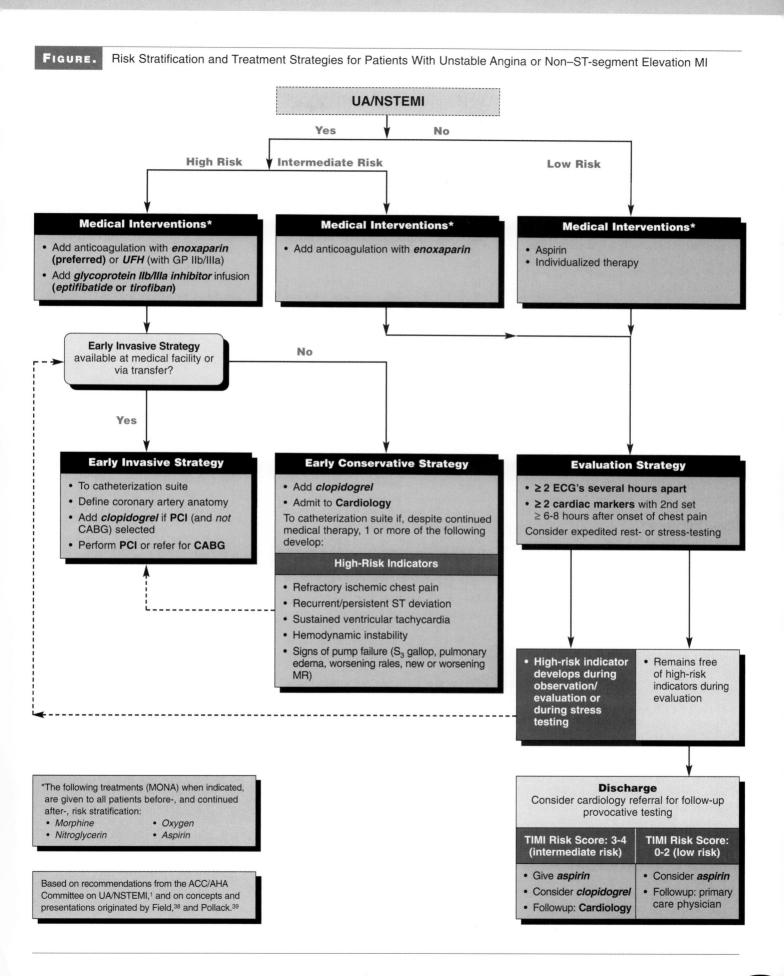

References

1. Braunwald E, Antman EM, Beasley JW, Califf RM, Cheitlin MD, Hochman JS, Jones RH, Kereiakes D, Kupersmith J, Levin TN, Pepine CJ, Schaeffer JW, Smith EE 3rd, Steward DE, Theroux P, Gibbons RJ, Alpert JS, Faxon DP, Fuster V, Gregoratos G, Hiratzka LF, Jacobs AK, Smith SC Jr. ACC/AHA guideline update for the management of patients with unstable angina and non-ST-segment elevation myocardial infarction—2002: summary article: a report of the American College of Cardiology/American Heart Association Task Force on Practice Guidelines (Committee on the Management of Patients With Unstable Angina). *Circulation.* 2002;106:1893-1900.

2. Eppler E, Eisenberg MS, Schaeffer S, Meischke H, Larson MP. 911 and emergency department use for chest pain: results of a media campaign. *Ann Emerg Med.* 1994;24:202-208.

3. Braunwald E. Unstable angina. A classification. *Circulation.* 1989;80:410-414.

4. Braunwald E. Unstable angina: an etiologic approach to management [editorial]. *Circulation.* 1998;98:2219-2222.

5. Braunwald E, Antman EM, Beasley JW, Califf RM, Cheitlin MD, Hochman JS, Jones RH, Kereiakes D, Kupersmith J, Levin TN, Pepine CJ, Schaeffer JW, Smith EE 3rd, Steward DE, Theroux P, Gibbons RJ, Alpert JS, Eagle KA, Faxon DP, Fuster V, Gardner TJ, Gregoratos G, Russell RO, Smith SC Jr. ACC/AHA guidelines for the management of patients with unstable angina and non-ST-segment elevation myocardial infarction: executive summary and recommendations. A report of the American College of Cardiology/American Heart Association task force on practice guidelines (committee on the management of patients with unstable angina). *Circulation.* 2000;102:1193-1209.

6. Braunwald E, Antman EM, Beasley JW, Califf RM, Cheitlin MD, Hochman JS, Jones RH, Kereiakes D, Kupersmith J, Levin TN, Pepine CJ, Schaeffer JW, Smith EE 3rd, Steward DE, Theroux P, Gibbons RJ, Alpert JS, Faxon DP, Fuster V, Gregoratos G, Hiratzka LF, Jacobs AK, Smith SC Jr. ACC/AHA 2002 guideline update for the management of patients with unstable angina and non-ST-segment elevation myocardial infarction--summary article: a report of the American College of Cardiology/American Heart Association task force on practice guidelines (Committee on the Management of Patients With Unstable Angina). *J Am Coll Cardiol.* 2002;40:1366-1374.

7. Braunwald E, Antman EM, Beasley JW, Califf RM, Cheitlin MD, Hochman JS, Jones RH, Kereiakes D, Kupersmith J, Levin TN, Pepine CJ, Schaeffer JW, Smith EE, III., Steward DE, Theroux P, Alpert JS, Eagle KA, Faxon DP, Fuster V, Gardner TJ, Gregoratos G, Russell RO, Smith SC Jr. ACC/AHA guidelines for the management of patients with unstable angina and non-ST-segment elevation myocardial infarction. A report of the American College of Cardiology/American Heart Association Task Force on Practice Guidelines (Committee on the Management of Patients With Unstable Angina). *J Am Coll Cardiol.* 2000;36:970-1062.

8. Braunwald E, Califf RM, Cannon CP, Fox KA, Fuster V, Gibler WB, Harrington RA, King SB 3rd, Kleiman NS, Theroux P, Topol EJ, Van de Werf F, White HD, Willerson JT. Redefining medical treatment in the management of unstable angina. *Am J Med.* 2000;108:41-53.

9. Braunwald E, Jones RH, Mark DB, Brown J, Brown L, Cheitlin MD, Concannon CA, Cowan M, Edwards C, Fuster V, et al. Diagnosing and managing unstable angina. Agency for Health Care Policy and Research. *Circulation.* 1994;90:613-622.

10. Antman EM, Cohen M, Bernink PJ, McCabe CH, Horacek T, Papuchis G, Mautner B, Corbalan R, Radley D, Braunwald E. The TIMI risk score for unstable angina/non-ST elevation MI: A method for prognostication and therapeutic decision making. *JAMA.* 2000;284:835-842.

11. de Lemos JA, Antman EM, Gibson CM, McCabe CH, Giugliano RP, Murphy SA, Coulter SA, Anderson K, Scherer J, Frey MJ, Van Der Wieken R, Van De Werf F, Braunwald E. Abciximab improves both epicardial flow and myocardial reperfusion in ST-elevation myocardial infarction: observations from the TIMI 14 trial. *Circulation.* 2000;101:239-243.

12. de Lemos JA, Antman EM, Giugliano RP, Morrow DA, McCabe CH, Cutler SS, Charlesworth A, Schroder R, Braunwald E. Comparison of a 60- versus 90-minute determination of ST-segment resolution after thrombolytic therapy for acute myocardial infarction. In TIME-II Investigators. Intravenous nPA for Treatment of Infarcting Myocardium Early-II. *Am J Cardiol.* 2000;86:1235-1237, A1235.

13. Cannon CP, Weintraub WS, Demopoulos LA, Vicari R, Frey MJ, Lakkis N, Neumann FJ, Robertson DH, DeLucca PT, DiBattiste PM, Gibson CM, Braunwald E. Comparison of early invasive and conservative strategies in patients with unstable coronary syndromes treated with the glycoprotein IIb/IIIa inhibitor tirofiban. *N Engl J Med.* 2001;344:1879-1887.

14. Cohen M, Demers C, Gurfinkel EP, Turpie AG, Fromell GJ, Goodman S, Langer A, Califf RM, Fox KA, Premmereur J, Bigonzi F. A comparison of low-molecular-weight heparin with unfractionated heparin for unstable coronary artery disease. Efficacy and Safety of Subcutaneous Enoxaparin in Non-Q-Wave Coronary Events Study Group. *N Engl J Med.* 1997;337:447-452.

15. Scirica BM, Cannon CP, Antman EM, Murphy SA, Morrow DA, Sabatine MS, McCabe CH, Gibson CM, Braunwald E. Validation of the thrombolysis in myocardial infarction (TIMI) risk score for unstable angina pectoris and non-ST-elevation myocardial infarction in the TIMI III registry. *Am J Cardiol.* 2002;90:303-305.

16. Morrow DA, Antman EM, Snapinn SM, McCabe CH, Theroux P, Braunwald E. An integrated clinical approach to predicting the benefit of tirofiban in non-ST elevation acute coronary syndromes. Application of the TIMI Risk Score for UA/NSTEMI in PRISM-PLUS. *Eur Heart J.* 2002;23:223-229.

17. American Heart Association in collaboration with International Liaison Committee on Resuscitation. Guidelines 2000 for Cardiopulmonary Resuscitation and Emergency Cardiovascular Care: International Consensus on Science, Part 7: the Era of Reperfusion: Section 1: Acute Coronary Syndromes (Acute Myocardial Infarction). *Circulation.* 2000;102(suppl I): I172-I203.

18. Boden WE, O'Rourke RA, Crawford MH, Blaustein AS, Deedwania PC, Zoble RG, Wexler LF, Kleiger RE, Pepine CJ, Ferry DR, Chow BK, Lavori PW. Outcomes in patients with acute non-Q-wave myocardial infarction randomly assigned to an invasive as compared with a conservative management strategy. Veterans Affairs Non-Q-Wave Infarction Strategies in Hospital (VANQWISH) Trial Investigators. *N Engl J Med.* 1998;338:1785-1792.

19. Yusuf S, Flather M, Pogue J, Hunt D, Varigos J, Piegas L, Avezum A, Anderson J, Keltai M, Budaj A, Fox K, Ceremuzynski L. Variations between countries in invasive cardiac procedures and outcomes in patients with suspected unstable angina or myocardial infarction without initial ST elevation. OASIS (Organisation to Assess Strategies for Ischaemic Syndromes) Registry Investigators. *Lancet.* 1998;352: 507-514.

20. Ryan TJ, Antman EM, Brooks NH, Califf RM, Hillis LD, Hiratzka LF, Rapaport E, Riegel B, Russell RO, Smith EE 3rd, Weaver WD, Gibbons RJ, Alpert JS, Eagle KA, Gardner TJ, Garson A Jr., Gregoratos G, Smith SC Jr. 1999 update: ACC/AHA guidelines for the management of patients with acute myocardial infarction. A report of the American College of Cardiology/American Heart Association Task Force on Practice Guidelines (Committee on Management of Acute Myocardial Infarction). *J Am Coll Cardiol.* 1999;34:890-911.

21. Wallentin L, Lagerqvist B, Husted S, Kontny F, Stahle E, Swahn E. Outcome at 1 year after an invasive compared with a non-invasive strategy in unstable coronary-artery disease: the FRISC II invasive randomised trial. FRISC II Investigators. Fast Revascularisation during Instability in Coronary artery disease. *Lancet.* 2000;356:9-16.

22. FRISC II Investigators. Invasive compared with non-invasive treatment in unstable coronary-artery disease: FRISC II prospective randomised multicentre study. FRagmin and Fast Revascularisation during InStability in Coronary artery disease Investigators. *Lancet.* 1999;354:708-715.

23. Brieger DB, Mak KH, Kottke-Marchant K, Topol EJ. Heparin-induced thrombocytopenia. *J Am Coll Cardiol.* 1998;31:1449-1459.

24. Ohman EM, Kleiman NS, Gacioch G, Worley SJ, Navetta FI, Talley JD, Anderson HV, Ellis SG, Cohen MD, Spriggs D, Miller M, Kereiakes D, Yakubov S, Kitt MM, Sigmon KN, Califf RM, Krucoff MW, Topol EJ. Combined accelerated tissue-plasminogen activator and platelet glycoprotein IIb/IIIa integrin receptor blockade with Integrilin in acute myocardial infarction: results of a randomized, placebo-controlled, dose-ranging trial. IMPACT-AMI Investigators. *Circulation.* 1997;95:846-854.

25. Klein LW, Wahid F, VandenBerg BJ, Parrillo JE, Calvin JE. Comparison of heparin therapy for < or = 48 hours to > 48 hours in unstable angina pectoris. *Am J Cardiol.* 1997;79:259-263.

26. Antman EM, Giugliano RP, Gibson CM, McCabe CH, Coussement P, Kleiman NS, Vahanian A, Adgey AA, Menown I, Rupprecht HJ, Van der Wieken R, Ducas J, Scherer J, Anderson K, Van de Werf F, Braunwald E. Abciximab facilitates the rate and extent of thrombolysis: results of the thrombolysis in myocardial infarction (TIMI) 14 trial. The TIMI 14 Investigators. *Circulation.* 1999;99: 2720-2732.

27. GUSTO Investigators, Hasdai D, Holmes DR Jr, Califf RM, Thompson TD, Hochman JS, Pfisterer M, Topol EJ. Cardiogenic shock complicating acute myocardial infarction: predictors of death. GUSTO Investigators. Global Utilization of Streptokinase and Tissue-Plasminogen Activator for Occluded Coronary Arteries. *Am Heart J.* 1999;138:21-31.

28. Antman EM, Kereiakes DJ. Antithrombotic therapy in unstable angina/non-ST elevation myocardial infarction: the evolving role of low-molecular-weight heparin. *J Invasive Cardiol.* 2000;12(suppl E):E1-E4.

29. Young JJ, Kereiakes DJ, Grines CL. Low-molecular-weight heparin therapy in percutaneous coronary intervention: the NICE 1 and NICE 4 trials. National Investigators Collaborating on Enoxaparin Investigators. *J Invasive Cardiol.* 2000;12 Suppl E:E14-E18.

30. Bozovich GE, Gurfinkel EP, Antman EM, McCabe CH, Mautner B. Superiority of enoxaparin versus unfractionated heparin for unstable angina/non-Q-wave myocardial infarction regardless of activated partial thromboplastin time. *Am Heart J.* 2000;140:637-642.

31. Kereiakes DJ, Grines C, Fry E, Esente P, Hoppensteadt D, Midei M, Barr L, Matthai W, Todd M, Broderick T, Rubinstein R, Fareed J, Santoian E, Neiderman A, Brodie B, Zidar J, Ferguson JJ, Cohen M. Enoxaparin and abciximab adjunctive pharmacotherapy during percutaneous coronary intervention. *J Invasive Cardiol.* 2001;13:272-278.

32. Kong DF, Califf RM, Miller DP, Moliterno DJ, White HD, Harrington RA, Tcheng JE, Lincoff AM, Hasselblad V, Topol EJ. Clinical outcomes of therapeutic agents that block the platelet glycoprotein IIb/IIIa integrin in ischemic heart disease. *Circulation.* 1998;98:2829-2835.

33. Boersma E, Pieper KS, Steyerberg EW, Wilcox RG, Chang WC, Lee KL, Akkerhuis KM, Harrington RA, Deckers JW, Armstrong PW, Lincoff AM, Califf RM, Topol EJ, Simoons ML. Predictors of outcome in patients with acute coronary syndromes without persistent ST-segment elevation. Results from an international trial of 9461 patients. The PURSUIT Investigators. *Circulation.* 2000;101:2557-2567.

34. Topol EJ, Byzova TV, Plow EF. Platelet GPIIb-IIIa blockers. *Lancet.* 1999;353:227-231.

35. Topol EJ, Mark DB, Lincoff AM, Cohen E, Burton J, Kleiman N, Talley D, Sapp S, Booth J, Cabot CF, Anderson KM, Califf RM. Outcomes at 1 year and economic implications of platelet glycoprotein IIb/IIIa blockade in patients undergoing coronary stenting: results from a multicentre randomised trial. EPISTENT Investigators. Evaluation of Platelet IIb/IIIa Inhibitor for Stenting. *Lancet.* 1999;354:2019-2024.

36. Mehta SR, Yusuf S, Peters RJ, Bertrand ME, Lewis BS, Natarajan MK, Malmberg K, Rupprecht H, Zhao F, Chrolavicius S, Copland I, Fox KA. Effects of pretreatment with clopidogrel and aspirin followed by long-term therapy in patients undergoing percutaneous coronary intervention: the PCI-CURE study. *Lancet.* 2001;358:527-533.

37. Yusuf S, Zhao F, Mehta SR, Chrolavicius S, Tognoni G, Fox KK. Effects of clopidogrel in addition to aspirin in patients with acute coronary syndromes without ST-segment elevation. *N Engl J Med.* 2001;345:494-502.

38. Field JM. In: Kern KB, ed. *Cardiology Clinics: Emergency Cardiovascular Care.* Philadelphia, Pa: WB Saunders; 2002:137-157.

39. Pollack CV Jr, Cohen M. In: Pollack CV Jr, ed. *CEVAT Panel Reports.* Atlanta, Ga: American Health Consultants; 2002:1-20.

Advanced Acute Coronary Syndromes Part 3: Complications of ACS: Shock, Pulmonary Edema, and Hypotension

Introduction

Shock is a clinical condition characterized by a sustained and significant reduction in blood flow and oxygen delivery to some organs and tissues. It may be caused by one or more of the following conditions:

- Arrhythmias

- Inadequate intravascular volume relative to the vascular space

- Myocardial failure

- Inappropriate vascular resistance or maldistribution of blood flow

The clinician can use these etiologic mechanisms to characterize shock and to identify the appropriate focus of therapy:

- Arrhythmic shock → Antiarrhythmic therapy

- Hypovolemic shock → Volume therapy

- Cardiogenic shock → Support of pump function

- Distributive shock → Vasoactive drug therapy

An etiologic approach to shock often oversimplifies the problem. Any patient with severe or sustained shock will likely require some support of heart rate and rhythm, titration of fluid therapy to optimize intravascular volume, support of pump function, and manipulation of vascular resistance and distribution of blood flow. All patients with severe or sustained shock will have some myocardial failure.

This part of Chapter 2 describes complications of acute coronary syndromes: shock, pulmonary edema, and hypotension. The first section, "Cardiogenic Shock Complicating AMI," summarizes the pathophysiology and treatment of cardiogenic shock associated with AMI, emphasizing therapy unique to patients with these conditions. The second section, "The Acute Pulmonary Edema, Hypotension, and Shock Algorithm," details initial evaluation and stabilization of any patient with pulmonary edema and shock. This section contains more information about treatment decisions based on the initial response to therapy.

Cardiogenic Shock Complicating AMI

Infarction of 40% or more of the left ventricular myocardium usually results in cardiogenic shock and death. Although the incidence of cardiogenic shock has decreased in recent trials, mortality still averages 50% to 70%.[1-3] This section reviews the pathophysiology and management of cardiogenic shock in the patient with AMI.

Pathophysiology and Hemodynamics of Cardiogenic Shock

Myocardial infarction may result in hemodynamic instability and congestive heart failure. Cardiac output is the product of stroke volume and heart rate. When the ventricular ejection fraction falls, the stroke volume (ie, the amount of blood ejected with each heartbeat) usually decreases and cardiac output falls. To compensate, heart rate increases and the ventricle may dilate and increase end-diastolic volume. Tachycardia is an acute compensation for sudden reduction in stroke volume (eg, large MI). Ventricular dilation or remodeling occurs over days to months and results in an increase in end-diastolic volume. This increase in end-diastolic volume (increased ventricular *preload*) may help maintain stroke volume near normal levels despite the fall in ejection fraction. Paradoxically, reduced ejection fraction and ventricular dilation are prognostic indicators of increased survival in septic shock syndrome.

As an example, a patient's ejection fraction falls from 50% to 25% (normal is 50% to 70%). If the patient's end-diastolic volume was initially 100 mL and remains at 100 mL, his stroke volume will fall from 50 to 25 mL when the ejection fraction decreases. But if the patient's ventricle dilates and the ventricular end-diastolic volume increases from 100 to 160 mL, stroke volume may fall from 50 mL to 40 mL (a fall of 20%) despite the substantial fall in ejection fraction.

As noted, tachycardia also may help maintain cardiac output despite a fall in ejection fraction and stroke volume. But all of these compensatory changes are likely to increase myocardial oxygen consumption. They also can worsen ischemia in viable or distant myocardium and extend infarction. In some cases (eg, large anterior MI), a reduction in heart rate with β-blockade improves outcome. Blockade of excess sympathetic and neurohumoral stimulation reduces myocardial oxygen consumption. In other situations, called compensatory tachycardia, β-blockade can be life-threatening. For example, in pericardial tamponade stroke volume is critically dependent on the tachycardia.

When left ventricular end-diastolic pressure (LVEDP) increases substantially (>25 to 30 mm Hg), pulmonary edema develops. If right ventricular end-diastolic pressure (RVEDP) increases, systemic edema will be observed. A fall in cardiac output also triggers an adrenergic response, producing tachycardia and peripheral vasoregulatory changes that try to redistribute blood flow. Constriction of arteries to the skin, kidneys, and gut redistributes blood flow away from these tissues to maintain blood flow to the brain and heart. But this systemic vasoconstriction may create increased left ventricular *afterload,* impeding left ventricular ejection. As cardiac output continues to fall, hypotension and lactic acidosis develop. This combination of pulmonary edema with signs of inadequate systemic perfusion is the hallmark of cardiogenic shock.

The patient with LV dysfunction often has a cardiac index (cardiac output corrected for body surface area) less than 2.5 L/min per m^2, a pulmonary capillary wedge pressure greater than 18 to 20 mm Hg, and a systolic blood pressure less than 100 mm Hg. When the cardiac index falls to 2.2 L/min per m^2 and SBP falls to 90 mm Hg, frank signs of poor peripheral perfusion are usually present.

Treatment of Cardiogenic Shock Associated With AMI

The mortality rate of AMI associated with cardiogenic shock is 50% or more in virtually every outcome report.[3-9] Initial therapy for LV dysfunction includes oxygen administration, intravenous administration of nitrates to reduce cardiac preload and afterload, and diuresis (see "Box 3. First-Line Treatment," below). Morphine is also

an excellent adjunct agent if the patient has continuing ischemia.

If the patient becomes markedly hypotensive, avoid or discontinue vasodilators and administer vasoactive drugs to increase arterial tone (vasopressors), improve blood pressure, and redistribute cardiac output. If the patient does not respond to initial therapies, be prepared to perform additional diagnostic studies, initiate advanced hemodynamic monitoring, and provide advanced therapies. Mechanical circulatory assistance with intra-aortic balloon counterpulsation is an effective adjunct with reperfusion therapy in selected patients. Results from the GUSTO-I[10] and SHOCK trials[3] suggest that an aggressive, invasive approach increases survival for patients with cardiogenic shock and AMI.

When possible, triage high-risk patients with AMI and cardiogenic shock or refer them to facilities with cardiac catheterization suites and interventional capability. Consider triage or transfer for patients with a large anterior wall infarct, CHF, or pulmonary edema. Defer fibrinolytic therapy if percutaneous coronary intervention is *rapidly* available and anticipated door-to-balloon-inflation time is ≤60 minutes. If you cannot ensure transfer within a time that would allow rapid PCI, administer fibrinolytics if there are no contraindications to their use; then transfer the patient. If the patient fails to reperfuse or remains clinically unstable, undertake angioplasty for failed lysis, a procedure often referred to as rescue angioplasty.

In hospitals without interventional capabilities or an on-site interventional team, proceed with fibrinolytic administration. If normal coronary flow is not re-established (TIMI III flow), coronary angiography and rescue PCI should be performed if at all possible.[11] Note that fibrinolytic therapy has not been shown to consistently improve outcome in patients with cardiogenic shock, and it may have several limitations.[11,12] The small number of patients in clinical trials limits the strength of the evidence supporting these recommendations.

With increasing use of both fibrinolytic therapy and PCI, controversy arose over which technique was the better method of reperfusion. Retrospective and registry trial evidence has shown that for patients with AMI and cardiogenic shock, an aggressive early strategy of PCI is superior to medical therapy with fibrinolytics:

■ The GUSTO-I investigators reported that mortality was lower in patients with cardiogenic shock treated with an aggressive PCI strategy than in similar patients given fibrinolytic therapy.[13]

■ Investigators from around the globe have reported higher survival rates for cardiogenic shock patients who undergo revascularization instead of fibrinolysis.[10]

■ In the US Second National Registry of Myocardial Infarction, the mortality rate in patients with AMI and shock was lower in those treated with PCI as a primary strategy than in those treated with fibrinolytics.[14]

■ In a large registry of patients with shock, mortality was lower in AMI patients who received early revascularization with either PCI or CABG.[15]

■ Multiple investigators have reported reduced mortality in patients with cardiogenic shock and AMI who received intra-aortic balloon pumping (IABP) followed by cardiac catheterization and revascularization with PCI or CABG (when anatomy was suitable).[16-19]

The controversy surrounding optimal therapy was resolved by the randomized, controlled SHOCK trial (**SH**ould We Emergently Revascularize **O**ccluded Coronaries for **C**ardiogenic Shoc**K**). This study compared early revascularization using IABP plus PTCA or CABG with early medical stabilization using fibrinolytic therapy.[3] Mortality at 6 months[3] and at 1 year of follow-up[8] was significantly lower in the early revascularization group than in the early medical therapy group (number needed to treat was approximately 8 at both time points). But this benefit occurred only in patients *less than 75 years of age.* The investigators recommend rapid transport of patients in cardiogenic shock, particularly those less than 75 years old, to interventional facilities.[3]

In 1999 the ACC/AHA Committee on Management of Acute Myocardial Infarction made PCI a Class I recommendation for patients with ACS and shock who are less than 75 years old.[20] Resuscitation experts reviewed and endorsed these recommendations at the international Guidelines 2000 Conference.[21,22] The current recommendations of the international ECC guidelines are as follows:

- Provide early triage or transfer to cardiovascular facilities with cardiac catheterization suites and interventional capability.

- When possible, transfer patients at high risk for mortality or severe LV dysfunction with signs of shock, pulmonary congestion, heart rate >100 bpm *and* SBP <100 mm Hg to a facility capable of performing cardiac catheterization and rapid revascularization (PCI or CABG). For patients younger than 75 years, this is a *Class I* recommendation.

- PCI, including angioplasty with stent placement, is a *Class I* recommendation for patients <75 years of age with acute coronary syndromes and signs of shock.

- Use of IABP and diagnostic cardiac catheterization and coronary revascularization with PCI or CABG (if anatomy is suitable) may reduce mortality.[16,18,19,23,24]

- The healthcare provider can use a checklist to identify patients who have contraindications to fibrinolytic therapy (see Volume 1, Chapter 17). If contraindications to fibrinolytic therapy exist, consider transfer to a cardiac intervention facility for reperfusion *(Class IIa).*

The Acute Pulmonary Edema, Hypotension, and Shock Algorithm

The Acute Pulmonary Edema, Hypotension, and Shock Algorithm (see Figure) illustrates the management of patients who present with these clinical problems. The following sections explain management of these patients in greater detail.

Box 1. Clinical Signs

Shock and pulmonary edema are medical emergencies. Signs of shock include inadequate tissue perfusion (diminished peripheral pulses, cool extremities, delayed capillary refill, decreased urine output, and lactic acidosis). With CHF signs of systemic and pulmonary venous congestion are present. Pulmonary edema produces tachypnea, labored respirations, rales, dyspnea, cyanosis, and hypoxemia. Frothy sputum may also be present. Rescuers should identify these conditions and begin treatment as soon as possible.

Box 2. Acute Pulmonary Edema

If signs of acute pulmonary edema are present (see list in previous paragraph), proceed to Box 3 of the algorithm. If the patient has no signs of acute pulmonary edema, proceed to Boxes 6, 8, and 14 as needed.

Box 3. First-Line Actions

First-Line Actions:

- Oxygen and intubation as needed
- Nitroglycerin SL
- Furosemide IV 0.5 to 1 mg/kg
- Morphine IV 2 to 4 mg

If the patient's blood pressure is adequate, help the patient sit upright with the legs dependent. This position increases lung volume and vital capacity, diminishes the work of breathing, and decreases venous return to the heart. You may also administer morphine to dilate veins and arteries and reduce cardiac preload and afterload. Rotating tourniquets provides no clinical benefit and is now considered obsolete.

Provide oxygen, establish IV access, and begin cardiac monitoring (ACLS providers treat "oxygen-IV-monitor" as a single word). Monitor oxyhemoglobin saturation with pulse oximetry, although results may be inaccurate and misleading if peripheral perfusion is poor. Oxyhemoglobin saturation does not provide information about hemoglobin concentration, oxygen content, ventilation, or acid-base status. You may need to evaluate hemoglobin and hematocrit and obtain an arterial sample for blood gas analysis when the patient reaches the Emergency Department.

Oxygen and Possible Intubation

Deliver oxygen at high flow rates, starting at 5 or 6 L/min by mask. Nonrebreathing masks with reservoir bags can provide oxygen concentrations of 90% to near 100%. You may need to use a bag-mask to provide assisted ventilation if the patient's ventilation is inadequate. If the patient is breathing spontaneously, you can provide continuous positive airway pressure by mask (mask must create a tight seal against the face).

Be prepared to intubate the patient who has significant respiratory distress or respiratory failure. A need for intubation is particularly likely in the following situations:

- PaO_2 cannot be maintained above 60 mm Hg despite 100% oxygen.
- Signs of cerebral hypoxia (eg, lethargy or confusion) develop.
- PCO_2 increases progressively.
- Respiratory acidosis develops.

Verify successful intubation using primary and secondary confirmation techniques. *Note:* Pulmonary edema should not interfere with detection of exhaled CO_2 in the trachea. If copious respiratory secretions are present, however, an esophageal detector device may fail to reinflate despite correct placement of the tube in the trachea. This failure may lead to the inaccurate conclusion that the tube is in the esophagus when it is accurately placed in the trachea. Once the patient is intubated, mechanical ventilation with positive end-expiratory pressure can improve oxygenation.

Nitroglycerin

If SBP is adequate (usually >90 to 100 mm Hg) and the patient has no serious signs or

FIGURE. Acute Pulmonary Edema, Hypotension, and Shock Algorithm

1 Clinical Signs: Shock, hypoperfusion, congestive heart failure, acute pulmonary edema
Most likely problem?

2 Acute Pulmonary Edema

6 Volume Problem

8 Pump Problem

14 Rate Problem

Bradycardia
See Vol. 1,
Chapter 14

Tachycardia
See Vol. 1,
Chapters
15 and 16

3 First-Line Actions
• *Oxygen* and intubation as needed
• *Nitroglycerin* SL
• *Furosemide* IV 0.5 to 1 mg/kg
• *Morphine* IV 2 to 4 mg

7 Administer
• *Fluids*
• *Blood transfusions*
• *Cause-specific interventions*
Consider vasopressors

9 Blood pressure?

Systolic BP
BP defines 2nd line of action
(See below)

10 Systolic BP
<70 mm Hg
Signs or symptoms of shock

11 Systolic BP
70 to 100 mm Hg
Signs or symptoms of shock

12 Systolic BP
70 to 100 mm Hg
No signs or symptoms of shock

13 Systolic BP
>100 mm Hg

• *Norepinephrine*
0.5 to 30 µg/min IV

• *Dopamine*
5 to 15 µg/kg per minute IV

• *Dobutamine*
2 to 20 µg/kg per minute IV

• *Nitroglycerin*
10 to 20 µg/min IV
Consider
• *Nitroprusside* 0.1 to 5 µg/kg per minute IV

4 Second-Line Actions—Acute Pulmonary Edema
• Nitroglycerin or nitroprusside if BP >100 mm Hg
• Dopamine if BP 70 to 100 mm Hg, signs or symptoms of shock
• Dobutamine if BP >100 mm Hg, no signs or symptoms of shock

5 Further Diagnostic and Therapeutic Considerations
• Identify and treat reversible causes
• Pulmonary artery catheterization
• Intra-aortic balloon pump
• Angiography and PCI
• Additional diagnostic studies
• Surgical interventions
• Additional drug therapy

symptoms of shock, then IV nitroglycerin is the drug of choice for acute pulmonary edema. Nitroglycerin reduces pulmonary congestion by dilating the venous capacitance vessels, reducing preload. It also dilates systemic arteries, decreasing systemic vascular resistance. This effect can reduce afterload and increase cardiac output.

Nitroglycerin may initially be administered by sublingual tablets, oral spray (isosorbide oral spray is an acceptable alternative), or the intravenous route. You can give 2 of the standard 0.4 mg tablets every 5 to 10 minutes provided SBP remains greater than 90 to 100 mm Hg and the patient has no clinical signs of tissue hypoperfusion (shock). You should not give nitroglycerin to hypotensive patients with signs of shock. Typically they cannot tolerate vasodilatation. In such patients clinicians should first support the circulation by treating underlying rate, volume, or pump problems. Withhold nitroglycerin until the patient's hemodynamic status improves (looks more good than bad).

Do not administer nitroglycerin to patients who are known to have used sildenafil citrate (Viagra) within the previous 24 hours.[25,26] In these patients nitroglycerin can cause severe hypotension refractory to vasopressors. Use nitroglycerin with caution (if at all) if the patient has an inferior wall AMI with possible right ventricular involvement.[27] Patients with RV dysfunction are very dependent on maintenance of RV filling pressures to maintain cardiac output and blood pressure.

Furosemide

Furosemide has long been a mainstay in the treatment of acute pulmonary edema. It has a biphasic action. First, within approximately 5 minutes it causes an immediate decrease in venous tone and an increase in venous capacitance. These changes lead to a fall in left ventricular filling pressure (preload) that may improve clinical symptoms. Second, furosemide produces diuresis within 5 to 10 minutes of IV administration. The diuresis need not be marked to be effective. If the patient is

not already taking furosemide, the typical dose is 0.5 to 1 mg/kg given as a slow IV bolus over 1 to 2 minutes. If the response to this dose is inadequate after about 20 minutes, you may give another bolus of 2 mg/kg. If the patient is already taking oral furosemide, the clinical rule of thumb is to administer an initial dose that is twice the daily oral dose. If no effect occurs within about 20 minutes, double the initial dose. You may need to use higher doses if the patient has massive fluid retention, refractory heart failure, or renal insufficiency.

Recent clinical trials have been conducted with nesiritide, a recombinant human brain natriuretic peptide, in patients hospitalized with decompensated congestive heart failure. Compared with placebo and "standard therapy," nesiritide was associated with improved hemodynamic function, decreased dyspnea and fatigue, and better global clinical status.[28]

Morphine Sulfate

Morphine sulfate remains a part of the therapy for acute pulmonary edema, although recent research questions its effectiveness, especially outside the hospital. Morphine dilates the capacitance vessels of the peripheral venous bed. This dilatation reduces venous return to the central circulation and diminishes ventricular preload. Morphine also reduces afterload by causing mild arterial vasodilatation. It also has a sedative effect. More effective vasodilators are now available, so that morphine is considered an acceptable adjunct rather than a drug of choice for acute pulmonary edema.

Box 4. Second-Line Actions

Second-Line Actions:

- Nitroglycerin or nitroprusside if BP >100 mm Hg

- Dopamine if BP 70 to 100 mm Hg, signs or symptoms of shock

- Dobutamine if BP >100 mm Hg, no signs or symptoms of shock

Patients who respond to first-line actions for pulmonary edema may not require additional therapy. If additional therapy is indicated, base your second-line actions on the patient's systolic blood pressure and clinical response.

If SBP is >100 mm Hg, you can use a vasodilator to reduce ventricular preload and afterload. IV nitroglycerin is listed as both a first- and second-line agent because establishing IV access takes time. You may administer sublingual nitroglycerin until IV access is achieved and then give IV nitroglycerin. Although the sublingual form of nitroglycerin is more convenient and more readily available, IV nitroglycerin is a potent vasodilator and the mainstay of treatment. Clinicians can accurately titrate the dose of IV nitroglycerin while monitoring the patient's clinical and hemodynamic status.

The precautions noted under first-line actions apply. Avoid use of nitroglycerin in patients who: have taken Viagra within the previous 24 hours; with hypotension (SBP <90 mm Hg); with extreme bradycardia (HR <50 bpm); with tachycardia; and use with caution in patients with an inferior wall AMI with possible RV involvement. Nitroprusside is an alternative drug to treat hypertension.

Intravenous nitroglycerin may be initiated at a rate of 10 µg/min through continuous infusion with nonabsorbing tubing. Increase by 5 to 10 µg every 3 to 5 minutes until a symptom or blood pressure response is noted. If no response is seen at 20 µg/min, incremental increases of 10 µg/min and later 20 µg/min can be used. As the symptoms and signs of acute pulmonary edema or cardiac ischemia begin to resolve, there is no need to continue upward titration of nitroglycerin simply to obtain a fall in blood pressure. When blood pressure reduction is a therapeutic goal, reduce the dosage when the blood pressure begins to fall. Frequently recommended limits for blood pressure reduction are 10% of baseline level in normotensive patients and 30% reduction in hypertensive patients.[21]

If SBP is >100 mm Hg and signs of shock are present, a dopamine infusion is recommended. If SBP is 70 to 100 mm Hg and the patient has no signs of shock, a dobutamine infusion is recommended for normotensive pump failure and to improve cardiac output or distribution of blood flow.

Subsequent sections (Boxes 10 through 13) provide more details about vasoactive drug therapy for patients with various levels of hypotension.

Box 5. Further Diagnostic and Therapeutic Considerations

- Identify and treat reversible causes (consider 6 H's and 6 T's)
- Pulmonary artery catheterization (controversial; see below)
- Intra-aortic balloon pump (bridge to surgery)
- Angiography and PCI (if drugs fail)
- Additional diagnostic studies
- Surgical interventions (valve surgery, CABG, heart transplantation)
- Additional drug therapy:
  — Inamrinone 0.75 mg/kg, then 5 to 15 µg/kg per minute if BP >100 mm Hg (if other drugs fail)
  — Inhaled β-agonists (if wheezing)
  — Fibrinolytic therapy (for acute ST-elevation MI)
  — Antiarrhythmic therapy and rate control (for atrial fibrillation, supraventricular tachycardias)

Reserve these third-line actions for patients with pump failure and acute pulmonary edema who are resistant to first- and second-line actions or who develop specific complications. Whenever the patient does not respond to initial therapy, the ACLS provider should try to identify and treat reversible causes. The provider can use the memory aid of the *6 H's and 6 T's* (see this volume, Chapter 1: "Introduction to ACLS for the Experienced Provider").

Critical care experts have used hemodynamic monitoring based on pulmonary artery catheterization for decades to enable precise tracking of hemodynamic variables and evaluation of response to therapy. Controversy began to arise in the 1990s about observations of increased morbidity and mortality in patients monitored with pulmonary artery catheterization. This led to a call by some experts[29] for a moratorium on its use and the assembly of multispecialty experts to develop consensus guidelines in 1996,[30-44] and again in 2000.[45]

But critical care providers must know how to insert and maintain the catheter and how to interpret the calculated variables.[31] Insertion of a pulmonary artery catheter is recommended when the initial hemodynamics are unclear and a change in therapy would result. No benefit, and in some cases increased mortality, has been demonstrated with the routine or indiscriminate use of pulmonary artery catheters.

Used with skill and clinical acumen, hemodynamic monitoring using pulmonary artery catheterization offers value to selected patients, but the use of the catheter remains controversial.[46-62] The recent publication of a major, multicenter clinical trial that "found no benefit to therapy directed by pulmonary-artery catheter over standard care in elderly, high-risk surgical patients requiring intensive care"[46] is sure to rekindle the debates.[63]

Fibrinolytic agents have a limited role in patients with AMI and pump failure. These patients are better served by mechanical reperfusion (PCI/CABG) and support (IABP). Selected patients with multivessel disease or structural complications of MI will be candidates for acute surgical procedures such as CABG and repair or replacement of heart valves. An intra-aortic balloon pump, ventricular assist device (usually not acutely), or even a total artificial heart (not acutely) can successfully serve as a bridge to support the patient until surgery can be performed or nonsurgical recovery occurs. PCI can be lifesaving for patients in cardiogenic shock: investigators have

reported survival rates as high as 50% when PCI was performed within the first 18 hours.[3] These rates are much higher than the rates with fibrinolytic therapy or aortic balloon counterpulsation alone or in combination.

Clinicians may use *inamrinone* for severe CHF refractory to diuretics, vasodilators, and conventional inotropes. This drug is a phosphodiesterase III inhibitor with both inotropic and vasodilatory effects. Give it intravenously in a loading dose of 0.75 mg/kg over 10 to 15 minutes; follow that infusion with a continuous infusion of 5 to 15 µg/kg per minute titrated to clinical effect. Optimal use requires hemodynamic monitoring.

The Cardiovascular Quadrad: A Conceptual Model

ECC providers need a conceptual tool to help understand and treat hypotension and shock. Such a tool is particularly helpful during the initial phase of a cardiovascular emergency, when invasive monitoring is usually unavailable.

The *Cardiovascular Quadrad* conceptualizes the cardiovascular system as having 4 main components:

1. Tank volume (intravascular volume relative to the vascular space)
2. Tank resistance (vasomotor tone, peripheral vascular resistance, and capillary permeability)
3. Pump (cardiac function)
4. Heart rate and rhythm

As a conceptual model, the Cardiovascular Quadrad provides a simple framework for assessment of the patient, clinical problem solving, and medical decision making. It will help the clinician identify the factors that may be producing hypotension, clarify the mechanisms of shock, provide a problem list, suggest appropriate therapies, and help prevent errors. It also can help clinicians discriminate between difficult clinical problems, such as hypotension due to an arrhythmia (see Volume 1, Chapters 13 through 16) and hypotension associated with trauma or other special resuscitation situations (see Chapter 4 in this volume).

In this model there are only 4 general causes of hypotension:

1. A *tank volume* problem (inadequate intravascular volume relative to the vascular space)

2. A *tank resistance* and vascular permeability problem (inappropriate vascular resistance or capillary permeability)

3. A *pump* problem (poor myocardial function)

4. A *rate* or *rhythm* problem (heart rate is too slow, too fast, or ineffective)

The clinician must often answer these questions in terms of *probabilities* rather than certainties. The clinician, for example, may need to begin therapy after concluding that a patient has a *probable* tank problem, a *possible* pump problem, and a *definite* rate or rhythm problem. You can easily determine heart rate and rhythm by counting the heart rate and obtaining a rhythm strip from a cardiac monitor. But pump, volume, and vascular resistance problems can be difficult to confirm without hemodynamic monitoring. Experienced clinicians can, however, make a reasonable assessment of the probability of these problems using the history, physical examination, and other available information even before hemodynamic monitoring is instituted.

Box 6. Evaluate Intravascular Volume and Vascular Resistance (Tank Volume and Tank Resistance)

The clinical term used to discuss intravascular volume is cardiac *preload;* the term used to discuss systemic vascular resistance is cardiac *afterload.* Think of preload as stretch placed on the myocardium ("loading") by the volume in the ventricle just before it begins to contract (ventricular end-diastolic volume). Although echocardiography can accurately assess end-diastolic volume, we cannot readily measure this volume at the bedside in the nonoperative

clinical setting. In practice, clinicians monitor ventricular end-diastolic *pressure* via central venous pressure (surrogate for right ventricular end-diastolic pressure) and pulmonary artery wedge pressure (surrogate for left ventricular end-diastolic pressure). Once a contraction begins, the ventricle encounters resistance ("load" or "impedance") to the contraction. This resistance is called *afterload.*

The tank contains fluid and is surrounded by vascular smooth muscle (making it "adjustable"). When evaluating intravascular volume (fluid status) and vasomotor tone (vascular resistance), the provider should consider whether the tank is "too full" (volume overloaded), "too empty" (hypovolemic), "too large" (vasodilated), or "too small" (vasoconstricted). You should consider tank volume relative to the vascular space.

Volume problems can be of 2 types: absolute or relative. An *absolute* volume problem is due to an actual fluid deficit. A *relative* volume problem occurs when the volume of circulating blood is inadequate relative to vascular tone, size of the tank, and vascular permeability. Bleeding, vomiting, diarrhea, polyuria, decreased volume intake, and dehydration can cause absolute volume loss. Vasodilation (systemic vascular resistance is too low), vasoconstriction (systemic vascular resistance is too high), and redistribution of fluid to third spaces (such as the lung or interstitial tissues) can produce relative volume loss. Anaphylactic shock is an example of a condition that can cause both absolute and relative volume loss: tank size increases because of vasodilatation, and there is an actual loss of fluid from the vascular compartment due to a capillary leak.

To evaluate right ventricular end-diastolic pressure, measure the central venous pressure (CVP). Clinical signs of a high CVP include jugular venous distention, hepatomegaly, ascites, and dependent edema.

Evaluate left ventricular end-diastolic pressure by measuring the pulmonary artery wedge pressure using a pulmonary artery

catheter. Clinical signs of a high pulmonary venous pressure include tachypnea, dyspnea, and evidence of pulmonary edema. Pulmonary edema may be caused by either high pulmonary venous pressure or increased capillary permeability (capillary leak).

A pulmonary capillary occlusion pressure (or pulmonary artery wedge pressure) of 18 mm Hg is optimal for patients with AMI (normal left ventricular end-diastolic pressure ≤12 mm Hg). Most patients with an AMI, and especially those with a right ventricular infarct, will have better cardiac output with a "full tank" rather than with normal filling pressures. That is, the stroke volume and cardiac output will improve if the ventricular muscle is stretched before it contracts. When myocardial function is poor, a filling pressure of about 18 mm Hg results in better cardiac output according to the Frank-Starling law.

Note: The signs of hypovolemia may be subtle. Be alert for occult volume or vascular resistance problems. If the lungs are clear and there is no evidence of pump failure, provide a fluid challenge if you suspect hypovolemia.

Box 7. Administer Fluids, Consider Vasopressors

If you suspect absolute or relative hypovolemia in a patient with signs of shock, administer fluids. Base your choice of fluid on the suspected cause of hypovolemia:

- **Fluids:** Administer isotonic crystalloids (normal saline or lactated Ringer's) 250 to 500 mL.

- **Blood:** If hemorrhage has occurred, administer blood or packed red blood cells (general rule: 5 to 10 mL/kg packed RBCs at 5 to 10 mL/min).

- **Cause-specific interventions:** Base the volume and content of fluids on the cause of fluid loss. In general you will administer isotonic crystalloid for acute volume resuscitation. But to replace specific fluid losses, you will try to match the fluid lost in volume and content. For example, you may administer more hypotonic fluid to replace volume loss from increased urine output in diabetes insipidus, but you would administer fluid that is more isotonic to replace fluid lost with vomiting and diarrhea.

Closely monitor the patient's respiratory function throughout fluid administration. Be prepared to provide assisted ventilation and intubation as needed. *You should expect pulmonary edema and respiratory distress to be worse after fluid administration.*

If hypotension is present after volume administration, consider administration of vasopressors (eg, epinephrine, norepinephrine, or vasopressin). For more information see below and Volume 1, Chapter 11: "Drugs for Cardiac Output and Peripheral Vascular Resistance."

If you are uncertain about whether the patient requires volume administration, it is reasonable to administer a "test" bolus of 250 to 500 mL and monitor the patient's response. If the patient's clinical appearance and blood pressure improve, you may administer additional fluid.

Box 8. Evaluate Pump Function

By definition any patient with signs of shock and AMI has a pump problem. Still, most patients with acute infarcts do not present with clinically significant pump failure. For a patient to develop hypotension or shock from a pump problem, there must be significant ventricular dysfunction with a reduced ejection fraction.

Pump failure can produce high ventricular end-diastolic pressures and adrenergic compensatory signs of tachycardia and vasoconstriction with attempts to redistribute blood flow. Right ventricular failure and high RVEDP produce high systemic venous pressure (CVP). Left ventricular failure and high LVEDP produce high pulmonary venous pressure and acute pulmonary edema. Pump failure can also produce clinical signs of inadequate cardiac output (hypotension, weak pulses, fatigue, weakness, dizziness, delayed capillary refill, and lactic acidosis).

Clinicians should try to determine the specific cause of pump failure because appropriate therapy can be lifesaving. Emergency surgery, for example, can repair acute valvular dysfunction due to acute rupture of chordae tendineae, papillary muscle dysfunction, or rupture of the intraventricular septum. In these conditions surgery should not be delayed for "medical" stabilization. As another example, bicarbonate administration can stop arrhythmias caused by tricyclic antidepressant overdose. And patients with β-blocker or calcium channel blocker overdose may need high doses of vasopressors to improve blood pressure and cardiac output (see Chapter 3 in this volume).

Pump problems can be primary or secondary. Primary pump problems, such as those caused by an AMI or drug overdose, may be diagnosed if adequate information about the patient's history is available. But it is easy to overlook secondary pump problems unless you consider the clinical setting and the total clinical picture. Remember that when one system or component fails, the others may follow. Whatever the initial problem, virtually all patients in shock will develop a pump problem as the heart is depleted of essential substrates such as oxygen, glucose, and adenosine triphosphate.

Box 9. Evaluate Systolic Blood Pressure

Select drug therapy to support cardiac output. Base your choice of drug on the patient's systolic blood pressure and the presence or absence of shock:

- SBP <70 mm Hg with signs or symptoms of shock

- SBP 70 to 100 mm Hg with signs or symptoms of shock

- SBP 70 to 100 mm Hg with *no* signs or symptoms of shock

- SBP >100 mm Hg

This approach assumes that hypovolemia has been or is being corrected and that pump failure is present.

Unless it is strikingly low, SBP alone is not a reliable and sensitive indicator of the presence of shock. Clinicians should always evaluate blood pressure in light of signs of systemic perfusion and trends in response to therapy. If you do not carefully correlate SBP with clinical signs and symptoms, you may fail to recognize shock. You should also evaluate blood pressure in light of the patient's *typical* blood pressure. A blood pressure of 140/80 mm Hg may be normal for one patient, relatively high for another, and relatively low for a third patient. A "normal" BP can provide inexperienced clinicians with a false sense of security.

Box 10. SBP <70 mm Hg With Signs or Symptoms of Shock

Patients in this subgroup are usually in profound shock. Norepinephrine infusion is recommended because it has both β$_1$-adrenergic (inotropic) and α-adrenergic (vasoconstrictive and vasopressor) effects even at low doses.

The recommended dose of norepinephrine is 0.5 to 30 µg/min continuous IV infusion; titrate to achieve the desired clinical response. Continue this infusion until systolic pressure rises to approximately 70 mm Hg or higher. Keep in mind that if the solution extravasates, the α-adrenergic effects of norepinephrine can injure soft tissues. If extravasation occurs, promptly infiltrate the area locally (inject directly into the soft tissues) with 10 mg of phentolamine, an α-blocking agent.

Box 11. SBP 70 to 100 mm Hg With Signs or Symptoms of Shock

By definition patients in this subgroup are in shock. Because the patient's hypotension is mild to moderate, signs of shock may be mild or moderate. But these patients may deteriorate quickly if you do not support the blood pressure and effectively treat causes of myocardial dysfunction. A continuous infusion of IV dopamine is recommended. Dopamine can provide dopaminergic effects (increased renal, coronary, and mesenteric perfusion) at low and moderate doses, β_1-adrenergic (inotropic) effects at moderate doses, and α-adrenergic (vasoconstrictive) effects at higher doses. Begin the infusion at approximately 5 µg/kg per minute; titrate up to approximately 15 µg/kg per minute to optimize blood pressure and systemic perfusion.

If an infusion dose of more than 20 µg/kg per minute of dopamine is required to maintain arterial BP, consider switching to a drug with more significant vasopressor effects, such as norepinephrine. Experienced clinicians may decide to use both dopamine and norepinephrine to exploit the unique properties of each.

Box 12. SBP 70 to 100 mm Hg With No Signs or Symptoms of Shock

By definition patients in this group are hypotensive but *not* in shock. Nonetheless their systolic blood pressure is borderline. They also may have inadequate cardiac output even in the absence of overt signs of shock.

You may think of patients in this group as being "more good than bad." Although the patient is hypotensive and probably has impaired cardiac output, perfusion to vital organs is adequate (if not optimal).

The recommended adrenergic agent for such patients is IV dobutamine delivered by continuous infusion. Start the infusion at 2 µg/kg per minute; titrate as needed to approximately 20 µg/kg per minute. Note that dobutamine has β-adrenergic effects, so it provides β_1 (inotropic) effects and β_2 (vasodilatory) effects. It has no significant α-adrenergic (vasoconstrictive) effects. But it is an excellent inotrope and can improve contractility without increasing cardiac work and myocardial oxygen consumption as much as dopamine.

Box 13. SBP >100 mm Hg

Patients in this group have clinically significant pump failure but normal systolic blood pressure. For these patients administer IV nitroglycerin at 10 to 20 µg/min or IV nitroprusside at 0.1 to 5 µg/kg per minute. Most emergency physicians prefer nitroglycerin in these patients because it is easier to administer and produces better coronary artery dilatation (which is good for coronary ischemia if present). Note the precautions mentioned earlier for use of nitroglycerin in patients who have taken Viagra within the previous 24 hours and in patients with an inferior wall MI with possible RV involvement (see "Nitroglycerin" and "Box 4. Second-Line Actions").

Closely monitor the patient's clinical appearance and vital signs during administration of any vasodilator. Be prepared to reduce or discontinue the infusion and administer volume if hypotension develops.

Nitroglycerin and nitroprusside can be used in combination. Experienced providers should use this combination in special situations.

Box 14. Evaluate Heart Rate and Rhythm

The last element in the Cardiovascular Quadrad is heart rate. Evaluate the heart rate with the cardiac rhythm. If the *ventricular rate* is normal, a rhythm problem alone is unlikely to cause hypotension. For example, a patient with third-degree AV block has a serious rhythm problem. But if the *ventricular rate* is adequate, the AV block alone is unlikely to be the cause of hypotension.

It is important to consider whether the heart rate is *appropriate* for the blood pressure. In general a patient with shock and hypotension should have a compensatory tachycardia. A "normal" heart rate in the presence of severe hypotension or shock is a potentially ominous sign of inadequate compensation. It may indicate that further deterioration is imminent. Keep in mind that the most appropriate treatment for such a patient is to treat the underlying problem (eg, hypovolemia or pump failure), not to try to increase heart rate with drugs or a pacemaker.

For more information about treatment of arrhythmias, see Volume 1, Chapter 12: "Pharmacology 2: Agents for Control of Rate and Rhythm," Chapter 14: "Bradycardias: Atrioventricular Blocks and Emergency Pacing," and Chapter 15: "Narrow-Complex Supraventricular Tachycardias."

Summary

- For treatment of patients with acute pulmonary edema, hypotension, and shock, some general rules help to guide therapy. For patients with AMI and cardiogenic shock, consider cardiac catheterization, intra-aortic balloon counterpulsation, PCI, or CABG if anatomy is suitable. Although the mortality rate in these patients is high, these procedures offer patients with cardiogenic shock the best chance of survival. Consider EMS triage or transfer to a facility with a cardiac catheterization suite with interventional capabilities.

- For any patient with shock, try to identify and correct any underlying clinical problems while supporting pump function and blood pressure. If you know which system is failing, treat the failing system. Without invasive hemodynamic monitoring it may be difficult to assess the effectiveness of intravascular volume relative to the vascular space, vascular resistance, and pump function (tank volume, tank resistance, pump). You may need to make an initial assessment based on probabilities and formulate a treatment strategy accordingly.

- If you do not know which component of the Cardiovascular Quadrad is causing or contributing to the hypotension or shock, it may be helpful to follow these rules of thumb:

  — Treat any clinically significant heart rate or rhythm problems.

  — If the lungs are clear and there is no evidence of CHF or pulmonary edema, administer fluids.

  — Consider use of an inotrope to increase contractility and improve pump function.

  — Consider use of a vasopressor to increase vasomotor tone.

— Consider use of a vasodilator to reduce ventricular preload or afterload.

■ Do not use vasopressors to treat hypovolemic shock unless you have provided or are providing adequate volume replacement. Use vasopressors to increase systemic vascular resistance in patients with adequate circulating blood volume. If you are unsure if volume is needed, it is reasonable to try a test volume infusion.

References

1. Hasdai D, Holmes DR Jr, Topol EJ, Berger PB, Criger DA, Hochman JS, Bates ER, Vahanian A, Armstrong PW, Wilcox R, Ohman EM, Califf RM. Frequency and clinical outcome of cardiogenic shock during acute myocardial infarction among patients receiving reteplase or alteplase. Results from GUSTO-III. Global Use of Strategies to Open Occluded Coronary Arteries. *Eur Heart J.* 1999;20:128-135.

2. Single-bolus tenecteplase compared with front-loaded alteplase in acute myocardial infarction: the ASSENT-2 double-blind randomised trial. Assessment of the Safety and Efficacy of a New Thrombolytic Investigators. *Lancet.* 1999;354:716-722.

3. Hochman JS, Sleeper LA, Webb JG, Sanborn TA, White HD, Talley JD, Buller CE, Jacobs AK, Slater JN, Col J, McKinlay SM, LeJemtel TH. Early revascularization in acute myocardial infarction complicated by cardiogenic shock. SHOCK Investigators. Should We Emergently Revascularize Occluded Coronaries for Cardiogenic Shock. *N Engl J Med.* 1999;341:625-634.

4. Goldberg RJ, Gore JM, Alpert JS, Osganian V, de Groot J, Bade J, Chen Z, Frid D, Dalen JE. Cardiogenic shock after acute myocardial infarction. Incidence and mortality from a community-wide perspective, 1975 to 1988. *N Engl J Med.* 1991;325:1117-1122.

5. Bengtson JR, Kaplan AJ, Pieper KS, Wildermann NM, Mark DB, Pryor DB, Phillips HR III, Califf RM. Prognosis in cardiogenic shock after acute myocardial infarction in the interventional era. *J Am Coll Cardiol.* 1992;20:1482-1489.

6. Hasdai D, Califf RM, Thompson TD, Hochman JS, Ohman EM, Pfisterer M, Bates ER, Vahanian A, Armstrong PW, Criger DA, Topol EJ, Holmes DR Jr. Predictors of cardiogenic shock after thrombolytic therapy for acute myocardial infarction. *J Am Coll Cardiol.* 2000;35:136-143.

7. Hochman JS, Boland J, Sleeper LA, Porway M, Brinker J, Col J, Jacobs A, Slater J, Miller D, Wasserman H, et al. Current spectrum of cardiogenic shock and effect of early revascularization on mortality. Results of an International Registry. SHOCK Registry Investigators. *Circulation.* 1995;91:873-881.

8. Hochman JS, Sleeper LA, White HD, Dzavik V, Wong SC, Menon V, Webb JG, Steingart R, Picard MH, Menegus MA, Boland J, Sanborn T, Buller CE, Modur S, Forman R, Desvigne-Nickens P, Jacobs AK, Slater JN, LeJemtel TH. One-year survival following early revascularization for cardiogenic shock. *JAMA.* 2001;285:190-192.

9. Itoh T, Fukami K, Oriso S, Umemura J, Nakajima J, Obonai H, Hiramori K. Survival following cardiogenic shock caused by acute left main coronary artery total occlusion. A case report and review of the literature. *Angiology.* 1997;48:163-171.

10. Holmes DR Jr, Califf RM, Van de Werf F, Berger PB, Bates ER, Simoons ML, White HD, Thompson TD, Topol EJ. Difference in countries' use of resources and clinical outcome for patients with cardiogenic shock after myocardial infarction: results from the GUSTO trial. *Lancet.* 1997;349:75-78.

11. Califf RM, Bengtson JR. Cardiogenic shock. *N Engl J Med.* 1994;330:1724-1730.

12. Bates ER, Topol EJ. Limitations of thrombolytic therapy for acute myocardial infarction complicated by congestive heart failure and cardiogenic shock. *J Am Coll Cardiol.* 1991; 18:1077-1084.

13. Berger PB, Holmes DR Jr, Stebbins AL, Bates ER, Califf RM, Topol EJ. Impact of an aggressive invasive catheterization and revascularization strategy on mortality in patients with cardiogenic shock in the Global Utilization of Streptokinase and Tissue Plasminogen Activator for Occluded Coronary Arteries (GUSTO-I) trial. An observational study. *Circulation.* 1997;96:122-127.

14. Tiefenbrunn AJ, Chandra NC, French WJ, Gore JM, Rogers WJ. Clinical experience with primary percutaneous transluminal coronary angioplasty compared with alteplase (recombinant tissue-type plasminogen activator) in patients with acute myocardial infarction: a report from the Second National Registry of Myocardial Infarction (NRMI- 2). *J Am Coll Cardiol.* 1998;31:1240-1245.

15. Lee L, Erbel R, Brown TM, Laufer N, Meyer J, O'Neill WW. Multicenter registry of angioplasty therapy of cardiogenic shock: initial and long-term survival. *J Am Coll Cardiol.* 1991;17:599-603.

16. Ohman EM, Califf RM, George BS, Quigley PJ, Kereiakes DJ, Harrelson-Woodlief L, Candela RJ, Flanagan C, Stack RS, Topol EJ. The use of intraaortic balloon pumping as an adjunct to reperfusion therapy in acute myocardial infarction. The Thrombolysis and Angioplasty in Myocardial Infarction (TAMI) Study Group. *Am Heart J.* 1991;121:895-901.

17. Sanborn TA, Sleeper LA, Bates ER, Jacobs AK, Boland J, French JK, Dens J, Dzavik V, Palmeri ST, Webb JG, Goldberger M, Hochman JS. Impact of thrombolysis, intra-aortic balloon pump counterpulsation, and their combination in cardiogenic shock complicating acute myocardial infarction: a report from the SHOCK Trial Registry. SHould we emergently revascularize Occluded Coronaries for cardiogenic shocK? *J Am Coll Cardiol.* 2000;36: 1123-1129.

18. Ishihara M, Sato H, Tateishi H, Kawagoe T, Shimatani Y, Kurisu S, Sakai K. Intraaortic balloon pumping as adjunctive therapy to rescue coronary angioplasty after failed thrombolysis in anterior wall acute myocardial infarction. *Am J Cardiol.* 1995;76:73-75.

19. Grines CL. Aggressive intervention for myocardial infarction: angioplasty, stents, and intra-aortic balloon pumping. *Am J Cardiol.* 1996; 78:29-34.

20. Ryan TJ, Antman EM, Brooks NH, Califf RM, Hillis LD, Hiratzka LF, Rapaport E, Riegel B, Russell RO, Smith EE 3rd, Weaver WD, Gibbons RJ, Alpert JS, Eagle KA, Gardner TJ, Garson A Jr, Gregoratos G, Smith SC Jr. 1999 update: ACC/AHA guidelines for the management of patients with acute myocardial infarction. A report of the American College of Cardiology/American Heart Association Task Force on Practice Guidelines (Committee on Management of Acute Myocardial Infarction). *J Am Coll Cardiol.* 1999;34:890-911.

21. American Heart Association in collaboration with International Liaison Committee on Resuscitation. Guidelines 2000 for Cardiopulmonary Resuscitation and Emergency Cardiovascular Care: International Consensus on Science, Part 7: The Era of Reperfusion: Section 1: Acute Coronary Syndromes (Acute Myocardial Infarction). *Circulation.* 2000;102:I172-I203.

22. Aufderheide TP, Bossaert LL, Field J, Herlitz J, Leizorovicz A, Littrell KA, Ornato JP, Peberdy MA, Ribichini F. Cardiopulmonary resuscitation and emergency cardiovascular care. Acute coronary syndromes. *Ann Emerg Med.* 2001;37:S163-S181.

23. Nanas JN, Nanas SN, Kontoyannis DA, Moussoutzani KS, Hatzigeorgiou JP, Heras PB, Makaritsis KP, Agapitos EB, Moulopoulos SD. Myocardial salvage by the use of reperfusion and intraaortic balloon pump: experimental study. *Ann Thorac Surg.* 1996;61:629-634.

24. Talley JD, Ohman EM, Mark DB, George BS, Leimberger JD, Berdan LG, Davidson-Ray L, Rawert M, Lam LC, Phillips HR, Califf RM. Economic implications of the prophylactic use of intraaortic balloon counterpulsation in the setting of acute myocardial infarction. The Randomized IABP Study Group. Intraaortic Balloon Pump. *Am J Cardiol*. 1997;79:590-594.

25. Kloner RA, Zusman RM. Cardiovascular effects of sildenafil citrate and recommendations for its use. *Am J Cardiol*. 1999;84:11N-17N.

26. Webb DJ, Muirhead GJ, Wulff M, Sutton JA, Levi R, Dinsmore WW. Sildenafil citrate potentiates the hypotensive effects of nitric oxide donor drugs in male patients with stable angina. *J Am Coll Cardiol*. 2000;36:25-31.

27. Arora RR, Timoney M, Melilli L. Acute myocardial infarction after the use of sildenafil. *N Engl J Med*. 1999;341:700.

28. Colucci WS, Elkayam U, Horton DP, Abraham WT, Bourge RC, Johnson AD, Wagoner LE, Givertz MM, Liang CS, Neibaur M, Haught WH, LeJemtel TH. Intravenous nesiritide, a natriuretic peptide, in the treatment of decompensated congestive heart failure. Nesiritide Study Group. *N Engl J Med*. 2000;343:246-253.

29. Dalen JE, Bone RC. Is it time to pull the pulmonary artery catheter? *JAMA*. 1996;276:916-918.

30. Ahrens TS. Is nursing education adequate for pulmonary artery catheter utilization? *New Horiz*. 1997;5:281-286.

31. Pulmonary Artery Catheter Consensus Conference. Chicago, Illinois, December 6-8, 1996. *New Horiz*. 1997;5:173-296.

32. Chalfin DB. The pulmonary artery catheter: economic aspects. *New Horiz*. 1997;5:292-296.

33. Hollenberg SM, Hoyt J. Pulmonary artery catheters in cardiovascular disease. *New Horiz*. 1997;5:207-213.

34. Ivanov RI, Allen J, Sandham JD, Calvin JE. Pulmonary artery catheterization: a narrative and systematic critique of randomized controlled trials and recommendations for the future. *New Horiz*. 1997;5:268-276.

35. Kelso LA. Complications associated with pulmonary artery catheterization. *New Horiz*. 1997;5:259-263.

36. Kirton OC, Civetta JM. Do pulmonary artery catheters alter outcome in trauma patients? *New Horiz*. 1997;5:222-227.

37. Leibowitz AB, Beilin Y. Pulmonary artery catheters and outcome in the perioperative period. *New Horiz*. 1997;5:214-221.

38. Nelson LD. The new pulmonary artery catheters: continuous venous oximetry, right ventricular ejection fraction, and continuous cardiac output. *New Horiz*. 1997;5:251-258.

39. Papadakos PJ, Vender JS. Training requirements for pulmonary artery catheter utilization in adult patients. *New Horiz*. 1997;5:287-291.

40. Parker MM, Peruzzi W. Pulmonary artery catheters in sepsis/septic shock. *New Horiz*. 1997;5:228-232.

41. Sprung CL, Eidelman LA. The issue of a U.S. Food and Drug Administration moratorium on the use of the pulmonary artery catheter. *New Horiz*. 1997;5:277-280.

42. Sprung CL, Eidelman LA. Ethical issues of clinical trials for the pulmonary artery catheter. *New Horiz*. 1997;5:264-267.

43. Thompson AE. Pulmonary artery catheterization in children. *New Horiz*. 1997;5:244-250.

44. Trottier SJ, Taylor RW. Physicians' attitudes toward and knowledge of the pulmonary artery catheter: Society of Critical Care Medicine membership survey. *New Horiz*. 1997;5:201-206.

45. Bernard GR, Sopko G, Cerra F, Demling R, Edmunds H, Kaplan S, Kessler L, Masur H, Parsons P, Shure D, Webb C, Weidemann H, Weinmann G, Williams D. Pulmonary artery catheterization and clinical outcomes: National Heart, Lung, and Blood Institute and Food and Drug Administration Workshop Report. Consensus Statement. *JAMA*. 2000;283:2568-2572.

46. Sandham JD, Hull RD, Brant RF, Knox L, Pineo GF, Doig CJ, Laporta DP, Viner S, Passerini L, Devitt H, Kirby A, Jacka M. A randomized, controlled trial of the use of pulmonary-artery catheters in high-risk surgical patients. *N Engl J Med*. 2003;348:5-14.

47. Avery JK. Loss prevention case of the month. Frequent complication overlooked. *Tenn Med*. 2001;94:475-476.

48. Dalen JE. The pulmonary artery catheter-friend, foe, or accomplice? *JAMA*. 2001;286:348-350.

49. Stocking JE, Lake CL. The role of the pulmonary artery catheter in the year 2000 and beyond. *J Cardiothorac Vasc Anesth*. 2000;14:111-112.

50. Asteri T, Tsagaropoulou I, Vasiliadis K, Fessatidis I, Papavasi-Liou E, Spyrou P. Beware Swan-Ganz complications. Perioperative management. *J Cardiovasc Surg (Torino)*. 2002;43:467-470.

51. Sakka SG, Reinhart K, Wegscheider K, Meier-Hellmann A. Is the placement of a pulmonary artery catheter still justified solely for the measurement of cardiac output? *J Cardiothorac Vasc Anesth*. 2000;14:119-124.

52. Antle DE. Ensuring competency in nurse repositioning of the pulmonary artery catheter. *Dimens Crit Care Nurs*. 2000;19:44-51.

53. Williams G, Grounds M, Rhodes A. Pulmonary artery catheter. *Curr Opin Crit Care*. 2002;8:251-256.

54. Lefrant JY, Muller L, Bruelle P, Pandolfi JL, L'Hermite J, Peray P, Saissi G, de La Coussaye JE, Eledjam JJ. Insertion time of the pulmonary artery catheter in critically ill patients. *Crit Care Med*. 2000;28:355-359.

55. Ivanov R, Allen J, Calvin JE. The incidence of major morbidity in critically ill patients managed with pulmonary artery catheters: a meta-analysis. *Crit Care Med*. 2000;28:615-619.

56. Fontes M, Barash PG. Pulmonary artery catheter under the microscope. *Crit Care Med*. 2000;28:891-892.

57. Afessa B, Spencer S, Khan W, LaGatta M, Bridges L, Freire AX. Association of pulmonary artery catheter use with in-hospital mortality. *Crit Care Med*. 2001;29:1145-1148.

58. Cruz K, Franklin C. The pulmonary artery catheter: uses and controversies. *Crit Care Clin*. 2001;17:271-291.

59. Needham D, Santos Cd C. Toronto Critical Care Medicine Symposium, 18-20 October 2001, Canada: research breakthroughs are not enough. *Crit Care*. 2001;5:329-330.

60. Manikon M, Grounds M, Andrew R. The pulmonary artery catheter. *Clin Med*. 2002;2:101-104.

61. Spodick DH. Pulmonary artery catheterization in the ICU/critical care unit: indications and contraindications remain objectively undefined. *Chest*. 2001;119:999-1000.

62. Arcand G, Denault A, Belisle S, Tremblay N, Blain R, Couture P, Sheridan P, Sahab P, Searle N, Taillefer J. The appropriateness of the pulmonary artery catheter in cardiovascular surgery. *Can J Anaesth*. 2002;49:1001-1002; Author Reply 1002-1003.

63. Parsons PE. Progress in research on pulmonary-artery catheters. *N Engl J Med*. 2003;348:66-68.

Advanced Acute Coronary Syndromes Part 4: "Atypical" ACS and Life-Threatening, Non-ACS Causes of Chest Pain

Overview

This part of Chapter 2 presents the differential diagnosis of acute chest pain. It reviews atypical presentations of ACS and the classical descriptions of symptoms of serious or life-threatening noncardiac causes of chest pain.

Patients presenting with chest pain are rapidly screened for life-threatening causes. The initial ECG and further clinical assessment will identify patients with ST-segment deviation eligible for reperfusion or aggressive antiplatelet and antithrombin therapy. Often the question of an acute coronary syndrome persists. For some of these patients a noncardiac cause of chest pain is identified, such as pneumonia or musculoskeletal pain, or a non-ACS cardiovascular cause is found such as aortic dissection or pericarditis. These patients are treated appropriately and discharged from the protocol. The possibility of an acute coronary syndrome remains in a large group of patients with normal or nonspecific ECG changes.

Challenges to ACS Risk Stratification With ECG

What Are Nonspecific ECG Changes?

ST-Segment Changes

The ECG is not a perfect test for myocardial ischemia or infarction. ST-segment elevation, for example, can be due to AMI, pericarditis, or normal variations called early repolarization. Cardiac ischemia is identified when ST-segment depression is present. In the past, arbitrary limits of ST-segment deviation were based on clinical data or trials with thresholds established to obtain adequate sensitivity (detect patients with disease) and specificity (identify patients who likely do not have the disease and will not benefit from therapy).

ST-segment depression often represents ischemia, and 0.5 to 1 mm of horizontal (flat) depression persisting for 0.04 second after the J point is used to define this abnormality. Some clinical trials have used earlier measurements (0.02 second after the J point) to increase sensitivity. Others have used less (0.06 second after the J point) to increase specificity. Clinical algorithms for acute chest pain used ST-segment depression measured 0.04 second after the J point as representative and easy to measure (it is one horizontal small box on the ECG).

Recently clinical trials found that 0.5 mm of ST depression was as predictive as 1 mm.[1-4] Although this 0.5-mm ST-deviation threshold has not yet been subjected to the ECC Evidence Evaluation Process, it is the threshold recommended in the ACC/AHA Guidelines[5] and the ACC/AHA Guidelines Update,[6] and the material in this text has been changed to reflect this threshold.

T-Wave Changes

T waves may normally be present in lead III (and occasionally in lead II), and these T waves are often incorrectly interpreted as indicating ischemia.

T-wave inversions that do reflect ischemia involve a widening of the normal QRS axis and T-wave vector for an individual ECG. This change occurs with ischemia and may also be associated with a prolonged QTc interval. This diagnosis may be difficult for pattern ECG readers to make. But remember that T waves are normally upright in the leads that have dominant R waves (more of the QRS above baseline than below it). T-wave abnormalities may be difficult to identify unless a previous tracing is available for comparison. In outcome studies of ACS, T-wave abnormalities alone are not helpful in diagnosis or prognosis.

Dynamic T-wave changes are important indicators of ischemia in patients with acute chest pain. In such patients the finding of widening of the angle between the QRS axis and the T-wave axis and resolution of this abnormality with rest or nitroglycerin is indicative of ischemia. To detect these dynamic changes, you must obtain an ECG *before* administration of nitroglycerin in patients with suspected ACS. Typical response to nitrates (in several minutes) is suggestive but not diagnostic of cardiac ischemia. If you fail to obtain an ECG tracing when the patient is in pain and a repeat ECG after resolution of the pain, you may miss a diagnostic abnormality. T waves suspicious for ischemia are defined in the ACC/AHA Guidelines[5,6] as T waves that are ≥2 mm inverted in leads with dominant R waves.

Nondiagnostic ECGs

Cardiologists vary widely in their criteria for diagnosis of nonspecific ST-segment and T-wave changes. Also, criteria may differ for some clinical situations. For example, ischemic ST-segment deviation in ACS is measured at 0.04 second after the J point. A cardiologist performing a treadmill test measures ST-segment deviation at a point that is 0.08 second after the J point and does not count T waves at all.

A normal or nondiagnostic ECG has the following characteristics:

- ST depression <0.5 mm, measured 0.04 second after the J point

- Upright T waves in leads with dominant R waves (normal) *or*

- T-wave inversion <2 mm in leads with dominant R waves

Sequential Evaluation of Chest Pain

Why can't the clinical history sort patients with life-threatening causes of chest pain immediately? Isn't chest pressure or heaviness *ACS,* and tearing or ripping migratory chest pain *aortic dissection?*

As new diseases are recognized, clinicians and pathologists often identify the "classic" symptoms characteristic of the disease in the first patients reported. Over time, however, it is often apparent that these classic presentations actually occur in the minority of patients. The classic pain of aortic dissection, for example, is present in the minority of patients at initial presentation (see below).

To add to the challenge of disease recognition, many disorders share symptoms. For this reason evaluation requires review of the patient's history, physical examination, and selected diagnostic tests. Ultimately the provider's clinical judgment and a rational selection of tests should increase the likelihood of a correct diagnosis, minimize the risks of missing a problem, and keep the costs of health care reasonable. It would be unreasonable and would increase the cost of health care to

perform a transthoracic echocardiogram, aortic angiogram, CT scan of the chest, $\dot{V}/\dot{Q}$ scan, and coronary angiogram for every patient with chest pain. Remember the following caveats for evaluation of chest pain:

- The initial evaluation is performed to identify the most likely cause of chest pain.

- The subsequent evaluation continues this process and risk-stratifies the patient for adverse clinical events and treatment benefits.

- The majority of patients with chest pain require ongoing evaluation. In many patients you will not be able to establish a definite cause for chest pain. A continuing evaluation revisits the differential diagnosis before discharge.

- Even when you use a continuing process, many patients will not have a "final diagnosis" but will be deemed at low risk for ACS. These patients require early follow-up and access to care if symptoms recur or worsen.

Who Is at Low Risk for ACS?

Patients considered at low risk for ACS are those with

- No recurrent chest pain during evaluation

- No diabetes

- No congestive heart failure on clinical exam or chest x-ray

- No cardiac marker increase

- No diagnostic ECG changes (ie, the patient has a normal or nondiagnostic ECG on at least 2 ECGs)

If these criteria are met, patients are classified at low risk for MACE and are considered to have possible angina. Patients can be considered for discharge if the ECG is normal, the clinician thinks that the likelihood of ACS is low, and the patient has follow-up and functional testing available in 48 to 72 hours. These patients are only a small percentage of those presenting with chest pain. The rest are assessed with a stress test before discharge. The timing and type of stress or functional study varies

with institutional preferences and local expertise in these tests. Protocols have included routine exercise stress testing, exercise and dobutamine stress testing, and exercise and pharmacologic nuclear studies. If the resources are available, ED nuclear perfusion imaging rapidly triages patients for aggressive management or discharge.

The following sections discuss the variable presentations of the life-threatening mimics of ACS and review the common diagnostic tests and general evaluation protocols used to identify these problems. On first presentation the life-threatening/ serious causes of chest pain are

- ST-segment elevation MI (STEMI)

- Non–ST-segment elevation MI (NSTEMI) and high-risk unstable angina

- Acute pulmonary embolism

- Aortic dissection

- Pericardial effusion (pericarditis) with pretamponade or tamponade physiology

- Tension pneumothorax

- Ruptured esophagus (Boerhaave syndrome)

ACS But Does Not Present Like ACS

Volume 1, Chapter 17 and Parts 1 and 2 of this chapter provide information about the most common symptomatic presentations of ACS. The most common cause of ACS is rupture of an atherosclerotic plaque with subsequent platelet adhesion and aggregation, thrombus formation, and arterial occlusion (intermittent, partial, or complete). The patient's condition may evolve into STEMI, NSTEMI, or unstable angina (UA).

An "atypical" patient does not experience the familiar pattern of severe central substernal chest pressure or tightness, typical radiation, and frequent associated symptoms of diaphoresis and shortness of breath. Instead this patient experiences only a variation of usual symptoms or "atypical" symptoms. Pain, if any, is not described as a pressure or tightness, is of a different nature (quality) than usual, in a different location, for a different duration, or of a different intensity.

Clinical observation and research have identified several groups of patients who tend to experience an ACS in a so-called "atypical" manner with "atypical" symptoms. Chest discomfort is the predominant symptom of ACS in men and women. But women, the elderly, and diabetic patients have an increased frequency of atypical chest pain and presenting symptoms. Women presenting with MI typically present about 1 hour later than men, in part due to more atypical symptoms, including epigastric pain, shortness of breath, nausea, and fatigue.

Evaluation of women with chest pain is particularly difficult. In all age groups the prevalence of angina pectoris is higher in women than in men, and angina is the most common manifestation of coronary artery disease (CAD) in women. But the incidence of associated CAD varies widely, and atypical manifestations of acute ischemic syndromes occur with increased frequency. The variability in presentation and differences from men are multifactorial in cause and are due in part to different pathophysiology and perhaps different somatic pain thresholds.

What Is the Difficulty in Evaluating Chest Pain in Women?

Several factors make evaluation of chest pain in women difficult:

- Premenopausal women have a low likelihood of CAD and commonly present with typical angina. The low incidence of positive angiograms in these women has led to a perception that their chest pain is benign and *noncardiac*. This misperception leads to underassessment of women with chest pain, so women with chest pain are less likely than men to be tested for CAD and less likely to be treated for CAD.

- There is also a perception that if CAD is present in women that its course is more benign than the course of CAD

in men. In fact, the prognosis of women with CAD is similar to that of men, but women often have more angina and disability than men (see Table 1).

When Atypical Symptoms Occur, What Is Different in Women?

Atypical symptoms in women often include the following:

- More angina at rest, occurring at night or precipitated by mental rather than physical stress.

- Symptoms may include shortness of breath, fatigue, palpitations, presyncope, sweating, nausea, or vomiting.

- Atypical angina rates do not differ in women with or without CAD.

Not ACS But Presents Like ACS

The ACLS provider may encounter patients who present with many of the typical chest pain signs and symptoms reported by ACS patients but who are in fact experiencing another problem altogether. Some of these "ACS mimics" are relatively benign (eg, costochondritis or gastroesophageal reflux disease), but several are severe and life-threatening, and the ACLS provider must be able to identify them. There are numerous non-ACS causes of chest pain. The 4 most frequent potentially fatal non-ACS causes of chest pain are

- Aortic dissection

- Pericardial effusion and tamponade

- Massive or submassive acute pulmonary embolism

- Spontaneous tension pneumothorax

ACLS providers must be alert for these and other less common life-threatening ACS mimics. Consider these differential diagnoses during initial patient assessment and throughout the clinical evaluation. The prudent ACLS provider will try to rule out these noncoronary causes of chest pain while trying to establish the diagnosis of ACS. If you think the patient has ACS but the patient fails to respond to initial therapy, you should again consider these non-ACS causes of chest pain.

ACS That Does Not Present Like ACS
ACS Symptoms for Women, the Elderly, and Diabetics

Women,[7-9] the elderly,[10] and insulin-dependent diabetics who develop ACS often do not present with the classic pattern of severe, crushing substernal chest pain or discomfort, nausea, diaphoresis, and pain radiating into the jaw, neck, or lateral aspect of the left arm. In fact, many middle-aged men with ACS do not present with this pattern.

Although chest discomfort occurs in the majority of patients with acute ischemia, the "typical" ACS symptom *complex* is not a particularly sensitive indicator for ACS. In one large study[11] of all patients presenting to an Emergency Department with typical ischemic symptoms, only 54% developed an ACS. In addition, the patients who did develop an ACS described a rich variety of symptoms: 43% had burning or indigestion, 32% had a "chest ache,"

TABLE 1. Angina in Women and Men

	Women	Men
Presentation of CAD	Angina (65%)	ACS (63%)
Most common cause of angina	Noncardiac	CAD
Significant CAD	≤50%	80%
Follow-up	Increases with age	Plateau (55-65 y)

and 20% had "sharp" or "stabbing" pain; 42% could not provide specific descriptors of their pain. The pain was partially pleuritic in 12%.

The ACS symptom complex for women, the elderly, and diabetics may vary greatly. These patients tend to describe their symptoms in one or more of the following ways:

- Uncomfortable "pressure," "fullness," "ache," "discomfort," "squeezing," or "pushing out" in the center of the chest lasting several minutes (typical angina quality).

- An ache or discomfort that may or may not be felt in the center of the chest but that seems to spread up to and across the shoulders, neck, arms, jaw, or back; between the shoulder blades; or into the epigastrium, upper left or right quadrant. The discomfort in the chest is less troublesome to the patient than the pain in the areas of spread. This pattern of symptom localization *outside* the chest was found to be most characteristic of women patients evaluated in the WISE study.[12]

- Chest discomfort or ache in itself may be minor. The patient is bothered more by associated lightheadedness, fainting, sweating, nausea, or shortness of breath. This is another example of the dominance of symptoms outside the chest.

- A global feeling of distress, anxiety ("something is wrong" or "something is just not right"), or impending doom.

Obviously these atypical symptoms are nonspecific and occur in many patients without acute myocardial ischemia. The clinical challenge is to consider acute ischemia in the appropriate patient setting. CAD is rare in *premenopausal women*. Their pretest likelihood of CAD is so low that signs and symptoms have little predictive value. In fact, the low pretest likelihood of CAD significantly increases the false-positive rate of diagnostic stress tests. Indiscriminate use of these tests can have adverse effects. For example, coronary angiography is the gold standard for evaluation of coronary anatomy and occlusive CAD but this test can have significant complications:

- Consider that the pretest likelihood of CAD is 1 in 300 000 for a 30- to 35-year-old woman, and the risk of a major complication from invasive coronary angiography is 1 in 3000.

- Also, a negative coronary angiogram may lead to the conclusion that symptoms are noncardiac in origin. In fact, in a significant group of women their symptoms represent microvascular angina and endothelial dysfunction.[12]

Diabetic patients may present without chest pain but with complaints of simple weakness, fatigue, or severe prostration. Anginal equivalents such as shortness of breath, syncope, and lightheadedness may be their only symptoms. In diabetics with neuropathy these presentations have often been attributed to altered pain and neural perception.

As a specific indicator of non-ACS chest pain, *reproducible chest wall tenderness* has long been used to rule out AMI. But this practice should have been abandoned years ago. In some studies 20% to 30% of people with confirmed AMI reported chest tenderness on palpation. When this tenderness is "localized" by the patient using 1 or 2 fingers in an atypical location, acute ischemia is unlikely but cannot be completely excluded.

Some combinations of chest pain symptoms are almost never caused by an ACS. For example, sharp, stabbing chest pain that increases with a deep breath is *respirophasic* pain that may be *either* musculoskeletal or pleuritic. Such pain that changes with position or is exactly reproducible by palpation is almost never due to an ischemic syndrome. This is particularly true if the patient has no history of CAD.

The Concept of Chest Pain (Anginal) "Equivalents"

Many patients with ACS present with signs and symptoms that have been termed *ischemic equivalents* or *anginal equivalents*. It is important to note that these patients are *not* having atypical chest pain as described above. These are patients who seldom offer complaints of "pain" in the chest, below the sternum, or elsewhere, and the healthcare provider may not be able to elicit a report of such pain. Instead patients may present with a symptom or sign that reflects the effects of the ischemia on left ventricular function or electrical stability.

Patients with anginal equivalents *are* experiencing an ACS. They require the same assessment, treatment, and decision making as any other patient with STEMI or UA/NSTEMI. Note that this phenomenon of ischemic equivalents occurs much more frequently in patients having UA/NSTEMI than in patients having STEMI. Diabetic patients and the elderly are most likely to present with these symptoms. With advancing age, the elderly are more likely to present with diaphoresis.

Some of the more common chest pain equivalent symptoms experienced by these ACS patients are shortness of breath, dyspnea on exertion, weakness, fatigue, palpitation, and lightheadedness or near-syncope with exercise.

The most common signs of anginal equivalents are acute pulmonary edema or pulmonary congestion, cardiomegaly, and a third heart sound. Ventricular arrhythmias can cause symptoms in these patients. Ventricular extrasystoles, nonsustained VT, and symptomatic VT or VF have been documented. Ventricular ectopy that *increases* with activity (most will suppress at increased sinus rates) is suspicious for ischemia. Atrial fibrillation is uncommonly an ischemic presentation.

Life-Threatening, Non-ACS Causes of Chest Pain

The "Immediate Life Threat" Concept

Physicians and nurses in emergency and critical care medicine are taught to frequently ask the question "Is this patient about to die?" Translated into practice this tenet means that the clinician should always evaluate the patient's chief complaints while keeping a prioritized list of life-threatening "differential diagnoses" under consideration.

This list is prioritized with a focus on identifying an immediate life threat. The healthcare professional evaluating a chief complaint of chest pain should consider whether the underlying cause is an ACS. In concert with these thoughts the provider should try to ask "What else could this patient have that has serious or life-threatening implications?"

The routine evaluation of the patient with possible ACS includes elements such as ECG, chest radiography, vital signs, physical exam, detailed history taking, and testing for cardiac markers that will help identify or rule out these life threats.

The Differential Diagnosis of Chest Pain

Table 2 lists the most important causes of acute chest pain (or chest pain equivalents) not caused by ACS. Note the 3 divisions of the table:

- Serious, immediate threat to life

- Serious, potential for significant morbidity

- Other common causes, less potential for immediate morbidity

This chapter discusses only the 4 most common life-threatening causes of acute chest pain not caused by ACS. These conditions share the common symptom of chest discomfort. Note that each condition is in the differential diagnoses of the other. The responsible physician who diagnoses ACS or 1 of these 4 problems should also take steps to exclude the other problems in this differential diagnosis. This exclusion can take the form of additional history, observation, or targeted testing based on evolving findings and clinical judgment.

The Rule-Out Fallacy

During evaluation of a patient with chest pain, the responsible clinician attempts to

rule in or rule out any life-threatening problems in the differential diagnosis. But none of these life threats can be ruled out with absolute confidence. Although there are *positive* signs, symptoms, and diagnostic techniques that rule *in* or identify each of these diagnoses, there are no *negative* findings that definitively (100%) rule *out* each condition. This fact underscores an important point: healthcare providers should focus on both risk stratification and diagnosis during initial patient evaluation. As the evaluation proceeds and an initial strategy is defined, the risks and benefits of testing and treatment are balanced against the probability and risk assessment of disease using clinical judgment and prudent assessment.

Aortic Dissection (Thoracic)

Signs and Symptoms

Aortic dissection is rare in comparison with ACS. The incidence of aortic dissection has been estimated at 5 to 30 per 1 million people per year; 4400 MIs occur per 1 million people per year. Severe pain is the most common presenting symptom of aortic dissection. Untreated aortic dissection is a lethal disease; 25% of patients die in the first 24 hours and 75% in 2 weeks.

Risk factors for aortic dissection include

- Hypertension (70% to 90% of patients)

- Male sex

- Advancing age (usually 6th or 7th decade)

- Marfan's syndrome

- Bicuspid aortic valve

- Aortitis

- Cocaine use

- Cardiac catheterization; prior CABG or aortic surgery

The typical patient is a male in his 70s with a history of hypertension, a predisposing factor in 70% to 90% of patients. Chest pain is the most frequent initial complaint caused by aortic dissection. This pain may

TABLE 2. Life-Threatening and Serious Causes of Non-ACS Chest Pain

- Serious, immediate threat to life
  1. Aortic dissection
  2. Acute pericardial effusion and tamponade
  3. Acute pulmonary embolism
  4. Tension pneumothorax
- Serious, potential for significant morbidity
  1. Peptic ulcer, perforated
  2. Esophageal rupture
  3. Acute pneumonia
  4. Aortic stenosis (chest pain, syncope, exertional dyspnea)
  5. Acute cholecystitis, cholelithiasis, ruptured gall bladder
  6. Acute pancreatitis
- Other common causes, less potential for immediate morbidity
  1. Gastroesophageal reflux disease
  2. Esophagitis, gastritis
  3. Hiatal hernia
  4. Musculoskeletal chest pain
  5. Costochondritis

be similar to that of ACS. In ascending and transverse aortic dissection, anterior chest pain is typical. Anterior chest pain also occurs in descending aortic dissection, but these patients also have more back and abdominal pain.[13]

More than 50% of patients with acute aortic dissection will describe their pain as "ripping" or "tearing." More often, though, the pain is described as sharp. Traditionally the pain is described as migratory (as the dissection plane advances), but a recent registry found this symptom in a minority (15%) of patients. But 90% of patients did describe this as the worst pain ever, a classic presentation. When you hear these terms used to describe pain, think *acute aortic dissection*. In a small number of patients, including some patients with Marfan's syndrome, aortic dissection may be painless.

The onset of the pain of aortic dissection is abrupt, and the pain is most severe at onset. Think *aortic dissection* when patients report sudden or abrupt pain that is most severe at the start. But remember that such pain neither confirms dissection nor rules out ACS.

The pain of aortic dissection may be migratory or may change in severity and location with time. The initial location of pain provides a valuable clue about the origin and extension of the dissection:

- Severe, substernal chest pain identical to the pain of STEMI is often associated with dissection of the aortic root or anterior aortic arch. Such a dissection can occlude flow to the coronary arteries (especially the right) and produce an acute STEMI. Do *not* give fibrinolytics to patients with STEMI and aortic dissection. Fibrinolytic therapy in these patients can produce disastrous consequences, including hemorrhagic death.

- Dissection into the aortic arch and the carotid and subclavian branches of the arch can cause pain in the neck or jaw.

- Pain in the intrascapular region is associated with dissection into the descending aorta. This pain can migrate to the back, diaphragm, flank, and groin.

Several problems may occur during acute dissection of the thoracic aorta:

- Acute STEMI or NSTEMI: Occlusion of the coronary arteries by the dissection causes ECG changes and increases in cardiac-specific markers.

- Acute cardiac tamponade: Dissection into the pericardial sac causes this condition. Tamponade may produce distant, muffled heart sounds, hypotension, electrical alternans, pulsus paradoxus, and distention of jugular veins. Note that if the patient is extremely hypotensive, it may be difficult to appreciate the presence of pulsus paradoxus.

- Blood pressure abnormalities: Asymmetrical pulses or left versus right blood pressure discrepancies may be observed.

- Auscultatory findings: New diastolic murmur (aortic insufficiency) or new or progressive bruits in carotid, brachial, or femoral arteries.

- Neurologic findings: Altered mental status and syncope (the most frequent neurologic signs); paresthesia, weakness, or paralysis of an extremity; signs of stroke, including hemiparesis or hemiparalysis; and Horner syndrome.

Approach to Diagnosis[14,15]

Chest Radiography

The chest radiograph is particularly helpful for patients with an ascending aortic dissection. A radiograph will show abnormalities in 80% of these patients.[13]

- Mediastinal widening (>8 cm seen on a portable anterior-posterior chest radiograph) is observed in 64% of patients diagnosed with aortic dissection.[13] Mediastinal widening is a nonspecific finding that may be caused by a wide variety of conditions, including tumor, lymphadenopathy, lymphoma, thyroid enlargement, and the tortuous aorta seen in patients with chronic hypertension. The recumbent position itself and a poor inspiratory film may produce mediastinal widening. In trauma patients only 3% of patients with a widened mediastinum will have aortic dissection using liberal criteria for angiography.

- If the aorta has a calcified intima, the dissection may displace the outer edge of the aorta more than 5 mm from the ring of calcium in the intima. This displacement produces the so-called ring sign. Though this sign is often absent, when it is observed it is highly diagnostic of a dissection.

- Other abnormalities associated with acute aortic dissection that may appear on the chest radiograph include left apical capping, deviation of the trachea, downward displacement of the left main bronchus, lateral esophageal deviation, and loss of the paratracheal stripe.

CT Scanning

When available, the helical CT study is the diagnostic tool of choice for aortic dissection in medical centers.[15] Contrast CT (helical or spiral) with 2- and 3-dimensional reconstructions detects more than 90% of acute dissections. The false-negative rate ranges from 0% to 10% in various studies.

Transthoracic Ultrasound

Transthoracic ultrasound (echocardiography) is a readily available, noninvasive diagnostic technique. It does not require the patient to leave the ED or patient care unit. It has acceptable sensitivity but confirms the diagnosis in only 80% of patients with aortic dissection. It is most accurate in detecting ascending and aortic root dissections.

A sensitivity of 80% is not sufficiently high. Further studies are necessary if clinical suspicion remains high despite negative ultrasound findings.

Transthoracic ultrasound can accurately detect the presence of cardiac tamponade or aortic regurgitation in patients with acute dissection.

Transesophageal Ultrasound

Transesophageal ultrasound (echocardiography—TEE) is superior to transthoracic ultrasound because it has extremely high sensitivity (detects 97% to 99% of aortic dissections) with an extremely low false-negative rate (<3%). Like transthoracic ultrasound, this technique does not require the unstable patient to leave the ED or critical care unit. Also like transthoracic ultrasound, a second diagnostic study is necessary if clinical suspicion remains high despite negative ultrasound findings. This technique can evaluate whether the coronary arteries are involved in the dissection and detect the presence of cardiac tamponade or aortic regurgitation.

Magnetic Resonance Imaging

Magnetic resonance imaging (MRI) detects more than 90% of aortic dissections, with a false-negative rate of 5%. MRI does not require contrast injection or radiation, but it is time-consuming and requires transport of potentially unstable patients away from the Emergency Department or critical care areas.

Aortography

Before current contrast-enhanced CT, aortography was the diagnostic gold standard and test of choice for aortic dissection. The need for this invasive test has decreased significantly. It is used primarily to resolve conflicting information from non-invasive studies when the clinical suspicion for dissection remains high. In selected patients, aortography and coronary angiography may be needed preoperatively to assess coronary anatomy. But angiography has drawbacks: the patient must be transported to a remote angiographic laboratory, and far worse, angiography has failed to identify intramural hematomas.

12-Lead ECG

If the acute aortic dissection occludes a coronary artery, it will produce ECG changes that closely mimic the ECG changes of ACS. The majority of patients with both conditions will have nondiagnostic ECGs with nonspecific changes. For this reason the ECG has little value in differentiating these 2 causes of chest pain.

The International Registry of Acute Aortic Dissection[13] recently reported the first choice of test for participating centers worldwide. Currently the initial imaging study of choice is CT (63%) followed by TEE (32%) of patients. A second imaging study was performed in over half the patients enrolled in this registry. TEE was used more often as the first imaging test at US centers. TEE has the advantage of bedside performance and immediate assessment of aortic regurgitation, coronary ostial involvement, pericardial effusion, and LV function. Limitations include the inability to image major arch vessels and track the dissection into the distal aorta.

Acute Pericarditis Effusion and Tamponade

Description[16]

This disease complex is often confused with ACS because it produces pain and ECG abnormalities that can be similar to those caused by ACS. It is important to

differentiate pericarditis from ACS, however, because fibrinolytic administration to patients with pericarditis can produce fatal hemorrhage since the inflamed pericardium will bleed easily. Heparin is also contraindicated except in a special form of postinfarction focal pericarditis.

The pericardial complex around the heart comprises the outer fibrous pericardium and a thin serous layer that adheres to the surface of the heart. Because of the close proximity of the serous pericardium to the heart, most instances of pericarditis are actually myopericarditis. This can further confuse the diagnosis because the myopericarditis may produce elevation of cardiac markers.

A potential space exists between the fibrous and the serous pericardial layers. Normally the space contains approximately 20 mL of plasmalike fluid. It can accommodate roughly 120 mL before pericardial pressure increases. If fluid accumulation continues, the pericardial pressure can rise sharply. This increased pressure results in a significant decrease in cardiac output and blood pressure. However, it is the *rate* of accumulation rather than absolute *volume* that is most important. Acute effusions, including hemopericardium from penetrating trauma, occur rapidly and can produce rapid decompensation. Cardiac rupture of the left ventricle following AMI also causes immediate fatal hemopericardium. The patient usually presents with the sudden onset of pulseless electrical activity. Survival is rare even with immediate pericardiocentesis and cardiac surgical availability.

Right ventricular perforation can occur following temporary pacer placement, pulmonary artery catheter insertion, and right ventricular biopsy. Right ventricular pressures are lower than left ventricular pressures, so survival following right ventricular perforation has been reported with prompt recognition and drainage.

Previously, idiopathic pericarditis was the primary cause of pericardial effusion and tamponade. But with the recent increase

in the number of cardiology interventions performed, the provider following these in-hospital patients must be able to detect and treat pericardial effusion as a potential complication of cardiac catheterization. Small guidewires are also used to track angioplasty balloons for dilation and stent placement. Microperforation of a coronary artery or dissection of the vessel may present with delayed tamponade after patients leave the catheterization suite, particularly if platelet inhibitors are administered after the procedure.

Cardiac tamponade refers to the hemodynamic effects of fluid accumulation in the pericardial sac.

The most common causes of pericardial effusions with tamponade are pericarditis, malignancy, uremia associated with renal failure, and tuberculosis (in geographic areas where it is endemic).[16] As noted above, hemopericardium is increasing in frequency, and tuberculous effusions are rare in developed countries.

- **Serous pericarditis** occurs in patients with inflammatory conditions, such as rheumatoid arthritis or lupus erythematosus.

- **Fibrous pericarditis** may develop in patients with AMI, Dressler's syndrome (postinfarction syndrome), trauma, uremia syndrome, rheumatoid arthritis, and infections. It also can develop after cardiac surgery.

- **Purulent or suppurative pericarditis** occurs with bacterial and viral infections.

Signs and Symptoms

Pericarditis

Chest pain is the most frequent symptom of acute pericarditis.[17,18] Patients may describe pericarditis with the same terms used to describe ACS, or the description may differ:

- Patients will describe the pain as sharp or stabbing. The pain is localized in the middle of the chest or below the sternum.

- Onset may be sudden or gradual. The pain may radiate to the back, neck, left arm, or left shoulder.

- Inspiration or movement can aggravate the pain. A unique feature of pericardial pain is that it typically increases when the patient lies supine and decreases when the patient sits and leans forward. This is believed to occur because the diaphragmatic surface of the pericardium is richly innervated. When the patient lies supine, the diaphragmatic surface of the heart comes into contact with this pericardial segment, creating more pain.

- Patients often have fever (low grade or intermittent), shortness of breath, cough, or painful swallowing. Patients with tuberculous pericarditis commonly have the fever, night sweats, and weight loss of tuberculosis infection.

A *pericardial friction rub* is present in about half of patients with pericarditis. The character of the rub often changes from one hour to the next, from heartbeat to heartbeat, and with changes in position. Many clinicians describe it as sounding like footsteps in crunchy snow or sandpaper rubbed together. It is loudest along the lower left border of the sternum and at the apex of the heart. The rub is best heard when the patient sits and leans forward or assumes the "hands-and-knees" position, bringing the anterior epicardium into contact with the inflamed pericardial segment.

Patients may have a low-grade fever, occasional premature atrial or ventricular beats, tachypnea and dyspnea, ascites, or hepatomegaly.

Cardiac Tamponade

As fluid accumulates in the pericardial sac, the patient may develop dyspnea, easy fatigue, anxiety, and other signs of hemodynamic compromise. The volume of fluid, the rate of fluid accumulation, and the compliance of the pericardial sac all affect the onset and severity of clinical consequences. Rapid or substantial fluid accumulation or a constrictive pericardium will produce more acute cardiovascular

deterioration than gradual fluid accumulation in the presence of a distensible pericardial sac.

Very few patients with pericardial tamponade demonstrate the 3 symptoms associated with tamponade that are known as *Beck's triad:* jugular venous distention, hypotension, and muffled or distant heart sounds.[19] The finding of clear lungs, hypotension, and jugular venous distention alerts trauma teams to the possible presence of traumatic hemopericardium with effusion.

Pulsus paradoxus is commonly present with tamponade. Pulsus paradoxus is a fall in systolic blood pressure ≥8 to 10 mm Hg during spontaneous inspiration. A fall in the SBP of more than 10 mm Hg is significant.[17] But providers need to know that acute airway disorders—rather than tamponade—are the most common causes of pulsus paradoxus. The name itself, *paradoxus,* is a misnomer. The pulse is actually not a paradox but an accentuation of the normal fall in SBP with inspiration. The difference is that the normal fall is not more than 10 mm Hg.

Approach to Diagnosis

Chest Radiography

The chest radiograph is of limited use in the diagnosis of pericarditis or pericardial tamponade because it may be normal even when tamponade is present. If the pericardium is constrictive or noncompliant, a small amount of fluid accumulation can cause tamponade yet not create an enlarged cardiac silhouette. If pericardial fluid accumulates gradually (chronic pericarditis) and the pericardium is compliant (distensible), the sac can accommodate 200 to 250 mL before it causes an enlarged cardiac silhouette. The enlarged silhouette appears globular in shape and may resemble a "water bottle." Amounts of 1 to 2 L have been found in hypothyroid patients, attesting to the ability of a normal pericardium to dilate with time.

Echocardiography

Echocardiography will detect the presence and volume of pericardial fluid and determine its significance.

- In a patient with pericarditis but no effusion, the heart will look normal.

- A *moderate* effusion will create an echo-free pericardial space (both anterior and posterior) of 10 to 20 mm in diastole. A pericardial space greater than 20 mm is *large*. It is important to recognize that a tamponade may be localized or loculated, causing critical impairment to filling, such as after cardiac surgery.

- Other echocardiographic features suggesting tamponade include right atrial and right ventricular collapse.

- Actual tamponade is indicated by a dilated inferior vena cava. During inspiration in the patient with tamponade, the inferior vena cava does not collapse, but the right ventricle does collapse. Right atrial pressure is very high (18 to 22 mm Hg) and correlates with jugular venous distention on clinical examination.

- Patients who are hypovolemic with tamponade may pose a diagnostic challenge. Administration of volume will often bring out more typical hemodynamics. This can be seen with volume resuscitation of a trauma patient or with use of a fluid challenge in the cardiac catheterization suite.

CT Scanning

Computed tomography provides more anatomic detail than other techniques, and it is less dependent on operator skill than the ultrasound. CT can detect calcification in the pericardium, which is diagnostic of constrictive pericarditis. CT scanning requires the use of contrast medium. In addition, it does not enable the assessment of hemodynamic parameters (eg, evaluation of cardiac anatomy and function) that is possible with echocardiography.

Magnetic Resonance Imaging

MRI provides the most anatomic detail for evaluation of the pericardium and pericardial sac, but it requires gated image acquisition. MRI may require as many as 250 regular heartbeats, precluding its use in patients with arrhythmias. Another disadvantage of MRI is that it requires transport of patients out of the Emergency Department or critical care unit.

12-Lead ECG

The 12-lead ECG can yield pathognomonic findings in both pericarditis and ACS.

- Four stages of ECG findings have been reported to occur in pericarditis, but all 4 stages occur in only about half of involved patients. These findings are diagnostic:

  — Stage 1: ST-segment elevation with ST segments that concave upward. This stage occurs within hours of the onset of pericarditis-associated chest pain. The elevation is frequently noted in all leads except V_1. ST-segment elevation may last several days.

  — Stage 2: T-wave flattening as the ST elevation returns to baseline.

  — Stage 3: T waves become inverted, but Q waves do not form.

  — Stage 4: The ECG gradually returns to normal.

- A separate finding, PR-segment depression, occurs in as many as 80% of patients with viral pericarditis.

- Cardiac tamponade may produce a diagnostic ECG pattern of *electrical alternans*. The amplitude (voltage) of each ECG complex (the P wave, QRS, and T wave) alternates from complex to complex. This pattern is caused by motion of the heart toward and away from the precordial leads. The motion is exacerbated by the large effusion. The heart "bobs" in the fluid, similar to a boat bobbing on the water.

It is important to remember that pericarditis and pericardial effusion may present with nonspecific ECG changes. Echocardiography can be a useful bedside tool to aid in the diagnosis, especially in the Emergency Department. In addition, ACS can mimic pericarditis and vice versa.

Following cardiac surgery, focal pericarditis can mimic anterior wall MI with ST-segment elevation in the precordial leads. Alternatively, an AMI from a large "wrap-around" LAD coronary artery can mimic pericarditis with changes in both the anterior and inferior leads because the LAD crosses the apex and supplies a significant portion of the inferior wall. This will produce typical ischemic symptoms, but the ECG can show findings consistent with both an anterior and inferior MI. Consideration of pericarditis may delay appropriate therapy for ACS (eg, fibrinolytics) in these patients. The use of echocardiography in the ED may be useful for the differential diagnosis.

Acute Pulmonary Embolism

Description

Pulmonary embolism (PE) is not a primary disease. It is a life-threatening complication of venous thrombosis, usually of the lower extremities. PE occurs when microthrombi manage to evade the body's intrinsic fibrinolytic system, and they enlarge and spread.

As these thrombi propagate, they become so large that they eventually break loose, traveling to the right heart and then into the pulmonary artery. When the embolus reaches a small enough artery, it blocks that pulmonary blood vessel. This interruption in blood flow produces effects both downstream (ventilation-perfusion mismatch, atelectasis, pain) and upstream (cor pulmonale, or right ventricular failure caused by pulmonary hypertension).[20,21] An international cooperative registry of pulmonary embolism, ICOPER, documented the serious nature of pulmonary thromboembolism with a 3-month mortality rate of 15%.[22]

Signs and Symptoms

You should consider the diagnosis of PE whenever you evaluate a patient with chest pain.[23] The symptoms and manifestations of PE, however, are often nonspecific, and the differential diagnosis is extensive. The

diagnosis is difficult and both underdiagnosis and overdiagnosis occur. Tachypnea is the most frequent presenting sign. In ICOPER 89% of patients were symptomatic and hemodynamically stable, and approximately 4% were unstable.[22] PE may cause these additional symptoms:

- Back, shoulder, or upper abdominal pain; chest wall tenderness.

- Syncope. The combination of syncope, dyspnea, and cyanosis usually indicates massive PE.

- Hemoptysis.

- Painful respirations, painful deep inspirations, pleuritic pain, new-onset wheezing.

- The classic triad for PE (hemoptysis, shortness of breath, and pleuritic chest pain) has little diagnostic value. It occurs in less than 20% of confirmed cases. This symptom complex is usually observed with smaller emboli that migrate to the lung periphery and cause pulmonary infarction and pleuritis. A small effusion may be present on chest x-ray. In one study of patients who died of massive PE, 60% had shortness of breath, 17% had chest pain, and 3% had hemoptysis.[24,25]

- Pleuritic pain or pain that varies with respirations should always raise a red flag. Of young, disease-free patients evaluated for isolated pleuritic pain, 21% were eventually found to have PE.[24,25]

Many patients with acute PE have no abnormal physical findings. Physical signs that may be present include

- New wheezing

- Pleural rub

- Spontaneous chest wall tenderness

Investigators have observed the following physical findings in patients with a diagnosed large PE (percentage of PE patients having the sign)[24,25]:

- Tachypnea, with RR >16/min (96%)
- Rales (58%)

- Accentuated S_2 (53%)
- Tachycardia, heart rate >100 bpm (44%)
- Fever >37.8°C (43%)
- Diaphoresis (36%)
- S_3 or S_4 gallop (34%)
- Signs or symptoms of thrombophlebitis (32%)
- Lower extremity edema (24%)
- Cardiac murmur (23%)
- Cyanosis (19%)

Approach to Diagnosis

A thorough discussion of the diagnosis of PE is beyond the scope of this discussion of non-ACS causes of chest pain. But a number of observations about the diagnosis of PE are relevant:

- So-called diagnostic cutoff values for arterial oxygen levels, alveolar-arterial oxygen gradients, and oxygen saturation values are useless in most clinical settings.[26] This observation applies to any diagnostic test for a condition that is normally distributed within a population but has a frequency less than 50%. In addition, the differential diagnosis of PE includes many conditions that compromise arterial oxygen tension and content, including chronic obstructive pulmonary disease, congestive heart failure, and pneumonia.

- White blood cell counts are often elevated; clotting is usually normal.

- The D-dimer by ELISA (enzyme-linked-immunosorbent assay) test has recently been used in the diagnosis of PE. D-dimer is a degradation product produced by proteolysis of the fibrin in a thrombus. The detection of D-dimer (positive D-dimer), however, is thought to be insufficiently sensitive and specific to alter evaluation or treatment for suspected PE. A positive D-dimer, for example, can occur in ACS and other conditions that activate the endogenous fibrinolytic system. The combination of a *negative* D-dimer result and a "low probability" clinical assessment can reliably exclude PE for many patients.[27-31]

- Chest radiographs are normal in the vast majority (>95%) of patients with acute PE.

- ECGs demonstrate the classic findings of PE (right heart strain, acute cor pulmonale) in only 20% of patients with PE. Approximately 25% of PE patients with pre- and postembolism ECGs have no changes at all. As with most diagnostic tests for PE, abnormalities are suggestive, but absence of abnormalities is not reassuring. Perhaps the most useful ECG finding is the presence of a tachycardia and signs of right heart strain. T-wave inversion in leads V_1 through V_4 is the most frequent ECG abnormality.[22] The classic S1Q3T3 sign (prominent S wave in lead I, widened Q wave in lead III, and T-wave inversion in lead III), a sign of acute right ventricular strain, occurs infrequently.

Several diagnostic tests are reliable for the detection of PE:

- Ventilation-perfusion ($\dot{V}/\dot{Q}$) scanning has been the most widely used test for diagnosis of PE. When the clinical probability of PE is high, the test is highly specific when positive. The clinical utility of the test is reduced by the frequent "indeterminant" reading. In the PIOPED trial, where pulmonary angiograms confirmed the diagnosis of PE, fewer than half of patients had high-probability lung scans.[32]

- Pulmonary angiography with IV contrast remains the gold standard for diagnosing acute PE. Pulmonary angiography can usually be performed safely in experienced hands. Most often, noninvasive tests obviate the need for angiography, and its use is confined to patients who remain at a high index of suspicion despite noninvasive testing. Pulmonary angiography is also used to confirm PE in patients under consideration for fibrinolytic therapy or mechanical intervention for life-threatening PE.[22]

- High-resolution helical or spiral CT angiography with IV contrast shows great promise.[33] This technique is being used with increasing frequency and

may soon rival or exceed ventilation-perfusion scanning. Spiral CT identifies major emboli in the proximal portion of the pulmonary vasculature. If the spiral CT is negative but a high index of clinical suspicion remains, contrast pulmonary angiography should still be performed to search for these small distal or fragmented emboli. Remember, it is usually the second or third thromboembolic event that is fatal.

- Some protocols use lower extremity ultrasonography to exclude residual life-threatening clots in this instance. As many as half of patients with pulmonary embolus, however, will have negative studies. Presumably this finding results from complete migration of the clot from the proximal venous system.

Why Are Troponins Positive in Some Patients With PE?

During the course of evaluation for ACS, patients have been identified with elevated cardiac markers and negative coronary angiograms. Investigation has found that troponins and occasionally CK-MB will elevate with PE. This finding correlates with a large PE and right ventricular dysfunction. The acute increase in right ventricular afterload imposed by submassive and massive PE causes right heart ischemia that can lead to subendocardial infarction.

Remember to revisit the differential diagnosis of chest pain as discussed above. If troponin-positive patients have normal coronary angiograms, consider the possibility of PE.

In this section 3 conditions other than MI have been noted to cause chest pain and elevated cardiac markers: PE, myocarditis, and myopericarditis.

What Can Early Recognition and Triage by ACLS Providers Do to Improve Outcome Beyond Traditional Therapy (Heparin)?

Risk stratification with echocardiography has now been introduced for patients with PE. Clinically about 5% of patients with PE present in shock and are candidates for fibrinolytic therapy or mechanical fragmentation techniques where available.

About 40% of patients with PE have RV dysfunction by transthoracic cardiac echocardiography (TTE). This is manifest as RV hypokinesis of variable degrees and normal arterial pressure. Some studies have shown that fibrinolytic therapy can rapidly improve RV function and lower the incidence of recurrent PE. Treatment of this patient group is currently controversial, but most experts would seriously weigh the risk-benefit treatment options if hemodynamics are borderline or tenuous cardiopulmonary comorbidity exists. At the very least, the finding of RV dysfunction alerts the provider to pay close attention to anticoagulation parameters and optimal adjunctive therapy.

Acute Tension Pneumothorax

Description

An injury to the lung parenchyma or a bronchus that produces an air leak can cause a tension pneumothorax. When a tension pneumothorax develops, air accumulates in the chest and pressure in the pleural space increases, compressing the lung on the involved side and pushing the heart and mediastinum to the opposite side.

The mediastinum can compress the opposite lung, causing collapse and worsening hypoxia. The pneumothorax compresses the heart and great vessels, impeding venous return and cardiac output. Hypotension and hypoxia can combine to produce hemodynamic collapse, shock, and death.

A pneumothorax can be primary or secondary. A primary pneumothorax is also called a spontaneous pneumothorax; it rarely causes tension pneumothorax, although it can cause acute chest pain.

Signs and Symptoms

The classic signs of tension pneumothorax are

- Decreased breath sounds, decreased chest expansion, and hyperresonance on the involved side.

- Shift of the mediastinum away from the side of the pneumothorax. This can cause decreased breath sounds in the chest opposite the side of the pneumothorax.

- Hypoxemia.

Additional signs of tension pneumothorax:

- Cardiovascular compromise. Jugular venous distention, hypotension, and signs of decreased cardiac output may be observed.

- Pulsus paradoxus may be present if venous return is substantially impaired.

- The patient who is breathing spontaneously will be dyspneic and tachypneic and may complain of chest pain.

Clinical circumstances also raise suspicion of a tension pneumothorax in certain patient groups:

- Recent insertion of a central venous catheter

- Any recent diagnostic procedure in the chest, lower neck, or upper abdomen

- Ventilated patients with underlying pulmonary disease or high peak inspiratory airway pressures

- Chest or multisystem trauma

- Following removal of chest tubes

Tension pneumothorax should be considered when the patient presents with acute chest pain:

- Chest pain occurs in more than 90% of conscious patients with tension pneumothorax.

- Shortness of breath occurs in 80%.

The diagnosis of a tension pneumothorax is a clinical and not a radiographic diagnosis. The ACLS provider should not wait to obtain a chest radiograph to make the diagnosis. The following clinical signs and symptoms of extreme compromise in cardiopulmonary function indicate the need for empiric needle decompression:

- Lung sounds that are decreased or even absent on one side

- Tracheal deviation (a very late finding)

- Distention of jugular veins

- Hypotension

- Pulsus paradoxus

- Respiratory distress or arrest

- Cyanosis

Approach to Diagnosis

An arterial blood gas analysis is not a diagnostic test for tension pneumothorax. But this information is useful for evaluating the extent of hypoxia.

As noted above, the diagnosis of a tension pneumothorax is made on the basis of clinical findings. When a tension pneumothorax causes acute cardiopulmonary deterioration, immediate needle decompression is needed. Immediate response to the needle decompression confirms the diagnosis.

Imaging studies may be used to diagnose a pneumothorax that is not compromising clinical status:

- **Chest radiography:** Radiographs are a useful and convenient tool to screen for the development of a pneumothorax following invasive procedures or in high-risk patients on ventilators.[34]

- **Computed tomography:** CT is sensitive enough for evaluation of small pneumothoraxes, pneumomediastinum, and underlying pulmonary disease or injury that might have caused the original pneumothorax.

References

1. Cannon CP, McCabe CH, Stone PH, Rogers WJ, Schactman M, Thompson BW, Pearce DJ, Diver DJ, Kells C, Feldman T, Williams M, Gibson RS, Kronenberg MW, Ganz LI, Anderson HV, Braunwald E. The electrocardiogram predicts one-year outcome of patients with unstable angina and non-Q wave myocardial infarction: results of the TIMI III Registry ECG Ancillary Study. Thrombolysis in Myocardial Ischemia. *J Am Coll Cardiol.* 1997;30:133-140.

2. Holmvang L, Luscher MS, Clemmensen P, Thygesen K, Grande P. Very early risk stratification using combined ECG and biochemical assessment in patients with unstable coronary artery disease (a thrombin inhibition in myocardial ischemia [TRIM] substudy). The TRIM Study Group. *Circulation.* 1998;98:2004-2009.

3. Savonitto S, Ardissino D, Granger CB, Morando G, Prando MD, Mafrici A, Cavallini C, Melandri G, Thompson TD, Vahanian A, Ohman EM, Califf RM, Van de Werf F, Topol EJ. Prognostic value of the admission electrocardiogram in acute coronary syndromes. *JAMA*. 1999; 281:707-713.

4. Diderholm E, Andren B, Frostfeldt G, Genberg M, Jernberg T, Lagerqvist B, Lindahl B, Venge P, Wallentin L. The prognostic and therapeutic implications of increased troponin T levels and ST depression in unstable coronary artery disease: the FRISC II invasive troponin T electrocardiogram substudy. *Am Heart J*. 2002;143: 760-767.

5. Braunwald E, Antman EM, Beasley JW, Califf RM, Cheitlin MD, Hochman JS, Jones RH, Kereiakes D, Kupersmith J, Levin TN, Pepine CJ, Schaeffer JW, Smith EE III, Steward DE, Theroux P, Alpert JS, Eagle KA, Faxon DP, Fuster V, Gardner TJ, Gregoratos G, Russell RO, Smith SC Jr. ACC/AHA guidelines for the management of patients with unstable angina and non-ST-segment elevation myocardial infarction. A report of the American College of Cardiology/American Heart Association Task Force on Practice Guidelines (Committee on the Management of Patients With Unstable Angina). *J Am Coll Cardiol*. 2000;36:970-1062.

6. Braunwald E, Antman EM, Beasley JW, Califf RM, Cheitlin MD, Hochman JS, Jones RH, Kereiakes D, Kupersmith J, Levin TN, Pepine CJ, Schaeffer JW, Smith EE III, Steward DE, Theroux P, Gibbons RJ, Alpert JS, Faxon DP, Fuster V, Gregoratos G, Hiratzka LF, Jacobs AK, Smith SC Jr. ACC/AHA 2002 guideline update for the management of patients with unstable angina and non-ST-segment elevation myocardial infarction—summary article: a report of the American College of Cardiology/American Heart Association Task Force on Practice Guidelines (Committee on the Management of Patients With Unstable Angina). *J Am Coll Cardiol*. 2002;40:1366-1374.

7. Peberdy M, Ornato J. Coronary artery disease in women. *Heart Dis Stroke*. 1992;1:315-319.

8. Douglas PS, Ginsburg GS. The evaluation of chest pain in women. *N Engl J Med*. 1996; 334:1311-1315.

9. Sullivan AK, Holdright DR, Wright CA, Sparrow JL, Cunningham D, Fox KM. Chest pain in women: clinical, investigative, and prognostic features. *BMJ*. 1994;308:883-886.

10. Solomon CG, Lee TH, Cook EF, Weisberg MC, Brand DA, Rouan GW, Goldman L. Comparison of clinical presentation of acute myocardial infarction in patients older than 65 years of age to younger patients: the Multicenter Chest Pain Study experience. *Am J Cardiol*. 1989;63:772-776.

11. Lee TH, Cook EF, Weisberg M, Sargent RK, Wilson C, Goldman L. Acute chest pain in the emergency room: identification and examination of low-risk patients. *Arch Intern Med*. 1985;145:65-69.

12. Lewis JF, Lin L, McGorray S, Pepine CJ, Doyle M, Edmundowicz D, Holubkov R, Pohost G, Reichek N, Rogers W, Sharaf BL, Sopko G, Merz CN. Dobutamine stress echocardiography in women with chest pain: pilot phase data from the National Heart, Lung, and Blood Institute Women's Ischemia Syndrome Evaluation (WISE). *J Am Coll Cardiol*. 1999; 33:1462-1468.

13. Hagan PG, Nienaber CA, Isselbacher EM, Bruckman D, Karavite DJ, Russman PL, Evangelista A, Fattori R, Suzuki T, Oh JK, Moore AG, Malouf JF, Pape LA, Gaca C, Sechtem U, Lenferink S, Deutsch HJ, Diedrichs H, Marcos y Robles J, Llovet A, Gilon D, Das SK, Armstrong WF, Deeb GM, Eagle KA. The International Registry of Acute Aortic Dissection (IRAD): new insights into an old disease. *JAMA*. 2000;283:897-903.

14. Sarasin FP, Louis-Simonet M, Gaspoz JM, Junod AF. Detecting acute thoracic aortic dissection in the emergency department: time constraints and choice of the optimal diagnostic test. *Ann Emerg Med*. 1996;28:278-288.

15. Moore AG, Eagle KA, Bruckman D, Moon BS, Malouf JF, Fattori R, Evangelista A, Isselbacher EM, Suzuki T, Nienaber CA, Gilon D, Oh JK. Choice of computed tomography, transesophageal echocardiography, magnetic resonance imaging, and aortography in acute aortic dissection: International Registry of Acute Aortic Dissection (IRAD). *Am J Cardiol*. 2002;89: 1235-1238.

16. Aikat S, Ghaffari S. A review of pericardial diseases: clinical, ECG and hemodynamic features and management. *Cleve Clin J Med*. 2000;67:903-914.

17. Bilchick KC, Wise RA. Paradoxical physical findings described by Kussmaul: pulsus paradoxus and Kussmaul's sign. *Lancet*. 2002; 359:1940-1942.

18. Hoit BD. Management of effusive and constrictive pericardial heart disease. *Circulation*. 2002;105:2939-2942.

19. Beck CS. Two cardiac compression triads. *JAMA*. 1935;104:714-716.

20. Podbregar M, Krivec B, Voga G. Impact of morphologic characteristics of central pulmonary thromboemboli in massive pulmonary embolism. *Chest*. 2002;122:973-979.

21. Konstantinides S, Geibel A, Olschewski M, Kasper W, Hruska N, Jackle S, Binder L. Importance of cardiac troponins I and T in risk stratification of patients with acute pulmonary embolism. *Circulation*. 2002;106: 1263-1268.

22. Goldhaber SZ. Pulmonary embolism. *N Engl J Med*. 1998;339:93-104.

23. Spittell JA Jr. Chest pain in patients with normal findings on angiography [letter]. *Mayo Clin Proc*. 2002;77:296.

24. The urokinase pulmonary embolism trial: a national cooperative study. *Circulation*. 1973;47(suppl II):II1-II108.

25. Bell WR, Simon TL, Stengle JM, Sherry S. The urokinase-streptokinase pulmonary embolism trial (phase II) results. *Circulation*. 1974;50:1070-1071.

26. Miller GH, Feied CF. Suspected pulmonary embolism: the difficulties of diagnostic evaluation. *Postgrad Med*. 1995;97:51-58.

27. Kline JA, Nelson RD, Jackson RE, Courtney DM. Criteria for the safe use of D-dimer testing in emergency department patients with suspected pulmonary embolism: a multicenter US study. *Ann Emerg Med*. 2002;39:144-152.

28. Sijens PE, Oudkerk M. Should patients be managed for suspected pulmonary embolism on the basis of pretest clinical probability and D-dimer results? [letter]. *Ann Intern Med*. 2002;136:781.

29. Kruip MJ, Slob MJ, Schijen JH, van der Heul C, Buller HR. Use of a clinical decision rule in combination with D-dimer concentration in diagnostic workup of patients with suspected pulmonary embolism: a prospective management study. *Arch Intern Med*. 2002;162:1631-1635.

30. Brown MD, Rowe BH, Reeves MJ, Bermingham JM, Goldhaber SZ. The accuracy of the enzyme-linked immunosorbent assay D-dimer test in the diagnosis of pulmonary embolism: a meta-analysis. *Ann Emerg Med*. 2002;40: 133-144.

31. Dunn KL, Wolf JP, Dorfman DM, Fitzpatrick P, Baker JL, Goldhaber SZ. Normal D-dimer levels in emergency department patients suspected of acute pulmonary embolism. *J Am Coll Cardiol*. 2002;40:1475-1478.

32. Value of the ventilation/perfusion scan in acute pulmonary embolism: results of the prospective investigation of pulmonary embolism diagnosis (PIOPED). The PIOPED Investigators. *JAMA*. 1990;263:2753-2759.

33. Carman TL, Deitcher SR. Advances in diagnosing and excluding pulmonary embolism: spiral CT and D-dimer measurement. *Cleve Clin J Med*. 2002;69:721-729.

34. Aleman C, Alegre J, Armadans L, Andreu J, Falco V, Recio J, Cervera C, Ruiz E, Fernandez de Sevilla T. The value of chest roentgenography in the diagnosis of pneumothorax after thoracentesis. *Am J Med*. 1999;107:340-343.

Toxicology in Emergency Cardiovascular Care

"Lily's consciousness cratered, her kidneys failed, and she became so perilously acidotic that her heart forgot even the most rudimentary steps of its once rhythmic and joyful dance."

—Katherine Stone.
Star Light, Star Bright.
MIRA books. 2002.

Highlights From the International *ECC* Guidelines 2000

- When appropriate, early consultation with a medical toxicologist or certified regional poison information center is highly recommended. Early consultation will enhance the care of victims with severe or unusual poisoning.[1,2]

- When indicated, refer severe or unusual poisoning victims to regional centers that specialize in the clinical care and treatment of patients with unusual poisonings.

- There is no convincing evidence that gastric lavage improves clinical outcome, and it may cause significant morbidity. International guidelines now recommend that gastric lavage be considered only for patients who present within 1 hour of ingestion of a potentially lethal amount of drug or toxin.[3]

- When patients are obtunded or comatose, perform rapid sequence intubation before gastric lavage to reduce the risk of aspiration pneumonia. There is no evidence that intubation is required in patients who can protect their airways, and the use of drugs traditionally employed in the "rapid sequence" technique may be unnecessary or even contraindicated.

- Reversal of benzodiazepine intoxication with flumazenil is more hazardous than reversal with other agents. Routine inclusion of flumazenil in "coma cocktail" protocols is not recommended.

General Considerations

Magnitude of the Problem: Fatal Poisonings

In the United States fatal poisonings account for 11% of all injury-related mortality, making poisoning the third most lethal injury. In 1995 there were an estimated 2.4 million poisoning exposures reported to US poison centers, 1 million Emergency Department visits (1% of all visits), 215 000 hospital admissions, and 18 549 deaths.[4-6] Although poisoning *exposures* are common, life-threatening or fatal poisonings are not, with only 7 deaths per 1000 reported poisoning exposures.

Lack of High-Level Evidence for Guidelines Development

A Toxicology Working Group of the American Heart Association ACLS and Pediatric Resuscitation Subcommittees developed the 2000 evidence-based and consensus-based guidelines.[7,8] The group's objectives were to identify the severe poisonings for which standard ECC guidelines may not be optimal or appropriate and to develop evidence-based guidelines for the management of those poisonings.

The infrequency of life-threatening poisonings and the lack of a systematic approach to management in US hospitals present obstacles to performance of high-quality clinical research. Because the research in this area consists primarily of small case series (level of evidence 5), animal studies (level of evidence 6), and reports on single cases (level of evidence 8), most recommendations made by the experts for the *ECC Guidelines 2000* and for the recommendations in this chapter are *Class IIb* or *Indeterminate* recommendations.[7,8]

Symptom-Based Therapy: Management of Respiratory Compromise

Airway and Respiratory Compromise

Airway and Respiratory Management in Opioid Poisoning

Lethal opioid poisoning eliminates airway protective reflexes and directly suppresses respiratory drive. Opioid poisoning provides the "default" model for a general approach to drug-induced airway and respiratory compromise. Although this chapter focuses on the effects of poisonings and drug overdoses on the *cardiovascular* system, respiratory failure is the most common cause of death in cases of overdose and poisoning.

Opioid Reversal

Before or After Tracheal Intubation?

In a patient with a clinically significant opioid overdose, healthcare providers have long taken the practical approach of performing tracheal intubation before giving naloxone. This sequence allowed the narcotizing effects of the opioid to serve as an intubation adjunct. In addition, intubation and ventilation allowed correction of hypercarbia before administration of naloxone. There is some data from animals and limited clinical experience[9,10] that if ventilation normalizes the arterial carbon dioxide tension *before* naloxone administration, the potential rise in epinephrine concentration associated with naloxone administration and its attendant potentially toxic effects are blunted. The practice of *routine intubation* before naloxone administration for treatment of severe opioid overdose is no longer recommended.

Specific ACLS recommendations for naloxone administration, tracheal intubation, and support of ventilation for opioid toxicity include the following:

■ When patients with suspected opioid overdose have *respiratory insufficiency plus a detectable pulse,* attempt opioid reversal *before* tracheal intubation.

■ Healthcare providers should support ventilation via bag and mask while preparing to administer naloxone. ACLS experts thought that existing evidence does not justify withholding naloxone until ventilation is initiated. This recommendation differs from the PALS recommendation to support ventilation to attempt to normalize the partial pressure of arterial CO_2 *before* naloxone - administration. In recent years in the United States, opioid use is associated with more drug-induced cardiopulmonary arrests that any other drug. The incidence of severe complications after opioid reversal is less than 2%.

■ Naloxone is the preferred reversal agent for opioid toxicity even though it has a shorter duration of effect (45 to 70 minutes) than heroin (4 to 5 hours).

■ Some experts note the theoretical advantages of the IM and SQ routes of naloxone administration over the IV route (ease of administration, reduced risk of needle puncture for healthcare personnel, and reduced severity of withdrawal for opioid addicts). Others contend, however, that all such patients should have IV access when possible because of the severity of their illness.

Endpoints for Opioid Reversal

■ The endpoint objectives for opioid reversal are adequate airway reflexes and ventilation, not complete arousal.

■ Acute, abrupt opioid withdrawal may increase the likelihood of severe complications, such as pulmonary edema, ventricular arrhythmias, and severe agitation and hostility.

Naloxone: Dose and Route

■ When naloxone is given in incremental doses of 0.1 mg, the average naloxone reversal dose is 0.2 mg IV.[11]

■ In emergencies a slow incremental rate of administration is less satisfactory. For these cases the recommended initial dose of naloxone is 0.4 to 0.8 mg IV or 0.8 mg IM or SQ.

■ The IM and SQ routes have advantages over the IV route: ease of administration, reduced risk of needle puncture for healthcare providers, and reduced severity of withdrawal for opioid addicts.

■ In communities where abuse of naloxone-resistant opioids is prevalent, larger initial doses of naloxone may be appropriate.

■ When opioid overdose is strongly suspected or in locations where "China white" (referring to fentanyl and its derivatives) abuse is prevalent, titration to total naloxone doses of 6 to 10 mg may be necessary.

Disposition After Arousal

■ The incidence of severe complications after opioid reversal is less than 2%.

■ It is recommended that opioid intoxicated patients aroused with naloxone be transported to the hospital, although some EMS systems, especially in Europe, allow selected patients aroused with naloxone to refuse transport to the hospital.

— The duration of action of naloxone is shorter than the duration of action

---

Debate From the Proceedings of the Evidence Evaluation and Guidelines 2000 Conferences

Topic 5: Use of Naloxone in Cases of Suspected Opioid-Induced Respiratory Failure Evaluation and Debate

Panelists believe that most healthcare providers should initiate both assisted ventilation and opioid reversal as soon as possible in patients with a suspected opioid overdose. At this time there is insufficient evidence to recommend withholding naloxone until ventilatory assistance has begun. In patients who have experienced a cardiac arrest as the result of a suspected opioid overdose, administration of naloxone during resuscitation may provide additional benefit to routine resuscitative measures. A lower initial dose of opioid antagonist is recommended because of the belief that it may result in less abrupt withdrawal, a less dramatic surge of catecholamines, and fewer complications. Because of possible poisoning from naloxone-resistant opioids such as synthetic or superpotent opioids, a total dose of 4 to 6 mg is recommended as the lower limit of the total naloxone challenge in a patient whose condition is refractory. The dosage recommendations are based on consensus rather than supportive evidence.

—Condensed from Albertson et al.[8]

of most opioids. Hence failure to continue care has occasionally led to serious consequences, such as severe re-narcotization or delayed pulmonary edema.[12,13]

— It is therefore recommended that following arousal, all patients be observed beyond the duration of the naloxone effect to ensure their safety.

Symptom-Based Therapy: Management of Cardiovascular Compromise Caused by Drugs or Toxins

Table 1 summarizes the altered vital signs that may be observed with drug-induced cardiovascular emergencies and lists both indicated and contraindicated therapies.

Hemodynamically Significant Bradycardia

Treatment

Atropine. Atropine is neither helpful nor harmful in the treatment of most drug-induced hemodynamically significant bradycardia. However, in the case of poisoning from cholinesterase inhibitors (organophosphates or carbamates or nerve agents), atropine may be lifesaving. The recommended starting adult dose for insecticide poisoning from cholinesterase inhibitors is 2 to 4 mg. In these cases doses well in excess of accepted maximums may be required.

Pacing. Electrical cardiac pacing is often effective in cases of mild to moderate drug-induced bradycardia. Start with transcutaneous pacing. Prophylactic transvenous pacing is not recommended because the tip of the transvenous catheter may trigger ventricular arrhythmias when the myocardium is irritable; this complication has been clearly linked to adverse outcomes in patients with digoxin toxicity. Transvenous pacing is needed if transcutaneous pacing fails or is poorly tolerated or if electrical capture is difficult to maintain.

In very severe poisonings, failure to capture may occur despite proper pacer electrode location and the highest pacemaker voltage output settings.

Vasopressors. In drug-induced bradycardia resistant to atropine and pacing, vasopressors with β-adrenergic agonist activity are indicated. See "Shock" (later in this chapter) for more information about the use of vasopressors in the management of drug-induced cardiovascular dysfunction.

Isoproterenol. Avoid isoproterenol for treatment of most drug-induced bradycardia. It may induce or aggravate hypotension and ventricular arrhythmias. In massive β-blocker poisoning, however, very-high-dose isoproterenol therapy has been reported to be effective.

Digoxin-specific Fab antibody fragments. This therapy is extremely effective for life-threatening ventricular arrhythmias or heart block due to digoxin and cardiac glycoside poisoning.[4]

Hemodynamically Significant Tachycardia

Treatment

Benzodiazepines. Benzodiazepines such as diazepam or lorazepam are generally safe and effective for treatment of symptomatic drug-induced tachycardia. Benzodiazepines are particularly helpful in the treatment of cocaine toxicity because they appear to attenuate the toxic cocaine myocardial and CNS effects.[14] Avoid using benzodiazepines in amounts that depress the level of consciousness and create the need for respiratory assistance.

Physostigmine. Physostigmine is a specific antidote for tachycardia and central anticholinergic syndrome due to *pure* anticholinergic poisoning. It should not be used in mixed tricyclic antidepressant poisoning.

Propranolol. A nonselective β-blocker such as propranolol may be effective in drug-induced tachycardia due to some poisonings, but β-blockers should not be used in the setting of cocaine intoxication, amphetamines, or ephedrine.

Precautions

Drug-induced tachycardia may induce myocardial ischemia, myocardial infarction, or ventricular arrhythmias and lead to high-output heart failure and shock. Avoid the more common therapies for supraventricular tachycardia such as adenosine and synchronized cardioversion; drug-induced supraventricular tachycardia is commonly recurrent or refractory. Avoid diltiazem and verapamil in poisoned patients with borderline hypotension; these drugs may precipitate more severe shock.

Wide-Complex Conduction Impairments

Treatment

Hypertonic saline and systemic alkalinization. Poisonings with sodium channel antagonists (membrane-stabilizing agents) result in prolonged ventricular conduction (increased QRS interval). Prolonged QRS and QT intervals predispose the heart to ventricular and other wide-complex tachycardias. Hypertonic saline and systemic alkalinization reverse these adverse electrophysiologic effects. This reversal prevents or terminates supraventricular tachycardias with aberrant conduction, and monomorphic and polymorphic ventricular tachycardia secondary to poisoning from many types of sodium channel blocking agents, such as tricyclic antidepressants.[15] Hypertonic sodium bicarbonate provides both hypertonic saline and systemic alkalinization. This therapy appears to provide benefit in several types of sodium channel blocker poisoning, such as tricyclic antidepressants and cocaine intoxication.

Treatment Goals of Systemic Alkalinization

In severe poisonings the goal of alkalinization therapy is an arterial pH of 7.50 to 7.55. Establish the target pH with repeated boluses of 1 to 2 mEq/kg sodium bicarbonate. Respiratory alkalosis can be induced as a temporizing measure until the appropriate degree of metabolic alkalosis can be attained with sodium bicarbonate. Maintain alkalinization by

TABLE 1. Drug-Induced Cardiovascular Emergencies or Altered Vital Signs*: Therapies to Consider† and Contraindicated Interventions

Drug-Induced Cardiovascular Emergency or Altered Vital Signs*	Therapies to Consider†	Contraindicated Interventions (or Use With Precaution)
Bradycardia	• Pacemaker (transcutaneous or transvenous) • Toxic drug—*calcium channel blocker:* NS, epinephrine, calcium salt? glucose/insulin? glucagon? • Toxic drug—*β-blocker:* NS, epinephrine, calcium salt? glucose/insulin? glucagon?	• Atropine (seldom helpful except for cholinesterase inhibitor poisonings) • Isoproterenol if hypotensive • Prophylactic transvenous pacing
Tachycardia	• Toxic drug—*sympathomimetics:* benzodiazepines, lidocaine, sodium bicarbonate, nitroglycerin, nitroprusside • Toxic drug—*tricyclic antidepressants:* sodium bicarbonate, hyperventilation, NS, magnesium sulfate, lidocaine • Toxic drug—*anticholinergics:* physostigmine	• β-blockers (almost never useful in drug-induced tachycardia) • Cardioversion (rarely indicated) • Adenosine (rarely indicated) • Calcium channel blockers (rarely indicated) • Physostigmine (if TCA overdose)
Impaired conduction/ ventricular arrhythmias	• Sodium bicarbonate • Lidocaine	• If TCA overdose: type 1_A antiarrhythmics (procainamide)
Hypertensive emergencies	• Toxic drug—*sympathomimetics:* benzodiazepines, lidocaine, sodium bicarbonate, nitroglycerin, nitroprusside, phentolamine	• β-blockers
Acute coronary syndrome	• Benzodiazepines • Lidocaine • Sodium bicarbonate • Nitroglycerin • Aspirin, heparin • Base reperfusion strategy on cardiac catheterization data	• β-blockers
Shock	• Toxic drug—*calcium channel blocker:* NS, epinephrine, norepinephrine, dopamine, calcium salt? glucose/insulin? glucagon? • Toxic drug—*β-blocker:* NS, epinephrine, norepinephrine, dopamine, calcium salt? glucose/insulin? glucagon? • If refractory to *maximal* medical therapy: consider circulatory assist devices	• Isoproterenol • Avoid calcium salts if digoxin toxicity is suspected
Acute cholinergic syndrome	• Atropine • Pralidoxime/obidoxime	• Succinylcholine
Acute anticholinergic syndrome	• Physostigmine	• Antipsychotics • Other anticholinergic agents
Opioid poisoning	• Naloxone • Assisted ventilation • Tracheal intubation	

*Unless stated otherwise, listed alterations of vital signs (bradycardia, tachycardia, tachypnea) are "hemodynamically significant."
†*Therapies to consider* should be based on specific indications.

infusion of an alkaline solution consisting of 3 ampules of sodium bicarbonate (150 mEq) plus 30 mEq KCL mixed in 850 mL of D_5W titrated to serum pH.

Ventricular Tachycardia/Fibrillation

Drug-induced VT and VF may be difficult to distinguish from drug-induced wide-complex conduction impairments. You should suspect the development of a drug-induced VT whenever a poisoned patient demonstrates a sudden conversion to a wider-complex rhythm with hypotension. By definition this condition is unstable tachycardia; cardioversion is indicated.

Treatment

Cardioversion or Defibrillation

Perform electrical cardioversion for drug-induced VT with pulses; attempt defibrillation for VF or pulseless VT.

Epinephrine

In sympathomimetic poisonings with refractory VF, the cost-benefit ratio of epinephrine in management is unknown. If epinephrine is used, increase the interval between doses and use only standard dose amounts (1 mg IV). Avoid high-dose epinephrine.

Antiarrhythmics

Antiarrhythmics are indicated in hemodynamically stable drug-induced VT, although there are few published articles to guide the choice of agents.

Lidocaine. For most types of drug-induced monomorphic VT or VF, and for VT/VF associated with cocaine-induced myocardial ischemia, lidocaine is the antiarrhythmic of choice. This consensus is based on limited published studies but extensive clinical experience.[16] When VF/VT develops immediately after cocaine use, most experts favor early use of sodium bicarbonate.[17,18]

Propranolol. In sympathomimetic poisonings (especially with cocaine) propranolol is contraindicated. This guideline is based on limited human studies in the cardiac catheterization suite and on animal survival studies.

Procainamide. Procainamide is contraindicated in poisonings from tricyclic antidepressants and other drugs with similar antiarrhythmic (Vaughan Williams type Ia$_{vw}$) properties.

Phenytoin. Phenytoin was previously recommended for VT induced by tricyclic antidepressant overdose. Subsequent studies questioned the efficacy and safety of this agent.[19,20]

Magnesium. Magnesium has demonstrated beneficial effects for drug-induced VT. But magnesium may aggravate drug-induced hypotension.[21,22]

Amiodarone. A handful of cases of refractory drug-induced ventricular tachycardia or fibrillation have been reported to respond to amiodarone. Because data is limited and amiodarone may worsen drug-induced hypotension and may have proarrhythmic effects, it should be used with caution if at all.

Torsades de Pointes

Mechanism

Torsades de pointes has been associated with both therapeutic and toxic exposures to many drugs. Contributing factors for torsades de pointes include hypoxemia, hypokalemia, and hypomagnesemia.

Treatment

There are 3 aspects of treatment for drug-induced torsades de pointes:

- Correction of hypoxemia, hypokalemia, and hypomagnesemia
- Electrical therapy
- Pharmacologic therapy

Support Oxygenation and Ventilation. Ensure that hypoxemia is corrected.

Magnesium. Magnesium is recommended for torsades de pointes even with normal blood magnesium levels (dose: 1 to 2 g diluted in 10 mL D_5W IV push).

Potassium. Even with normal potassium levels some toxicologists recommend potassium administration.

Lidocaine. Studies of lidocaine for torsades de pointes have shown mixed results (dose: 1 to 1.5 mg/kg IV push; consider second dose to maximum of 3 mg/kg).

Electrical (overdrive) pacing. Pacing at rates up to 100 to 120 bpm is often effective at terminating torsades de pointes.

Isoproterenol. Pharmacologic overdrive pacing using isoproterenol has been recommended for torsades de pointes. Begin at 2 to 10 µg/kg per minute; titrate to increase heart rate until VT is suppressed.

Level of Evidence

The safety and efficacy of many of these recommended therapies for drug-induced polymorphic VT have not been established by high levels of research. From the perspective of evidence-based guidelines, we have only low-level evidence (case reports, case series, and extrapolated data). For this reason these recommendations are considered *Class Indeterminate*. This class neither prohibits nor encourages clinical use. It merely acknowledges that many toxicologic approaches are "best assumptions" based on an understanding of the mechanisms of disease and consensus of experts. Administration of magnesium to treat torsades de pointes with known hypomagnesemia is a Class IIb recommendation.

Hypertensive Emergencies

Mechanism of Hypertension

Drug-induced hypertensive emergencies are often short-lived. Therapy is often not indicted because the hypertension rapidly resolves and may be followed by hypotension. Hypertensive emergencies frequently develop in patients with cocaine toxicity.

Treatment

Benzodiazepines. Most toxicology experts consider benzodiazepines the first-line therapy for hypertension in the setting of sympathomimetic overdose (eg, cocaine intoxication).

Nitroprusside. In drug-induced hypertensive emergencies refractory to benzodiazepines, use a short-acting antihypertensive such as nitroprusside as the second line of therapy.

Combined α-/β-blockade. A combination of α- and β-blockade can be achieved using phentolamine and a nonselective α-antagonist, such as labetalol. Most experts, however, now recommend against the use of any β-blocker if the hypertensive emergency is suspected to be caused by a sympathomimetic such as cocaine.

Precautions

Propranolol (a nonselective β-blocker) is contraindicated. It may block only β receptors, leaving unopposed α-adrenergic stimulation and worsening hypertension.[23]

Hypertension is often short lived. So aggressive therapy for a drug-induced hypertensive emergency is rarely needed and may contribute to worsening hypotension after the hypertension resolves.[24]

Shock

Mechanism of Shock

Drug-induced shock results from 1 of 3 mechanisms or from a combination of these factors:

- The drug induces a *decrease in intravascular volume.*

- The drug induces a *fall in systemic vascular resistance.*

- The drug induces *diminished myocardial contractility.*

Treatment

Drug-Induced Hypovolemic Shock (With Normal Systemic Vascular Resistance)

Fluid challenge. Initial treatment must include a fluid challenge to correct hypovolemia and optimize cardiac preload. If the offending agent is cardiotoxic, it will reduce the patient's ability to tolerate excess intravascular volume; volume therapy may lead to iatrogenic congestive heart failure with pulmonary edema. Be prepared to support oxygenation and ventilation.

Vasopressors (dopamine). If shock persists after an adequate fluid challenge, start a vasopressor. Evidence supports dopamine as an effective pressor agent in mild to moderate poisonings.[25] Most patients with

drug-induced shock, however, have decreased myocardial contractility and decreased systemic vascular resistance, and more potent vasoconstrictors may be needed.

Higher-dose vasopressors. Higher-dose vasopressors are indicated when drug-induced shock is unresponsive to volume loading and conventional doses of dopamine and other vasopressors. If possible, establish central hemodynamic monitoring with a pulmonary artery or central venous catheter, but do not delay treatment of hypotension. Optimize cardiac preload quickly; then use calculated cardiac output and systemic vascular resistance to guide selection and titration of a vasopressor and inotropic agent.

Drug-Induced Distributive Shock (Normal Volume With Decreased Systemic Vascular Resistance)

Norepinephrine or phenylephrine. With normal volume plus decreased systemic vascular resistance (distributive shock), use more potent vasoconstrictive agents with greater α-adrenergic effect (norepinephrine or phenylephrine). Increase the dose of the α-adrenergic vasopressor until the shock is adequately treated or adverse effects (eg, ventricular arrhythmias) begin to appear. Some poisoned patients require doses of vasopressors far above conventional doses, so-called "high-dose vasopressor therapy." Consider use of powerful vasoconstrictors such as *vasopressin* or *endothelin* in severely poisoned patients if other adrenergic agents produce ventricular arrhythmias before the shock is adequately treated. Note that little formal evidence supports this recommendation.

Drug-Induced Cardiogenic Shock (Low Cardiac Output, Low Systemic Vascular Resistance)

Inotropic and vasopressor agents. Drug-induced shock is most often characterized by both a low cardiac output and low systemic vascular resistance. Inotropic agents are often required. Agents used successfully in some studies include *inamrinone* and *dobutamine*, as well as *calcium, glucose, and insulin.*[26,27] Sometimes more than one agent is necessary. Although these agents can increase contractility and cardiac

output, they may also decrease systemic vascular resistance. Often a concomitant vasopressor such as *norepinephrine* is required.[28]

Cardiac Arrest

Mechanism

Cardiac arrest associated with drugs or poisonings may be associated with any of the "collapse" rhythms: asystole, pulseless electrical activity, or VF/pulseless VT.

Treatment

Prolonged CPR and Resuscitation

In ACLS cardiac resuscitation attempts are usually terminated after 20 to 30 minutes unless mitigating factors or signs of CNS viability are present. Resuscitation of patients with cardiac arrest caused by drug toxicity or poisoning warrants more prolonged resuscitative efforts. Recovery with good neurologic outcome has been reported in poisoned patients after prolonged CPR, sometimes for periods up to 3 to 5 hours.[29,30] The marked vasodilatation associated with many types of severe poisonings may account for CNS viability despite the prolonged resuscitation.

Circulatory Assist Devices

Intra-aortic balloon pumps and cardiopulmonary bypass. These circulatory assist devices have been used successfully in critical poisonings refractory to maximal medical care. These techniques, however, are expensive and manpower intensive and have significant associated morbidity. To be effective, these devices must be employed early in the resuscitative effort, before the irreversible effects of severe shock or cardiac arrest develop.

Perspective. If intra-aortic balloon pump support is planned, the patient must have an intrinsic cardiac rhythm because the balloon inflation is synchronized with the ECG to provide diastolic augmentation. Emergency cardiopulmonary bypass does not require an intrinsic rhythm and recent technologic advancements have made rapid application possible through peripheral vessels.

Brain Death and Organ Donation Criteria

Critical concept. Brain death criteria based only on an electroencephalogram (EEG) and neurologic examination are invalid during acute toxic encephalopathy. These brain death criteria apply only when drug levels are no longer toxic. In the presence of toxic drug levels, the only valid confirmatory test for brain death is absent cerebral blood flow.

Organ transplantation after a fatal poisoning from agents capable of causing severe end-organ damage, such as carbon monoxide, cocaine, and iron, is controversial. When organ function is carefully evaluated, successful transplantation of some organs from victims of fatal poisoning with *acetaminophen, cyanide, methanol,* and *carbon monoxide* is possible.[31] However, transplantation of known *target* organs following a fatal poisoning is unlikely to succeed. These target organs include the heart in carbon monoxide poisoning, the heart and liver in cocaine and iron poisonings, and the liver and kidneys in acetaminophen poisonings.

Acute Coronary Syndromes

Mechanism

In adults the most frequent cause of cocaine-induced hospitalization is an acute coronary syndrome (ACS) producing chest pain and a variety of cardiac rhythm disturbances. ACS results from ischemia caused by the combined effects of cocaine: stimulation of β-adrenergic myocardial receptors increases myocardial oxygen demand, and the α-adrenergic and 5-HT agonist actions of cocaine cause coronary artery constriction.

Treatment

Benzodiazepines and nitroglycerin. These agents are the first-line agents for treatment of cocaine-induced ACS. Nitroglycerin has been shown to reverse cocaine-induced vasoconstriction when studied in the cardiac catheterization suite.[32-36]

Phentolamine. Phentolamine, a potent pure α-blocker, has a nitroglycerin-like ability to reverse cocaine-induced vasoconstriction.[33-36] Consider *phentolamine* a second-line therapy.

Precautions

Though *labetalol* has been reported to be effective in case reports, use of this drug is controversial because it is a nonselective β-blocker.[37,38] Labetalol does not reverse coronary vasoconstriction.[34,36] *Propranolol* is contraindicated (Class III) because it has been shown to worsen cocaine-induced vasoconstriction in patients studied in the cardiac catheterization suite. *Esmolol,* despite being a selective β-blocker (β₁ but not β₂), has been shown to aggravate hypertension and also to induce hypotension.[39] Most toxicology experts consider not only propranolol but also esmolol, metoprolol, and labetalol to be contraindicated in the management of cocaine-induced ACS.[8]

Fibrinolytics. Fibrinolytics are rarely indicated in the management of drug-induced ACS,[40] and they are contraindicated if uncontrolled, severe drug-induced hypertension is present. Percutaneous interventions (angioplasty and stent placement) are better alternatives when coronary atherosclerosis is present. If emergency cardiac catheterization reveals thrombus without atherosclerotic disease, intracoronary thrombolysis can be performed.[8,14]

Summary of Symptom-Based Therapy: Management of Cardiovascular Compromise Caused by Drugs or Toxins

In treatment of acute poison-induced shock and cardiac arrest, the *standard ACLS protocols* may not be effective.[7] Care of severely poisoned patients can be enhanced by urgent consultation with a medical toxicologist. Alternative approaches that may be needed for treatment of poisonings include the following:

- The use of *higher doses* of drugs than usual

- The use of *drugs rarely given in cardiac arrest,* such as inamrinone, calcium, esmolol, glucagon, insulin, labetalol, esmolol, phenylephrine, physostigmine, and sodium bicarbonate

- More frequent use of *heroic measures* such as prolonged CPR and circulatory assist devices

- *Earlier consideration of organ donation* when resuscitative efforts from a critical poisoning are unsuccessful and brain death is expected

Management of Specific Poisonings

Table 2 summarizes potentially cardiotoxic drugs, the cardiovascular signs of toxicity they produce, and therapies to consider.

Calcium Channel Blocker and β-Blocker Toxicity: Overview

Major Toxicities of Calcium Channel Blockers and β-Blockers

Both calcium channel blockers and β-blockers have negative inotropic and negative chronotropic effects. Whereas calcium channel blockers possess varying degrees of direct vasodilatory properties,[41] β-blockers do not.[42]

Toxicity from calcium channel blockers and β-blockers can produce the following signs and symptoms:

- Hypotension

- Depression of myocardial contractility

- Bradycardias from depression of SA nodal, AV nodal, and intraventricular conduction; heart block

- Decreased level of consciousness, lethargy, or even coma[41,42]

- Seizures (which may be the initial sign of serious toxicity), usually due to hypoperfusion of the central nervous system[43-45]

- Hypoglycemia, hyperkalemia with β-blocker overdose

- Hyperglycemia associated with calcium channel blocker overdose[43,44]

TABLE 2. Potentially Cardiotoxic Drugs: Cardiopulmonary Signs* of Toxicity and Therapy to Consider†

*Unless stated otherwise, listed alterations of vital signs (bradycardia, tachycardia, tachypnea) are "hemodynamically significant."
†Specific *therapy to consider* should be based on specific indications. Therapies followed by "?" are *Class Indeterminate*.

Potentially Toxic Drugs: by Type of Agent	Cardiopulmonary Signs* of Toxicity	Therapy to Consider†
Stimulants (sympathomimetics) • Amphetamines • Methamphetamines • Cocaine • Phencyclidine (PCP) • Ephedrine	• Tachycardia • Supraventricular arrhythmias • Ventricular arrhythmias • Impaired conduction • Hypertensive crises • Acute coronary syndromes • Shock • Cardiac arrest	• Benzodiazepines • Lidocaine • Sodium bicarbonate • Nitroglycerin • Nitroprusside • Reperfusion strategy based on cardiac catheterization data • Phentolamine (α-adrenergic blocker) • No β-blockers
Calcium channel blockers • Verapamil • Nifedipine (and other dihydro-pyridines) • Diltiazem	• Bradycardia • Impaired conduction • Shock • Cardiac arrest	• NS boluses (0.5 to 1 L) • Epinephrine IV; or other α/β agonists • Pacemakers • Circulatory assist devices? • Calcium infusions? • Glucose/insulin infusion? • Glucagon?
β-Adrenergic receptor antagonists • Propranolol • Atenolol • Sotolol	• Bradycardia • Impaired conduction • Shock • Cardiac arrest	• NS boluses (0.5 to 1 L) • Epinephrine IV; or other α/β agonists • Pacemakers • Circulatory assist devices? • Calcium infusions? • Glucose/insulin infusion? • Glucagon?
Tricyclic antidepressants • Amitriptyline • Desipramine • Nortriptyline	• Tachycardia • Bradycardia • Ventricular arrhythmias • Impaired conduction • Shock • Cardiac arrest	• Sodium bicarbonate • Hyperventilation • NS boluses (0.5 to 1 L) • Magnesium sulfate • Lidocaine • Epinephrine IV; or other α/β agonists
Cardiac glycosides • Digoxin • Digitoxin • Foxglove • Oleander	• Bradycardia • Supraventricular arrhythmias • Ventricular arrhythmias • Impaired conduction • Shock • Cardiac arrest	• Restore total body K^+, Mg^{++} • Restore intravascular volume • Digoxin-specific antibodies (Fab fragments: *Digibind* or *DigiFab*) • Atropine • Pacemakers (use caution and monitor for ventricular arrhythmias) • Lidocaine • Phenytoin?

Potentially Toxic Drugs: by Type of Agent	Cardiopulmonary Signs* of Toxicity	Therapy to Consider†
Anticholinergics • Diphenhydramine • Doxylamine	• Tachycardia • Supraventricular arrhythmias • Ventricular arrhythmias • Impaired conduction • Shock, cardiac arrest	• Physostigmine
Cholinergics • Carbamates • Nerve agents • Organophosphates	• Bradycardia • Ventricular arrhythmias • Impaired conduction, shock • Pulmonary edema • Bronchospasm • Cardiac arrest	• Atropine • Decontamination • Pralidoxime • Obidoxime
Opioids • Heroin • Fentanyl • Methadone	• Hypoventilation (slow and shallow respirations, apnea) • Bradycardia • Hypotension • Miosis (pupil constriction)	• Naloxone • Assisted ventilation • Tracheal intubation • Nalmefene
Isoniazid	• Lactic acidosis with/without seizures • Tachycardia or bradycardia • Shock, cardiac arrest	• Pyridoxine (vitamin B_6)
Sodium channel blockers (Class I$_{VW}$ antiarrhythmics) • Procainamide • Disopyramide • Lidocaine • Propafenone • Flecainide	• Bradycardia • Ventricular arrhythmias • Impaired conduction • Seizures • Shock, cardiac arrest	• Sodium bicarbonate • Pacemakers • α- and β-agonist • Lidocaine • Hypertonic saline

- Sudden decompensation to profound shock within minutes[41-44]

- Cardiac arrest due to refractory heart block or PEA

- β-Blocker overdose may also cause a variety of arrhythmias, including torsades de pointes, ventricular fibrillation, heart block, and in rare cases, asystole

Time Course

Signs and symptoms of overdose from either group of agents typically develop within 2 to 4 hours of ingestion of regular release preparations.[41,42] Failure to develop symptomatology within 4 to 6 hours of regular release ingestion indicates that moderate to severe toxicity is unlikely to occur. Toxic effects of controlled release and long-acting preparations, however, may not be seen for up to 6 to 18 hours after ingestion.[41]

Common Therapy for Calcium Channel and β-Blocker Overdoses

The optimal therapy for calcium channel and β-blocker overdoses has not been clearly defined. Evaluations of all available therapies have reported variable results. Initial therapies recommended by consensus include the following:

- Administer oxygen and monitor airway and ventilation (particularly if level of consciousness is depressed or seizures develop).

- Provide continuous ECG monitoring and be prepared to treat symptomatic or unstable arrhythmias.

- Perform careful assessment of blood pressure and hemodynamic status.

- Establish vascular access with 2 large-bore catheters.

- If hypotension is present, give a fluid challenge of 500 to 1000 mL of normal saline.[43,44] Monitor closely for signs of myocardial dysfunction and development of pulmonary edema.

- Determine the blood glucose with a bedside rapid test.

- Consider activated charcoal for gastric decontamination in patients who are awake, alert, and present within 1 hour of the ingestion with only mild hemodynamic effects.[46,47]

- Perform rapid sequence intubation followed by gastric lavage in patients who present within 1 hour of the ingestion and have moderate to severe hemodynamic toxicity.

- Perform whole bowel irrigation when toxic quantities of time-released preparations have been consumed, medications are seen on the abdominal X-ray, and only if bowel sounds are still present.[46]

- Do not give syrup of ipecac. Ipecac has delayed onset and a propensity to worsen bradycardia through vomiting-induced increases in vagal tone. In addition, calcium blockers and β-blockers can cause rapid declines in hemodynamic stability, altered mental status, and seizures before ipecac can take effect.[48]

Specific Therapy for Calcium Channel Blocker Overdose

- Establish vascular access and treat myocardial dysfunction and hypotension:

  — Start with a *normal saline* fluid challenge, 1 to 2 boluses, 500 to 1000 mL each. Monitor for development of pulmonary edema. If hemodynamically significant signs and symptoms continue, add:

  — *Epinephrine* infusion 2 to 100 μg/min or another catecholamine-like vasopressor (*norepinephrine*). Catecholamine-type vasopressors are the first-line drug therapy for hemodynamically significant **hypotension** or **shock** due to calcium channel blocker toxicity.[49,50]

  — Consider *calcium chloride* 8 to 16 mg/kg (usually 5 to 10 mL or 0.5 to 1 g of a 10% solution from

10 mL vials with 100 mg/mL) if the shock fails to respond adequately to the fluid challenges and the epinephrine or norepinephrine infusion. Because the effectiveness of this approach has varied greatly in case reports, it has a Class of Recommendation of only IIb (level of evidence 5).[41,43,45,51,52]

  - Additional IV calcium (slow IV push or continued infusion) to a total dose of 1 to 3 g IV is appropriate for patients who experience a positive hemodynamic response to the initial calcium infusion.

  - Only limited supportive data exists for the use of calcium infusions in other types of drug-induced shock (Class Indeterminate; level of evidence 6).[41,43,45,51,52]

  - Epinephrine and other α_1-agonists may sensitize the vasculature to the effects of calcium.[53]

- *Treat refractory hemodynamically significant* **bradycardia** due to calcium channel blocker toxicity with *pacing* (either transvenous or transcutaneous).

- Additional therapies to consider:

  — *Circulatory assist devices,* such as the intra-aortic balloon pump, or extracorporeal membrane oxygenation (ECMO)[54] should be considered for patients refractory to *maximal* medical therapy. Such support can maintain viability until the drug effects diminish below a lethal level, particularly for young, otherwise healthy persons.[55-57]

  — *Glucose/insulin infusions:* Infusions of glucose and insulin have been used in treatment of calcium channel blocker overdose. Although this intervention is supported by animal studies[58,59] and limited cases series,[60,61] there is insufficient evidence (level of evidence 5 and 6) at this time to merit more than a *Class Indeterminate* recommendation.

  — *Glucagon:* Myocardial toxicity due to calcium channel blockers has

responded to glucagon in some animal studies[62] and in case reports.[63,64] It is acceptable to use glucagon (1 to 5 mg IV), but this is a *Class Indeterminate* recommendation.

Specific Therapy for β-Blocker Overdose

- Establish vascular access and treat myocardial dysfunction and hypotension:

  — Start with *normal saline* fluid challenges, 1 to 2 boluses 500 to 1000 mL.

  — *Vasopressors:* If hemodynamically significant hypotension is present, treat with a vasopressor with moderate to high α-adrenergic activity, such as *epinephrine,*[44] infused at 2 to 10 μg/min. In case reports and series,[27,28,65,66] norepinephrine, dobutamine, isoproterenol, and dopamine have been associated with success.

  — *Glucagon:* Glucagon is an inotropic agent that stimulates cyclic AMP in cardiac tissue via non-α, non-β receptors. In animal models[62] and some human case reports,[44] glucagon showed promise as a valuable agent in *mild-to-moderate* β-blocker–induced shock. In reports of patients with more severe shock, however, consistent efficacy data is lacking. It is acceptable to use glucagon in mild-to-moderate shock for patients unresponsive to vasopressors (1 to 5 mg IV). Note that glucagon, like most inotropes, can further reduce systemic vascular resistance, often requiring vasopressor adjuncts.[67]

  — *Isoproterenol:* Isoproterenol can be used carefully as an adjunct with an epinephrine infusion or in combination with other agents, though significant improvement is rare.[27,28,65,66] Do not use isoproterenol as a first-line agent.

  — *Calcium:* Calcium infusions (8 to 16 mg/kg, usually 5 to 10 mL or 0.5 to 1 g of a 10% solution from 10 mL vials with 100 mg/mL) may be of benefit in β-blocker–induced shock that is unresponsive to glucagon and epinephrine. Calcium, however, cannot be recommended specifically because of currently limited animal data[68] and conflicting clinical case reports.[66,69]

— *Treatment of refractory, hemodynamically significant bradycardia:* If hemodynamically significant bradycardia is present, add pacing (either transvenous or transcutaneous).[70]

■ *Additional therapies to consider:*

— *Atropine:* While not harmful, atropine is rarely effective in β-blocker–induced bradycardia or in reversing symptomatic heart block.

— *Circulatory assist devices:* As with calcium channel blocker overdose, circulatory assist devices[54] or extracorporeal circulation[71] may be effective for drug-induced shock that fails to respond to maximal medical therapy. This approach, however, must be started before irreversible end organ damage has occurred.

— *Glucose/insulin infusion:* Some success has been reported with glucose/insulin infusion in treatment of shock caused by β-blocker overdose.[72] This therapy may produce hypokalemia unless potassium is monitored with supplementation provided. The use of glucose and insulin for β-blocker toxicity remains a *Class Indeterminate* recommendation.

Cocaine Toxicity

Overview

Millions of people in the United States use cocaine. They inhale nasally or inject intravenously the crystalline form of the drug[73] or smoke the freebase form of the drug, commonly known as "crack."[74] Although arrhythmias and cardiac arrest from cocaine are relatively uncommon, cocaine use of any type by any route can cause disastrous complications.[73-81]

Cocaine Toxicity

Cocaine first stimulates the release and then blocks the reuptake of norepinephrine, epinephrine, dopamine, and serotonin[73,77] (see Figure 1). Cocaine abusers experience an elevation in blood pressure, tachycardia, and feelings of euphoria coupled with decreased fatigue. Cocaine toxicity is dose dependent. Nonetheless numerous seizures, myocardial infarctions, and deaths have occurred in both new and long-term users who have taken only small quantities of the drug.[73,76,82]

Cardiac Toxicity

Serious cocaine-induced cardiac toxicity stems from the direct effect of cocaine on the heart. Cocaine also provokes the central nervous system to stimulate the cardiovascular system.[83-87] The β-adrenergic effects of cocaine increase heart rate and myocardial contractility.[83,85] The α-adrenergic effects of cocaine decrease coronary blood flow and may induce coronary artery spasm.[35,36,85,86] Cocaine increases platelet adhesiveness, leading to increased risk of coronary thrombosis.[88] These mechanisms lead to decreased coronary artery perfusion at a time of increased myocardial oxygen demand. Hypoxia from pulmonary edema and acidosis from cocaine-induced seizures may exacerbate the cardiotoxicity of cocaine.[75,81,84]

Cocaine toxicity may cause thermoregulatory problems, including hyperpyrexia. A rise in the patient's body temperature can worsen existing tachycardia and neurologic symptoms. High ambient temperatures have also been associated with a significant increase in mortality in patients with cocaine toxicity.[14,89,90]

Treatment of Cocaine-Induced Arrhythmias

All patients with cocaine-induced central nervous system symptoms or cardiovascular complications require close observation. Treat fever and cool patients presenting with agitation, delirium, seizures, and elevated body temperature. If an arrhythmia or ACS is present, administer oxygen and provide continuous ECG monitoring.

FIGURE 1. Mechanism of cocaine toxicity. Reprinted with permission from *The New England Journal of Medicine.* 2001;345:351-358. Copyright 2001 Massachusetts Medical Society. All rights reserved.[14] Published correction appears in *N Engl J Med.* 2001;345:1432.

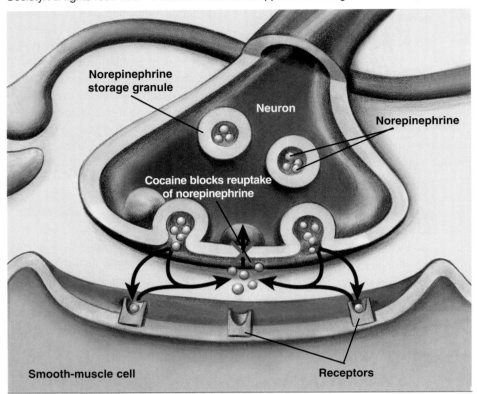

Norepinephrine storage granule

Neuron

Norepinephrine

Cocaine blocks reuptake of norepinephrine

Smooth-muscle cell

Receptors

Cocaine-Induced Supraventricular Arrhythmias

Cocaine-induced supraventricular arrhythmias include paroxysmal supraventricular tachycardia, rapid atrial fibrillation, and atrial flutter.[80] These arrhythmias are often short lived and seldom require therapy unless hemodynamic compromise is also present.[24,91,92]

Benzodiazepine. Treat persistent supraventricular arrhythmias in hemodynamically stable patients with a benzodiazepine, such as *diazepam* in a dose of 5 to 20 mg IV over 5 to 20 minutes. Benzodiazepines modulate the stimulatory effects of cocaine on the central nervous and cardiovascular systems, blunting the patient's hypersympathetic state.[93-95]

Cocaine-Induced Stable Ventricular Tachycardia

Nonarrest ventricular arrhythmias due to cocaine include ventricular ectopy, episodes of nonsustained ventricular tachycardia, and stable monomorphic and polymorphic VT.[84,85,96]

Benzodiazepine. Like supraventricular arrhythmias, ventricular ectopy and tachycardia are often transient and may require only careful observation. Most experienced clinicians will administer *benzodiazepine* in a titrated fashion (eg, *diazepam* 5 to 20 mg IV over 5 to 20 minutes).

Lidocaine. Many experts recommend lidocaine at the standard dose of 1 to 1.5 mg/kg for treatment of ventricular arrhythmias unresponsive to a titrated benzodiazepine. Cocaine, long-established as a legitimate anesthetic agent, has properties of a sodium channel blocker (Class I_{VW} antiarrhythmic). Lidocaine, acting as a similar sodium channel blocker (Class I_{VW} antiarrhythmic) competes with cocaine at the sodium channel, thus decreasing cocaine's effects. The decision to use lidocaine must be carefully weighed against the increased risk of seizure due to the synergistic toxic effects of lidocaine in the presence of cocaine.[94,97]

Sodium bicarbonate. There are experimental animal studies[17,98] and some human case reports[18,99] that support the use of sodium bicarbonate (1 to 2 mEq/kg) in the treatment of cocaine-induced ventricular fibrillation and ventricular tachycardia.[100] Most toxicologists agree that sodium bicarbonate should be used early in the management of ventricular tachycardias resulting from the use of cocaine.[14,100,101]

Defibrillation. As a precaution, have a defibrillator available at the bedside. Adhesive defibrillator pads can be pre-attached, and cardiac monitoring can be performed by conventional defibrillator/ monitors.

Cocaine-Induced Ventricular Fibrillation

Primary and Secondary ABCD Surveys

CPR and defibrillation. The steps of the Primary and Secondary ABCD Surveys apply to cocaine-induced VF arrest. These steps include CPR, up to 3 shocks, airway control, and IV access.

Epinephrine. The initial medication given after 3 unsuccessful shocks for VF arrest that is not associated with cocaine toxicity is an adrenergic agent, either *epinephrine* or *vasopressin.* Most experts agree that epinephrine is an appropriate vasoconstrictor to give in cocaine-induced VF arrest, even though the similar cardiovascular effects would argue otherwise. Little evidence exists to confirm either benefit or harm from an initial epinephrine dose of 1 mg. Clinicians should, however, increase the interval between subsequent doses of epinephrine to every 5 to 10 minutes and avoid high-dose epinephrine (>1 mg per dose) in patients with refractory VF.

Vasopressin. The *ECC Guidelines 2000* experts added *vasopressin* 40 U IV push × 1 as an acceptable alternative to epinephrine for VF arrest. Extrapolation from pharmacologic principles suggests that vasopressin should offer considerable advantages over epinephrine for refractory, cocaine-induced VF arrest. Because of the current absence of data, this recommendation is a *Class Indeterminate* recommendation.

For shock-refractory VF, give a lidocaine bolus of 1 to 1.5 mg/kg, and then reattempt defibrillation. Clinical evidence about the effect of lidocaine in cocaine toxicity is limited. The *ECC Guidelines 2000* experts added *amiodarone* as an acceptable alternative to lidocaine for conventional management of shock-refractory VF. Whether this amiodarone recommendation applies to cocaine-induced persistent VF is unknown. In the absence of relevant data, omit amiodarone.

Sodium bicarbonate. The evidence that supports the use of sodium bicarbonate (1 to 2 mEq/kg) in the treatment of cocaine-induced, stable ventricular tachycardia applies to cardiac arrest associated with ventricular fibrillation.[17,18,98,99] Give a first bolus of sodium bicarbonate after establishment of IV access and administration of epinephrine and lidocaine.[14,100,101]

Summary: Treatment of Cocaine-Induced Arrhythmias

General Treatment

- Administer oxygen.
- Correct elevated body temperature.
- Perform continuous ECG monitoring.
- Monitor neurologic status.

Supraventricular Arrhythmias Requiring Therapy

- *Diazepam* 5 mg IV, escalating as needed to 20 mg

Hemodynamically Stable Ventricular Tachycardia

- *Diazepam* 5 mg IV, escalating as needed to 20 mg
- If persistent, *lidocaine* 1 to 1.5 mg/kg IV
- Followed by *sodium bicarbonate* 1 to 2 mEq/kg IV

Ventricular Fibrillation

Ventricular fibrillation should initially be treated in standard fashion:

- *Attempt defibrillation with up to 3 shocks of 200 J, 200 to 300 J, 360 J or equivalent biphasic dose.*

- If VF persists, follow with *epinephrine* 1 mg IV, limited to a single dose or repeated in 5 to 10 minutes, or vasopressin 40 U IV push × 1.

- If VF persists, follow with *lidocaine* 1 to 1.5 mg/kg IV bolus.

- If VF persists, follow with *sodium bicarbonate* 1 to 2 mEq/kg IV.

Treatment of Cocaine-Induced Hypertension and Pulmonary Edema

Cocaine-Induced Hypertension

Cocaine toxicity can produce hypertensive emergencies through effects on the central nervous system and peripheral α-agonist stimulation.[73,77,84]

Benzodiazepine. Hypertensive patients should initially be treated with a benzodiazepine in an attempt to minimize the stimulatory effects of cocaine on the central nervous and cardiovascular systems.[87,94,95]

Nitroglycerin or nitroprusside. Patients who require additional therapy should be treated with a vasodilator such as nitroglycerin or nitroprusside in a titrated dose. Nitroglycerin is preferable in patients with superimposed chest pain.

Precautions

Do not use β-blocking agents such as *propranolol* or *esmolol*.[23,39] Both have the potential to raise blood pressure by antagonizing cocaine-induced β-receptor stimulation and allowing unopposed cocaine-induced α-receptor stimulation. Labetalol, with both α-blocker and β-blocker effects, has shown inferior results compared with *nitroglycerin* or *nitroprusside* and should be avoided.[37,102] A pure α-blocker such as phentolamine (1 mg every 2 to 3 minutes; up to 10 mg) may be used, although it too is not well studied for treatment of cocaine toxicity.[103]

Cocaine-Induced Pulmonary Edema

The effects of cocaine on pulmonary dynamics may result in pulmonary edema. Pulmonary edema may also occur secondary to a subarachnoid hemorrhage, from a cocaine-induced myocardial infarction, or as a consequence of additional drugs of abuse such as heroin.[75,81,104,105] Most patients respond to standard medical management. *Positive-pressure ventilation* with a continuous positive airway pressure (CPAP) mask or intubation supplemented by positive end-expiratory pressure (PEEP) will usually rapidly correct hypoxemia.

Treatment of Cocaine-Induced Chest Pain and ACS

See "FYI: Cardiovascular Complications of Cocaine Use" for a detailed discussion of this topic.

Cocaine-Induced Chest Pain

Chest pain is one of the most common complaints of cocaine users.[24,91,92] The vast majority of patients have only transient chest pain with no evidence of acute ischemia on their ECG. Clinicians should be aware that abnormal but nondiagnostic ECGs are common in young adults who use cocaine.[106]

Cocaine-Induced ACS

Although rare, acute myocardial infarctions (AMIs) do occur in cocaine users.[79,82,107,108] Most cocaine-related infarctions occur in patients who smoke cigarettes or who have other cardiac risk factors,[79,82,107] although some infarctions occur in active, healthy patients with no risk factors for ischemic heart disease.[79,107-109]

Cocaine-related myocardial ischemia should be treated with *oxygen, aspirin, nitrates,* and a titrated dose of a *benzodiazepine*.[33,95] β-Blockers should *not* be used because of the possibility of α-mediated vasospasm.[36] Because of its antispasm effects and its beneficial role in myocardial infarction, *magnesium* can also be used for cocaine-related ischemia and infarction.[110-112] *Morphine* should be administered for continued pain.

Fibrinolytic and Anticoagulant Therapy

Fibrinolytic therapy in conjunction with heparin has the potential to restore relatively normal coronary arterial flow to these predominantly young, previously healthy patients.[107] But use of fibrinolytics

FYI: Cardiovascular Complications of Cocaine Use

Cardiovascular Toxicity

Cocaine causes myocardial ischemia through complex pathophysiologic mechanisms.[14] Acutely cocaine results in coronary artery vasoconstriction, tachycardia, systemic arterial hypertension, increased myocardial oxygen demand, platelet aggregation, and in situ thrombus formation. In long-term cocaine users, atherosclerosis and left ventricular hypertrophy develop at an accelerated pace. These conditions can further exacerbate the oxygen supply-demand mismatch. Myocardial ischemia and infarction may occur in patients with or without underlying atherosclerotic disease.[113]

Cocaine-Associated ACS

The interval associated with highest risk of myocardial ischemia and infarction after cocaine use has not been established. The risk of myocardial infarction is increased 24-fold in the first hour after cocaine use.[114] Most cocaine-associated myocardial infarctions occur within 24 hours of cocaine use,[107] although spontaneous episodes of ST-segment elevation have been documented on ambulatory monitoring for up to 6 weeks after last use of cocaine.[115]

Evidence-Based Treatment?

The treatment of cocaine-associated ACS is methodologically difficult to study in randomized, controlled clinical trials. High quality, prospective, multicenter cohort evaluations have provided valuable information.[116,117] Most consensus recommendations, however, are supported by evidence of the following levels: level 5 (case series); level 7 (reasonable extrapolations from existing data), and level 8 (common sense, face validity, no evidence of harm).[118] The basis for most current recommendations comes from a knowledge of

successful therapies in patients with ACS unrelated to cocaine, animal investigations, and human volunteer studies, plus extrapolations from the known pathophysiologic mechanisms of cocaine-associated ACS.[14]

Treatment Differences: Cocaine-Related vs Cocaine-Unrelated ACS

Benzodiazepines. Benzodiazepines are recommended for patients with cocaine-associated ACS even though these agents are not routinely used in patients with ACS unrelated to cocaine.[7,14,91,119] In cocaine-induced ACS, benzodiazepines decrease central nervous system excitation and have a salutary effect on the centrally stimulated cardiovascular consequences of cocaine.[14]

β-Blockers. Despite the success of β-blockers in AMI unrelated to cocaine, they are contraindicated for cocaine-associated ACS (see next page).[36,39,120]

Fibrinolytics. Fibrinolytic therapy is standard for patients with AMI unrelated to cocaine. But these agents should be used with caution in patients with cocaine-associated AMI. There has been no demonstrated efficacy in this patient population.[121] Fibrinolytic agents have different risk-benefit profiles for patients with cocaine-related AMI than those reported in patients with AMI unrelated to cocaine.[121]

Emergency Treatment of Cocaine-Induced ACS

Emergency treatment of patients with cocaine-associated myocardial ischemia targets the acute pathophysiologic effects of the process. Attempts to reduce or reverse the coronary vasoconstriction, hypertension, tachycardia, and predisposition to thrombus formation are the mainstays of treatment. The objective is to improve coronary artery perfusion and oxygen delivery while reducing myocardial oxygen demand.

Benzodiazepines

Benzodiazepines protect the central nervous system while decreasing sympathetic outflow. Multiple animal experiments, widespread anecdotal experience, and one randomized controlled trial in humans support *diazepam* as the initial agent for treating all cocaine-intoxicated patients.[91,122-124] Benzodiazepines decrease sympathetic outflow, calming the patient and returning vital signs to the normal range. Additional direct effects on peripheral benzodiazepine receptors may counteract the vasoconstrictive properties of cocaine and its metabolite benzoylecgonine. One human randomized, controlled trial showed that diazepam had the same effect as nitroglycerin on chest pain resolution and cardiac performance.[124]

Nitroglycerin

Specific anti-ischemic therapy begins with *nitroglycerin*. Neither reduction in infarct size nor mortality benefit has been assessed following nitroglycerin in patients with cocaine-associated ACS. The *Class Indeterminate* recommendation for nitrates is based on experimental reversal of coronary vasoconstriction in humans and clinical relief of chest pain.[32,33,124]

Antiplatelet and Antithrombotic Agents

Attempts to decrease the acute coagulability of blood with *aspirin* or *heparin* are recommended with some support from clinical reports specific to cocaine users[88] (Class Indeterminate). The current understanding of the pharmacology of the agents suggests some value, as does the extensive clinical experience with ACS unrelated to cocaine.

Management of Refractory ACS

Patients with ischemia refractory to the above measures can be treated with either *phentolamine, calcium antagonists*, or *reperfusion therapy*, depending on the clinical circumstances.[7]

Phentolamine

Phentolamine blocks the α-adrenergic effects of cocaine and reverses the coronary vasoconstrictive effects of cocaine.[35] One case report showed efficacy in a patient with cocaine-associated chest pain.[103] Because phentolamine may result in hypotension, use of small incremental doses (1 mg every 2 to 3 minutes) is recommended.

Calcium Antagonists

Calcium channel blockers. Calcium channel blockers do not have a clear role to play in patients with cocaine-induced vascular ischemia.

The evidence. Data on the efficacy of calcium antagonists for the treatment of cocaine toxicity are contradictory.

- In a human cardiac catheterization model of cocaine toxicity, verapamil successfully reversed cocaine-induced coronary artery vasoconstriction.[125]

- In multicenter clinical trials in patients with ACS *not* associated with cocaine toxicity, researchers have found no benefit from calcium channel blockers on important outcomes such as survival.

- In studies of cocaine-poisoned animals pretreated with calcium channel blockers, investigators have observed favorable results for a variety of endpoints, such as better survival, fewer seizures, and fewer cardiac arrhythmias.[126-128] But in other studies investigators have found adverse effects.[129] Note that the positive results were reported only in animals that were *pre*-treated with calcium channel blockers. If the cocaine-poisoned animals were not pretreated with calcium channel blockers, *later* administration of calcium channel blockers showed no benefit.[129-131]

Fibrinolytic Agents: Continued Debate

In acute myocardial injury associated with cocaine toxicity, experts continue to debate the precise role to be played by fibrinolytic agents.[14,40,85,107,109,114,121,132] Opponents raise these concerns:

- AMI associated with cocaine use has a low mortality rate. ST-segment elevation as a "diagnostic test" for acute myocardial injury has a high false-positive rate in cocaine users. These patients can meet TIMI criteria for fibrinolytic therapy even though they are not having an AMI.[40,121,132]

Clinicians should reserve fibrinolytics for the following patients with cocaine toxicity:

- Patients with AMI confirmed by diagnostic changes in cardiac markers and ECGs

- Patients with presumed AMI for whom percutaneous interventions (angioplasty or stent placement) are unavailable

- Patients unresponsive to vasodilator therapy

- Patients with a low risk for cerebrovascular bleeding

- Patients with a low risk for the hemorrhagic complications of fibrinolytic agents

β-Adrenergic Antagonists (β-Blockers): Class III

Despite the success of β-blockers in patients with AMI unrelated to cocaine, β-blockers are contraindicated in recent cocaine users.[7] *Clinicians should not administer β-blockers or mixed α-/β-blockers such as labetalol to patients who have recently used cocaine.*

The Evidence

- β-Blockers increase central nervous system toxicity and exacerbate coronary artery vasospasm in animal models of cocaine toxicity.[122,123,133]

- Human case series show that β-blockers do not reverse the hypertensive and tachycardic effects of cocaine.[39]

- Studies in human volunteers show that β-blockers exacerbate cocaine-induced coronary artery vasoconstriction.[36,133]

- Scientific agreement has not been established on the role, if any, of either pure β- or mixed α-/β-blockers in the treatment of cocaine intoxication. *Labetalol*, a mixed α-/β-antagonist, has attracted considerable attention from toxicologists. Labetalol does not appear to offer any advantages over pure β-antagonists even though it produced no adverse outcomes in some cases[37,38,134] *The evidence does not support the use of labetalol:*

  — It has more β-adrenergic antagonist effects than α-adrenergic antagonist effects.

  — It leads to unopposed α effects with severe hypertension in patients with pheochromocytomas.

  — It increases the risk of seizure and death in animal models of cocaine toxicity.[131]

  — It does not reverse coronary artery vasoconstriction in humans.[34]

must be weighed against the high risk of hemorrhagic complications in patients who have had multiple episodes of uncontrolled hypertension due to "crack" smoking.[75,82] An additional concern is that up to half of all cocaine-related myocardial infarctions appear to be due to spasm, not thrombus.[79,107-109] Indications for fibrinolytic therapy must be reviewed in light of the fact that "false positive" ST-segment changes are common in cocaine users. These variant patterns include early repolarization and QRS complexes with elevated J points.[106] Before starting fibrinolytic therapy some clinicians require a diagnostic echocardiogram or demand evidence of infarction by a rapid assay technique of cardiac markers. These dilemmas have led many experts to recommend urgent cardiac catheterization so that the cardiologist can select the appropriate reperfusion strategy (fibrinolytics versus percutaneous coronary interventions).

Cyclic Antidepressants

Toxicity

When taken in excess the tricyclic antidepressants (TCAs) are among the most cardiotoxic agents in medicine.[135-143] Although TCAs rarely cause cardiovascular side effects when taken in therapeutic amounts, they are the number one cause of death from overdose in patients who arrive at the hospital alive.[111,144]

The toxic side effects of TCAs are due to the interplay of their 4 major pharmacologic properties.[135-141] Tricyclics

- Stimulate catecholamine release and then block reuptake at postganglionic synapses

- Have central and peripheral anticholinergic actions

- Inhibit potassium channels in myocardium and fast (voltage-dependent) sodium channels in brain and myocardium

- Have direct α-blocking actions

Major Signs of Tricyclic Toxicity

As a toxic dose of a tricyclic begins to take effect, the following signs appear:

- Alterations in mental status, including agitation, irritability, confusion, delirium, hallucinations, hyperactivity, seizures, and hyperpyrexia

- Sinus tachycardia (especially in association with a rightward QRS axis)[145]; SVT and hypertension may develop early after ingestion but are usually short lived because catecholamine depletion then develops

- Prolongation of the QT interval[145-148]

- Anticholinergic effects, such as delirium, mydriasis, urinary retention, and gastric atony[137,142,143]

More ominous signs that require immediate therapy are

- Coma

- Seizures

- QRS widening

- Wide-complex arrhythmias

- Ventricular arrhythmias[137-139,142]

- Preterminal sinus bradycardia and heart block

- Hypotension[138,149]

- Acidosis

The signs of significant TCA overdoses may be recalled by the memory aid "Three C's and an A": **C**oma, **C**onvulsions (Seizures), **C**ardiac arrhythmias, and **A**cidosis. Serum levels usually are not readily available and are of little prognostic or therapeutic value in acute overdoses.[142]

Time Course of TCA Toxicity

Most patients will manifest some sign of toxicity within 2 to 4 hours of ingestion. Patients who are asymptomatic after 6 hours of continuous monitoring, with no QT prolongation on the 12-lead ECG,[145,146,148] are at essentially no risk for toxicity.[137,142]

General Management of TCA Overdose

- Gastric decontamination with activated charcoal should be considered for all patients who present with an acute TCA overdose within 1 hour of ingestion.[47]

- Gastric lavage should be considered in all unconscious patients; particularly for patients who present within 1 to 2 hours of ingestion of a life-threatening quantity of a TCA.[46]

- Syrup of ipecac is unnecessary in the hospital care of patients, where superior gastric emptying techniques are readily available.[48]

Bicarbonate for TCA Overdose

Alkalinization With Sodium Bicarbonate

Alkalinization with sodium bicarbonate is the mainstay of therapy for severe TCA overdoses.[137,138,141,142,150-159]

- Alkalinization decreases the free, non-protein-bound form of the tricyclic molecule and overrides the tricyclic-induced sodium channel blockade of phase 0 of the action potential.[142,158,160]

- Alkalinization is not required in patients who have only a mild resting tachycardia or mild prolongation of the QT interval.

- Alkalinization (raising serum pH to 7.50 to 7.55) is indicated for patients with

  — Prolongation of the QRS to greater than 100 ms

  — Ventricular arrhythmias

  — Hypotension unresponsive to a saline bolus of 500 to 1000 mL

Alkalinization for the Unstable Patient With TCA Overdose

- Provide immediate hyperventilation to a pH of 7.50 to 7.55 for patients who present with seizures or inadequate respiratory function.[154]

- Give *sodium bicarbonate* 1 to 2 mEq/kg over 1 to 2 minutes.

- Follow with a *sodium bicarbonate* infusion of 3 ampules (150 mEq) plus KCl (30 mEq) mixed in 850 mL of D_5W, at an initial rate of 150 to 200 mL/h, titrated to keep pH 7.50 to 7.55.

- The initial goal of therapy is to raise the pH to 7.50 to 7.55 and to maintain that pH with confirmation by measurement of venous and arterial pH on a regular basis.

- Continue to infuse sodium bicarbonate until the patient's condition stabilizes (ie, QRS shortens to <100 ms, arrhythmias stop, and blood pressure returns to normal range).

Magnesium for TCA Overdose

Some patients may develop arrhythmias due to tricyclic actions on phase 2 of the action potential.[140,141,161]

- The phase 2 effects are initially manifest by a prolongation of the QT interval. But they may result in the torsades de pointes variant of VT.[21,161-165]

- Magnesium sulfate is the drug of choice for this select group of patients.[21,162,163,165]

- The dose of magnesium is 1 to 2 g diluted in 10 mL D_5W IV push in unstable patients (a total of 5 to 10 g IV may be used). Give this dose more slowly (over 1 to 5 minutes) in hemodynamically stable patients.[21,162,164]

TCA-Induced Cardiac Arrest

TCA overdose usually causes profound myocardial depression. When cardiac arrest develops, it is often associated with pulseless electrical activity.[138,142,158,166] The following recommendations apply to the treatment of TCA-induced cardiac arrest:

- Initiate the *Primary and Secondary ABCD Surveys.*

- Start *hyperventilation* as soon as advanced control of the airway is achieved.

- Administer *normal saline* at 1000 mL/h when IV access is obtained.

- Slow push *sodium bicarbonate* 1 to 2 mEq/kg over 1 to 2 minutes.

- Follow with a *sodium bicarbonate* infusion of 3 ampules (150 mEq) with 30 mEq KCl mixed in 850 mL D_5W at 150 to 200 mL/h.

- Add epinephrine 1 mg IV every 3 to 5 minutes if the patient does not respond to alkalinization and the saline infusion.

- Load with lidocaine 1 to 1.5 mg/kg; follow with a maintenance infusion of 1 to 4 mg/min. Nonresponders at this point should be treated with magnesium sulfate 1 to 2 g diluted in 10 mL D_5W IV push.[164] Procainamide should *not* be used in TCA-induced arrhythmias because of its tricyclic-like pharmacologic properties.[140,141]

The protocol for treating VF due to TCA overdose requires some modification of the standard ACLS Algorithm:

- Attempt defibrillation with up to 3 shocks in the standard fashion.

- Intubate, oxygenate, give epinephrine 1 mg or vasopressin (40 U IV × 1), and immediately attempt defibrillation at 360 J or equivalent biphasic energy dose.

- Rapidly alkalinize the patient by administering sodium bicarbonate 1 to 2 mEq/kg IV push. If bicarbonate is not readily available, perform hyperventilation to create respiratory alkalosis.

TCA-Induced Seizures and Hypotension

Seizures due to TCA overdose should be terminated immediately with benzodiazepines. Uncontrolled seizure activity results in hypoxia, acidosis, tachycardia, hypotension, and electrolyte fluxes. These responses increase morbidity and mortality from TCA overdose.[138,142,167]

- Hypotension usually responds to infusions of 500 to 1000 mL of normal saline.

- Alkalinization with sodium bicarbonate is recommended for nonresponders.

- Patients with refractory hypotension may be treated with dopamine or norepinephrine.[168-171]

Digitalis Overdose and Cardiac Toxicity

Digitalis-induced cardiac toxicity may develop in long-term users of this widely prescribed medication. It may also be due to an acute overdose in a previously healthy patient.

Signs and Symptoms of Digitalis Toxicity

Many of the early symptoms of digitalis intoxication are nonspecific signs of central nervous system and gastrointestinal toxicity. Fatigue, visual symptoms, weakness, nausea, vomiting, and abdominal pain are common.[172,173] Cardiac arrhythmias occur in the vast majority of patients with digitalis toxicity. The most common arrhythmias are ventricular ectopy and bradycardia, often in association with various degrees of heart block.[172,173] Some rhythm disturbances should immediately suggest digitalis intoxication. These disturbances include atrial tachycardia with high-degree AV block, nonparoxysmal accelerated junctional tachycardia, multifocal VT, new onset bigeminy, and regularized atrial fibrillation.[174]

Cardiac Toxicity of Digitalis

The cardiac toxicity of digitalis is due to the combination of its inhibitory effects on nodal conduction and its excitatory effects on individual atrial and ventricular fibers.[172,173] Life-threatening digitalis toxicity most often is due to

- Bradyarrhythmias with resultant congestive heart failure

- Malignant ventricular arrhythmias

- Hyperkalemia resulting from digitalis poisoning of the sodium-potassium adenosine triphosphatase pump[175-177]

General Approach to Treating Digitalis Toxicity

The treatment of arrhythmias due to digitalis toxicity is determined by the acuity of the overdose (ie, whether the overdose results from chronic therapy or acute ingestion) and the patient's hemodynamic function.

Management of Digitalis Toxicity Associated With Chronic Therapy

Digitalis intoxication in long-term users generally develops in association with hypokalemia, hypomagnesemia, dehydration, declining renal function, or loss of muscle mass.[173,178] Patients who take non–potassium-sparing diuretics are especially prone to developing toxicity. Cardiotoxicity in these patients is initially treated by

- Replenishing total body potassium

■ Replenishing total body magnesium stores[172]

■ Replacing volume with normal saline

If the patient with digitalis toxicity is hypokalemic, assume that he/she is also hypomagnesemic until proven otherwise.[179] The 3 modalities of rapid replacement of potassium, magnesium, and volume will usually correct most arrhythmias in long-term digitalis users within a few hours. For severe toxicity, consider use of digoxin-specific antibody (Fab fragments—see below).

General Management of Acute Digitalis Overdose

Gastric decontamination with activated charcoal. Emergency physicians should consider decontamination with activated charcoal in all patients with an acute digitalis overdose who present within 1 hour of ingestion.[46,47] Syrup of ipecac is not useful in the hospital care of patients with digitalis overdose; other gastric emptying techniques are available.[48]

Life-threatening digitalis overdose. In all *unconscious* patients perform rapid sequence intubation in preparation for orogastric lavage or administration of activated charcoal, or both. Some experts recommend gastric lavage for any patient seen within 1 to 2 hours of overdose with a life-threatening amount of digoxin, whether the patient is conscious or unconscious.[46] Exercise caution if gastric lavage is selected, because it may induce a vagal response that can cause or exacerbate digitalis toxicity. Many experts recommend administration of 0.5 mg of atropine before gastric lavage to blunt this vagal response.

General Management Precautions

Patients with digitalis toxicity are more prone to pacemaker-induced ventricular rhythm disturbances. Use of transvenous pacemakers should be highly selective.[168]

When arrhythmias develop, perform cardioversion or defibrillation when indicated. However, patients with digitalis toxicity may develop malignant ventricular arrhythmias or asystole after cardioversion. For

this reason, a lower initial cardioversion dose is used (see "Synchronized Cardioversion," below).

Patients with digitalis toxicity develop high levels of intracellular calcium, so do not administer additional calcium salts to these patients.[180] Hypokalemia and hypomagnesemia are risk factors for developing digitalis toxicity, although hyperkalemia may be present with acute severe toxicity (see below).

Management of Digitalis-Induced Symptomatic Bradycardias

Atropine. Patients with symptomatic bradycardia and heart block should initially receive atropine in doses starting at 0.5 mg IV. Because of the vagally mediated effects of digitalis, atropine may temporarily reverse digitalis intoxication.[172,181]

Digoxin-Specific Fab Fragment Therapy

The availability of digoxin-specific antibodies (Fab fragments) to treat severe chronic and acute toxicity has dramatically reduced morbidity and mortality from digitalis intoxication.[175,176,182,183] Fab fragments bind to free digoxin, resulting in an inactive compound that is excreted in the urine. Use of Fab fragments results in lower levels of free serum digoxin; this concentration gradient pulls free digoxin from myocardial tissue. Effects begin in minutes; complete reversal of digitalis-mediated effects most often occurs within 30 minutes of administration.[182] The high cost per vial of Fab fragment therapy must be weighed against the decreased need

for prolonged and expensive intensive care therapy.

Dosing of Fab Fragments

The specific dose of Fab fragments is determined by the patient's weight and serum digoxin level (if known) or in the case of acute toxicity, by the estimated milligrams ingested. Each 40-mg vial of Fab fragments binds 0.6 mg of digoxin (Table 3). Serum digoxin levels rise dramatically after Fab fragment therapy; thus the serum digoxin level should not be used to guide continuing therapy.[175,176]

In general, 3 to 5 vials are effective in patients with chronic intoxication. Hemodynamically significant bradyarrhythmias and life-threatening heart block in acute overdose require much greater quantities of Fab fragments. Use the dosing nomogram to determine the correct dose of antibody. Massive overdoses may require as many as 20 vials. There is no evidence to support attempts to totally correct elevated digoxin levels (ie, return the patient to a therapeutic level). Case reports suggest that this practice is frequently associated with undesirable outcomes.

Indications for Fab Fragment Therapy

The indications for Fab fragment therapy are digoxin toxicity in association with

■ Life-threatening arrhythmias refractory to conventional therapy

■ Shock or fulminant congestive heart failure

■ Hyperkalemia (K^+ >5 mEq/L)

TABLE 3. Adult Dose Estimate of Digibind (Fab Fragments in Number of Vials) From Steady-State Serum Digoxin Concentration

Patient Weight (kg)	Serum Digoxin Concentration (ng/mL) (Vials)						
	1	2	4	8	12	16	20
40	0.5	1	2	3	5	7	8
60	0.5	1	3	5	7	10	12
70	1	2	3	5	9	11	14
80	1	2	3	7	10	13	16
100	1	2	3	8	12	15	20

- Steady-state serum digoxin levels above 10 to 15 ng/mL in adults

- Cardiac arrest

- Acute ingestions greater than 10 mg in adults[183]

Management of Digitalis-Induced Ventricular Arrhythmias

Potassium, magnesium, and normal saline. Most episodes of digitalis toxicity–induced ventricular ectopy respond to simple administration of potassium, magnesium, and isotonic crystalloid.

Lidocaine. Lidocaine is the antiarrhythmic of choice if ventricular arrhythmias persist after administration of potassium, magnesium, and normal saline. Lidocaine acts rapidly and rarely causes acute toxicity when used in the recommended dose of 1 to 1.5 mg/kg.[172,173,181] Observe closely for early signs of lidocaine toxicity when placing elderly patients with congestive heart failure or renal impairment on a lidocaine maintenance infusion.

Phenytoin. In the past phenytoin was the preferred antiarrhythmic for digitalis-induced ventricular arrhythmias.[181] The advantages of phenytoin were that it caused fewer central nervous system side effects than lidocaine and few adverse effects on AV conduction.

Magnesium. A number of reports suggest that magnesium may be the initial drug of choice for digitalis-induced ventricular tachyarrhythmias.[184,185] A dose of 1 to 2 g of magnesium sulfate diluted in 10 mL of D_5W and given IV push over 1 to 5 minutes may be used as first-line therapy. Some providers use magnesium only in patients with ventricular tachyarrhythmias unresponsive to lidocaine or phenytoin. A continuous magnesium infusion of 1 to 2 g (8 to 16 mEq) of magnesium diluted in 50 to 100 mL D_5W given over one hour and then 0.5 to 1 g per hour may be required for continued arrhythmia suppression.

Patients with arrhythmias refractory to pharmacologic therapy should be treated with Fab fragment antibodies.[175,183]

Management of Digitalis-Induced Stable VT

Fab fragment antibodies. When digitalis toxicity induces stable ventricular tachycardia, Fab fragment antibodies combined with rapidly active antiarrhythmics are the treatment of choice.[172]

Lidocaine infusion. A lidocaine bolus of 1 to 1.5 mg/kg is the best initial antiarrhythmic therapy. If the patient responds, begin a lidocaine infusion of 1 to 4 mg/min until the Fab fragment therapy is effective.

Magnesium sulfate. Give magnesium sulfate 1 to 2 g (diluted in 10 mL D_5W) IV push over 1 to 2 minutes if there appears to be no response to the lidocaine. If a pharmacologic cardioversion occurs after the lidocaine and magnesium infusions, start a continuous magnesium infusion of 1 to 2 g (8 to 16 mEq) diluted in 50 to 100 mL D_5W for the next 30 to 60 minutes. This interval allows sufficient time for the Fab fragment to be administered and take effect. Patients with renal compromise may have developed digoxin-toxicity on a renal basis, and magnesium administration poses a risk for these patients of iatrogenic arrhythmias.

Management of Digitalis-Induced Unstable VT

Once digitalis-induced ventricular tachycardia becomes clinically unstable, the treatment priorities are

- Synchronized cardioversion

- Immediate administration of Fab fragment antibodies

- Lidocaine

- Magnesium sulfate

Synchronized Cardioversion

- Perform immediate cardioversion; start at low energy levels of 25 to 50 J because of the increased likelihood of postcountershock rhythm deterioration in patients with digitalis toxicity.[172,181]

- If no response, immediately reattempt cardioversion with 200 J; if no response, reattempt cardioversion with 300 J.

- Synchronized cardioversion attempts are preferable to unsynchronized shocks if the clinical situation allows the slightly longer time required to perform synchronized cardioversion. If setting up for synchronized cardioversion will require more than 30 to 60 seconds, provide unsynchronized shocks (attempt defibrillation).

Fab Fragment Antibodies

- Administer 10 to 20 vials of Fab fragments.

Lidocaine

- Give a loading dose of lidocaine of 1.5 mg/kg IV.

- If the patient responds to the lidocaine, begin a continuous infusion of 1 to 4 mg/min until the Fab fragment therapy becomes effective.

Magnesium Sulfate

- Give magnesium sulfate 1 to 2 g diluted in 10 mL D_5W IV push over 1 to 2 minutes if there appears to be no response to the lidocaine. Give up to 5 to 10 g over the next 2 to 5 minutes if there appears to be no response to the lidocaine.

- If a pharmacologic cardioversion occurs after the lidocaine and magnesium infusions, start a continuous magnesium infusion of 1 to 2 g (8 to 16 mEq) diluted in 50 to 100 mL D_5W for the next 30 to 60 minutes. This interval allows sufficient time for the Fab fragments to be administered and take effect.

Management of Digitalis-Induced VF

Two Major Variations in Standard ACLS Protocols

Ventricular fibrillation due to digitalis overdose requires some modifications of standard ACLS guidelines. The Primary and Secondary ABCD Surveys should evolve in the standard pattern through the 3 shocks and administration of epinephrine or vasopressin and a fourth shock. Modify antiarrhythmic therapy and administer Fab fragments as indicated below:

- *Lidocaine* 1 to 1.5 mg/kg IV push

- Then administer *magnesium sulfate* 1 to 2 g diluted in 10 mL D_5W IV push

■ *Fab fragment antibodies* 20 vials (or as many as available up to 20)

■ *While awaiting response to Fab fragment therapy:*

— *Magnesium sulfate* 1 to 2 g diluted in 10 mL D_5W IV push; repeat every minute, up to a total of 5 to 10 g

— *Lidocaine* 0.5 mg/kg IV push; repeat every 8 to 10 minutes, up to a total of 3 mg/kg

Attempt defibrillation approximately every 60 seconds until conversion is achieved or the arrest terminated. The Fab fragments take some time to bind to the digoxin in the body and bloodstream. When Fab fragments have been administered, more prolonged resuscitative efforts are indicated to allow time for the antibodies to be effective.

References

1. American Academy of Clinical Toxicology. Facility assessment guidelines for regional toxicology treatment centers. *J Toxicol Clin Toxicol.* 1993;31:211-217.

2. Poison information and treatment systems. American College of Emergency Physicians. *Ann Emerg Med.* 1996;28:384.

3. Vale JA. Position statement: gastric lavage. American Academy of Clinical Toxicology; European Association of Poisons Centres and Clinical Toxicologists. *J Toxicol Clin Toxicol.* 1997;35:711-719.

4. Fingerhut LA, Cox CS. Poisoning mortality, 1985-1995. *Public Health Rep.* 1998;113:218-233.

5. Litovitz TL, Felberg L, White S, Klein-Schwartz W. 1995 annual report of the American Association of Poison Control Centers Toxic Exposure Surveillance System. *Am J Emerg Med.* 1996;14:487-537.

6. McCaig LF, Burt CW. Poisoning-related visits to emergency departments in the United States, 1993-1996. *J Toxicol Clin Toxicol.* 1999;37:817-826.

7. Guidelines 2000 for Cardiopulmonary Resuscitation and Emergency Cardiovascular Care. Part 8: advanced challenges in resuscitation: section 2: toxicology in ECC. The American Heart Association in collaboration with the International Liaison Committee on Resuscitation. *Circulation.* 2000;102:223-228.

8. Albertson TE, Dawson A, de Latorre F, Hoffman RS, Hollander JE, Jaeger A, Kerns WR II, Martin TG, Ross MP. TOX-ACLS: toxicologic-oriented advanced cardiac life support. *Ann Emerg Med.* 2001;37:S78-S90.

9. Mills CA, Flacke JW, Flacke WE, Bloor BC, Liu MD. Narcotic reversal in hypercapnic dogs: comparison of naloxone and nalbuphine. *Can J Anaesth.* 1990;37:238-244.

10. Kienbaum P, Thurauf N, Michel MC, Scherbaum N, Gastpar M, Peters J. Profound increase in epinephrine concentration in plasma and cardiovascular stimulation after mu-opioid receptor blockade in opioid-addicted patients during barbiturate-induced anesthesia for acute detoxification. *Anesthesiology.* 1998;88:1154-1161.

11. Osterwalder JJ. Naloxone—for intoxications with intravenous heroin and heroin mixtures—harmless or hazardous? A prospective clinical study. *J Toxicol Clin Toxicol.* 1996;34:409-416.

12. Vilke GM, Buchanan J, Dunford JV, Chan TC. Are heroin overdose deaths related to patient release after prehospital treatment with naloxone? *Prehosp Emerg Care.* 1999;3:183-186.

13. Moss ST, Chan TC, Buchanan J, Dunford JV, Vilke GM. Outcome study of prehospital patients signed out against medical advice by field paramedics. *Ann Emerg Med.* 1998;1:247-250.

14. Lange RA, Hillis LD. Cardiovascular complications of cocaine use [published correction appears in *N Engl J Med.* 2001;345:1432]. *N Engl J Med.* 2001;345:351-358.

15. Brown TC. Tricyclic antidepressant overdosage: experimental studies on the management of circulatory complications. *Clin Toxicol.* 1976;9:255-272.

16. Shih RD, Hollander JE, Burstein JL, Nelson LS, Hoffman RS, Quick AM. Clinical safety of lidocaine in patients with cocaine-associated myocardial infarction. *Ann Emerg Med.* 1995;26:702-706.

17. Beckman KJ, Parker RB, Hariman RJ, Gallastegui JL, Javaid JI, Bauman JL. Hemodynamic and electrophysiological actions of cocaine. Effects of sodium bicarbonate as an antidote in dogs. *Circulation.* 1991;83:1799-1807.

18. Kerns W II, Garvey L, Owens J. Cocaine-induced wide complex dysrhythmia. *J Emerg Med.* 1997;15:321-329.

19. Mayron R, Ruiz E. Phenytoin: does it reverse tricyclic-antidepressant-induced cardiac conduction abnormalities? *Ann Emerg Med.* 1986;15:876-880.

20. Callaham M, Schumaker H, Pentel P. Phenytoin prophylaxis of cardiotoxicity in experimental amitriptyline poisoning. *J Pharmacol Exp Ther.* 1988;245:216-220.

21. Knudsen K, Abrahamsson J. Effects of magnesium sulfate and lidocaine in the treatment of ventricular arrhythmias in experimental amitriptyline poisoning in the rat. *Crit Care Med.* 1994;22:494-498.

22. Kline JA, DeStefano AA, Schroeder JD, Raymond RM. Magnesium potentiates imipramine toxicity in the isolated rat heart. *Ann Emerg Med.* 1994;24:224-232.

23. Ramoska E, Sacchetti AD. Propranolol-induced hypertension in treatment of cocaine intoxication. *Ann Emerg Med.* 1985;14:1112-1113.

24. Brody SL, Slovis CM, Wrenn KD. Cocaine-related medical problems: consecutive series of 233 patients. *Am J Med.* 1990;88:325-331.

25. Vernon DD, Banner W Jr, Garrett JS, Dean JM. Efficacy of dopamine and norepinephrine for treatment of hemodynamic compromise in amitriptyline intoxication. *Crit Care Med.* 1991;19:544-549.

26. Wolf LR, Spadafora MP, Otten EJ. Use of amrinone and glucagon in a case of calcium channel blocker overdose. *Ann Emerg Med.* 1993;22:1225-1228.

27. Love JN, Leasure JA, Mundt DJ. A comparison of combined amrinone and glucagon therapy to glucagon alone for cardiovascular depression associated with propranolol toxicity in a canine model. *Am J Emerg Med.* 1993;11:360-363.

28. Kollef MH. Labetalol overdose successfully treated with amrinone and alpha-adrenergic receptor agonists. *Chest.* 1994;105:626-627.

29. Southall DR, Kilpatrick SM. Imipramine poisoning: survival of a child after prolonged cardiac massage. *Br Med J (Clin Res Ed).* 1974;4:508.

30. Ramsay ID. Survival after imipramine poisoning. *Lancet.* 1967;2:1308-1309.

31. Hebert MJ, Boucher A, Beaucage G, Girard R, Dandavino R. Transplantation of kidneys from a donor with carbon monoxide poisoning. *N Engl J Med.* 1992;326:1571.

32. Hollander JE, Hoffman RS, Gennis P, Fairweather P, DiSano MJ, Schumb DA, Feldman JA, Fish SS, Dyer S, Wax P, et al. Nitroglycerin in the treatment of cocaine associated chest pain—clinical safety and efficacy. *J Toxicol Clin Toxicol.* 1994;32:243-256.

33. Brogan WCr, Lange RA, Kim AS, Moliterno DJ, Hillis LD. Alleviation of cocaine-induced coronary vasoconstriction by nitroglycerin. *J Am Coll Cardiol.* 1991;18:581-586.

34. Boehrer JD, Moliterno DJ, Willard JE, Hillis LD, Lange RA. Influence of labetalol on cocaine-induced coronary vasoconstriction in humans. *Am J Med.* 1993;94:608-610.

35. Lange RA, Cigarroa RG, Yancy CW Jr, Willard JE, Popma JJ, Sills MN, McBride W, Kim AS, Hillis LD. Cocaine-induced coronary-artery vasoconstriction. *N Engl J Med.* 1989;321:1557-1562.

36. Lange RA, Cigarroa RG, Flores ED, McBride W, Kim AS, Wells PJ, Bedotto JB, Danziger RS, Hillis LD. Potentiation of cocaine-induced coronary vasoconstriction by beta-adrenergic blockade. *Ann Intern Med.* 1990;112:897-903.

37. Gay GR, Loper KA. The use of labetalol in the management of cocaine crisis. *Ann Emerg Med.* 1988;17:282-283.

38. Dusenberry SJ, Hicks MJ, Mariani PJ. Labetalol treatment of cocaine toxicity. *Ann Emerg Med.* 1987;16:235.

39. Sand IC, Brody SL, Wrenn KD, Slovis CM. Experience with esmolol for the treatment of cocaine-associated cardiovascular complications. *Am J Emerg Med.* 1991;9:161-163.

40. Hoffman RS, Hollander JE. Thrombolytic therapy and cocaine-induced myocardial infarction. *Am J Emerg Med.* 1996;14:693-695.

41. Pearigen PD, Benowitz NL. Poisoning due to calcium antagonists. Experience with verapamil, diltiazem and nifedipine. *Drug Saf.* 1991;6:408-430.

42. Jackson CD, Fishbein L. A toxicological review of beta-adrenergic blockers. *Fundam Appl Toxicol.* 1986;6:395-422.

43. Erickson FC, Ling LJ, Grande GA, Anderson DL. Diltiazem overdose: case report and review. *J Emerg Med.* 1991;9:357-366.

44. Weinstein RS. Recognition and management of poisoning with beta-adrenergic blocking agents. *Ann Emerg Med.* 1984;13:1123-1131.

45. Horowitz BZ, Rhee KJ. Massive verapamil ingestion: a report of two cases and a review of the literature. *Am J Emerg Med.* 1989;7:624-631.

46. Kulig K. Initial management of ingestions of toxic substances. *N Engl J Med.* 1992;326:1677-1681.

47. Park GD, Spector R, Goldberg MJ, Johnson GF. Expanded role of charcoal therapy in the poisoned and overdosed patient. *Arch Intern Med.* 1986;146:969-973.

48. Wrenn K, Rodewald L, Dockstader L. Potential misuse of ipecac. *Ann Emerg Med.* 1993;22:1408-1412.

49. Oe H, Taniura T, Ohgitani N. A case of severe verapamil overdose. *Jpn Circ J.* 1998;62:72-76.

50. Proano L, Chiang WK, Wang RY. Calcium channel blocker overdose. *Am J Emerg Med.* 1995;13:444-450.

51. Ramoska EA, Spiller HA, Winter M, Borys D. A one-year evaluation of calcium channel blocker overdoses: toxicity and treatment. *Ann Emerg Med.* 1993;22:196-200.

52. Belson MG, Gorman SE, Sullivan K, Geller RJ. Calcium channel blocker ingestions in children. *Am J Emerg Med.* 2000;18:581-586.

53. Horowitz BZ, Rhee KJ. Massive verapamil ingestion: a report of two cases and a review of the literature. *Am J Emerg Med.* 1989;7:624-631.

54. Holzer M, Sterz F, Schoerkhuber W, Behringer W, Domanovits H, Weinmar D, Weinstabl C, Stimpfl T. Successful resuscitation of a verapamil-intoxicated patient with percutaneous cardiopulmonary bypass. *Crit Care Med.* 1999;27:2818-2823.

55. Evans JS, Oram MP. Neurological recovery after prolonged verapamil-induced cardiac arrest. *Anaesth Intensive Care.* 1999;27:653-655.

56. Parra DA, Totapally BR, Zahn E, Jacobs J, Aldousany A, Burke RP, Chang AC. Outcome of cardiopulmonary resuscitation in a pediatric cardiac intensive care unit. *Crit Care Med.* 2000;28:3296-3300.

57. Waxman AB, White KP, Trawick DR. Electromechanical dissociation following verapamil and propranolol ingestion: a physiologic profile. *Cardiology.* 1997;88:478-481.

58. Kline JA, Tomaszewski CA, Schroeder JD, Raymond RM. Insulin is a superior antidote for cardiovascular toxicity induced by verapamil in the anesthetized canine. *J Pharmacol Exp Ther.* 1993;267:744-750.

59. Kline JA, Leonova E, Raymond RM. Beneficial myocardial metabolic effects of insulin during verapamil toxicity in the anesthetized canine. *Crit Care Med.* 1995;23:1251-1263.

60. Yuan TH, Kerns WP II, Tomaszewski CA, Ford MD, Kline JA. Insulin-glucose as adjunctive therapy for severe calcium channel antagonist poisoning. *J Toxicol Clin Toxicol.* 1999;37:463-474.

61. Boyer EW, Shannon M. Treatment of calcium-channel-blocker intoxication with insulin infusion. *N Engl J Med.* 2001;344:1721-1722.

62. Zaritsky AL, Horowitz M, Chernow B. Glucagon antagonism of calcium channel blocker-induced myocardial dysfunction. *Crit Care Med.* 1988;16:246-251.

63. Adams BD, Browne WT. Amlodipine overdose causes prolonged calcium channel blocker toxicity. *Am J Emerg Med.* 1998;16:527-528.

64. Papadopoulos J, O'Neil MG. Utilization of a glucagon infusion in the management of a massive nifedipine overdose. *J Emerg Med.* 2000;18:453-455.

65. Kalman S, Berg S, Lisander B. Combined overdose with verapamil and atenolol: treatment with high doses of adrenergic agonists. *Acta Anaesthesiol Scand.* 1998;42:379-382.

66. Snook CP, Sigvaldason K, Kristinsson J. Severe atenolol and diltiazem overdose. *J Toxicol Clin Toxicol.* 2000;38:661-665.

67. Agusa ED, Wexler LL, Witzburg RA. Massive propranolol overdose: successful treatment with high dose isoproterenol and glucagon. *Am J Med.* 1986;180:755-757.

68. Love JN, Hanfling D, Howell JM. Hemodynamic effects of calcium chloride in a canine model of acute propranolol intoxication. *Ann Emerg Med.* 1996;28:1-6.

69. Pertoldi F, D'Orlando L, Mercante WP. Electromechanical dissociation 48 hours after atenolol overdose: usefulness of calcium chloride. *Ann Emerg Med.* 1998;31:777-781.

70. Kenyon CJ, Aldinger GE, Joshipura P, Zaid GJ. Successful resuscitation using external cardiac pacing in beta adrenergic antagonist-induced bradyasystolic arrest. *Ann Emerg Med.* 1988;17:711-713.

71. McVey FK, Corke CF. Extracorporeal circulation in the management of massive propranolol overdose. *Anaesthesia.* 1991;46:744-746.

72. Kerns W II, Schroeder D, Williams C, Tomaszewski C, Raymond R. Insulin improves survival in a canine model of acute beta-blocker toxicity. *Ann Emerg Med.* 1997;29:748-757.

73. Cregler LL, Mark H. Medical complications of cocaine abuse. *N Engl J Med.* 1986;315:1495-1500.

74. Jekel JF, Allen DF, Podlewski H, Clarke N, Dean-Patterson S, Cartwright P. Epidemic free-base cocaine abuse. Case study from the Bahamas. *Lancet.* 1986;1:459-462.

75. Mody CK, Miller BL, McIntyre HB, Cobb SK, Goldberg MA. Neurologic complications of cocaine abuse. *Neurology.* 1988;38:1189-1193.

76. Lowenstein DH, Massa SM, Rowbotham MC, Collins SD, McKinney HE, Simon RP. Acute neurologic and psychiatric complications associated with cocaine abuse. *Am J Med.* 1987;83:841-846.

77. Farrar HC, Kearns GL. Cocaine: clinical pharmacology and toxicology. *J Pediatr.* 1989;115:665-675.

78. Roth D, Alarcon FJ, Fernandez JA, Preston RA, Bourgoignie JJ. Acute rhabdomyolysis associated with cocaine intoxication. *N Engl J Med.* 1988;319:673-677.

79. Amin M, Gabelman G, Karpel J, Buttrick P. Acute myocardial infarction and chest pain syndromes after cocaine use. *Am J Cardiol.* 1990;66:1434-1437.

80. Barth CW III, Bray M, Roberts WC. Rupture of the ascending aorta during cocaine intoxication. *Am J Cardiol.* 1986;57:496.

81. Allred RJ, Ewer S. Fatal pulmonary edema following intravenous "freebase" cocaine use. *Ann Emerg Med.* 1981;10:441-442.

82. Gradman AH. Cardiac effects of cocaine: a review. *Yale J Biol Med.* 1988;61:137-147.

83. Goldfrank LR, Hoffman RS. The cardiovascular effects of cocaine. *Ann Emerg Med.* 1991;20:165-175.

84. Catravas JD, Waters IW. Acute cocaine intoxication in the conscious dog: studies on the mechanism of lethality. *J Pharmacol Exp Ther.* 1981;217:350-356.

85. Kloner RA, Hale S, Alker K, Rezkalla S. The effects of acute and chronic cocaine use on the heart. *Circulation.* 1992;85:407-419.

86. Billman GE. Mechanisms responsible for the cardiotoxic effects of cocaine. *FASEB J.* 1990;4:2469-2475.

87. Wilkerson RD. Cardiovascular effects of cocaine in conscious dogs: importance of fully functional autonomic and central nervous systems. *J Pharmacol Exp Ther.* 1988; 246:466-471.

88. Heesch CM, Wilhelm CR, Ristich J, Adnane J, Bontempo FA, Wagner WR. Cocaine activates platelets and increases the formation of circulating platelet containing microaggregates in humans. *Heart.* 2000;83:688-695.

89. Lowenstein DH, Massa SM, Rowbotham MC, Collins SD, McKinney HE, Simon RP. Acute neurologic and psychiatric complications associated with cocaine abuse. *Am J Med.* 1987;83:841-846.

90. Catravas JD, Waters IW. Acute cocaine intoxication in the conscious dog: studies on the mechanism of lethality. *J Pharmacol Exp Ther.* 1981;217:350-356.

91. Derlet RW, Albertson TE. Emergency department presentation of cocaine intoxication. *Ann Emerg Med.* 1989;18:182-186.

92. Rich JA, Singer DE. Cocaine-related symptoms in patients presenting to an urban emergency department. *Ann Emerg Med.* 1991; 20:616-621.

93. Jonsson S, O'Meara M, Young JB. Acute cocaine poisoning. Importance of treating seizures and acidosis. *Am J Med.* 1983;75: 1061-1064.

94. Gay GR. Clinical management of acute and chronic cocaine poisoning. *Ann Emerg Med.* 1982;11:562-572.

95. Silverstein W, Lewin NA, Goldfrank L. Management of the cocaine-intoxicated patient. *Ann Emerg Med.* 1987;16:234-235.

96. Isner JM, Estes NA III, Thompson PD, Costanzo-Nordin MR, Subramanian R, Miller G, Katsas G, Sweeney K, Sturner WQ. Acute cardiac events temporally related to cocaine abuse. *N Engl J Med.* 1986;315:1438-1443.

97. Derlet RW, Albertson TE, Tharratt RS. Lidocaine potentiation of cocaine toxicity. *Ann Emerg Med.* 1991;20:135-138.

98. Parker RB, Perry GY, Horan LG, Flowers NC. Comparative effects of sodium bicarbonate and sodium chloride on reversing cocaine-induced changes in the electrocardiogram. *J Cardiovasc Pharmacol.* 1999;34: 864-869.

99. Wang RY. pH-dependent cocaine-induced cardiotoxicity. *Am J Emerg Med.* 1999;17: 364-369.

100. Williams RG, Kavanagh KM, Teo KK. Pathophysiology and treatment of cocaine toxicity: implications for the heart and cardiovascular system. *Can J Cardiol.* 1996;12:1295-1301.

101. Noel B. Cardiovascular complications of cocaine use. *N Engl J Med.* 2001;345:1575; discussion 1576.

102. Briggs RS, Birtwell AJ, Pohl JE. Hypertensive response to labetalol in phaeochromocytoma. *Lancet.* 1978;1:1045-1046.

103. Hollander JE, Carter WA, Hoffman RS. Use of phentolamine for cocaine-induced myocardial ischemia. *N Engl J Med.* 1992;327:361.

104. Hoffman CK, Goodman PC. Pulmonary edema in cocaine smokers. *Radiology.* 1989;172:463-465.

105. Cucco RA, Yoo OH, Cregler L, Chang JC. Nonfatal pulmonary edema after "freebase" cocaine smoking. *Am Rev Respir Dis.* 1987; 136:179-181.

106. Gitter MJ, Goldsmith SR, Dunbar DN, Sharkey SW. Cocaine and chest pain: clinical features and outcome of patients hospitalized to rule out myocardial infarction. *Ann Intern Med.* 1991;115:277-282.

107. Hollander JE, Hoffman RS. Cocaine-induced myocardial infarction: an analysis and review of the literature. *J Emerg Med.* 1992;10: 169-177.

108. Smith HW III, Liberman HA, Brody SL, Battey LL, Donohue BC, Morris DC. Acute myocardial infarction temporally related to cocaine use. Clinical, angiographic, and pathophysiologic observations. *Ann Intern Med.* 1987;107:13-18.

109. Minor RL Jr, Scott BD, Brown DD, Winniford MD. Cocaine-induced myocardial infarction in patients with normal coronary arteries. *Ann Intern Med.* 1991;115:797-806.

110. Kimura T, Yasue H, Sakaino N, Rokutanda M, Jougasaki M, Araki H. Effects of magnesium on the tone of isolated human coronary arteries. Comparison with diltiazem and nitroglycerin. *Circulation.* 1989;79:1118-1124.

111. Mayer DB, Miletich DJ, Feld JM, Albrecht RF. The effects of magnesium salts on the duration of epinephrine-induced ventricular tachyarrhythmias in anesthetized rats. *Anesthesiology.* 1989;71:923-928.

112. Woods KL, Fletcher S, Roffe C, Haider Y. Intravenous magnesium sulphate in suspected acute myocardial infarction: results of the second Leicester Intravenous Magnesium Intervention Trial (LIMIT-2). *Lancet.* 1992; 339:1553-1558.

113. American Heart Association, International Liason Committee on Resuscitation. (Tox Section) Guidelines for Cardiopulmonary Resuscitation and Emergency Cardiovascular Care. *Circulation.* 2000;102:I-223-228.

114. Mittleman MA, Mintzer D, Maclure M, Tofler GH, Sherwood JB, Muller JE. Triggering of myocardial infarction by cocaine. *Circulation.* 1999;99:2737-2741.

115. Nademanee K, Gorelick DA, Josephson MA, Ryan MA, Wilkins JN, Robertson HA, Mody FV, Intarachot V. Myocardial ischemia during cocaine withdrawal. *Ann Intern Med.* 1989; 111:876-880.

116. Hollander JE, Hoffman RS, Gennis P, Fairweather P, DiSano MJ, Schumb DA, Feldman JA, Fish SS, Dyer S, Wax P, et al. Prospective multicenter evaluation of cocaine-associated chest pain. Cocaine Associated Chest Pain (COCHPA) Study Group. *Acad Emerg Med.* 1994;1:330-339.

117. Hollander JE, Shih RD, Hoffman RS, Harchelroad FP, Phillips S, Brent J, Kulig K, Thode HC Jr. Predictors of coronary artery disease in patients with cocaine-associated myocardial infarction. Cocaine-Associated Myocardial Infarction (CAMI) Study Group. *Am J Med.* 1997;102:158-163.

118. Cummins R. Evidence-Based Resuscitation Guidelines. In: Field J, ed. *2000 Handbook of Emergency Cardiovascular Care for Healthcare Providers.* Dallas: American Heart Association; 2000:1-2.

119. Hoffman RS, Hollander JE. Evaluation of patients with chest pain after cocaine use. *Crit Care Clin.* 1997;13:809-828.

120. Freemantle N, Cleland J, Young P, Mason J, Harrison J. β-Blockade after myocardial infarction: systematic review and meta regression analysis. *BMJ.* 1999;318:1730-1737.

121. Hollander JE, Burstein JL, Hoffman RS, Shih RD, Wilson LD. Cocaine-associated myocardial infarction. Clinical safety of thrombolytic therapy. Cocaine Associated Myocardial Infarction (CAMI) Study Group. *Chest.* 1995;107:1237-1241.

122. Spivey WH, Schoffstall JM, Kirkpatrick R. Comparison of labetalol, diazepam, and haloperidol for the treatment of cocaine toxicity in a swine model. *Ann Emerg Med.* 1990;19:467-468.

123. Guinn MM, Bedford JA, Wilson MC. Antagonism of intravenous cocaine lethality in nonhuman primates. *Clin Toxicol.* 1980;16: 499-508.

124. Baumann BM, Perrone J, Hornig SE, Shofer FS, Hollander JE. Randomized, double-blind, placebo-controlled trial of diazepam, nitroglycerin, or both for treatment of patients with potential cocaine-associated acute coronary syndromes. *Acad Emerg Med.* 2000;7: 878-885.

125. Negus BH, Willard JE, Hillis LD, Glamann DB, Landau C, Snyder RW, Lange RA. Alleviation of cocaine-induced coronary vasoconstriction with intravenous verapamil. *Am J Cardiol.* 1994;73:510-513.

126. Trouve R, Nahas GG, Maillet M. Nitrendipine as an antagonist to the cardiotoxicty of cocaine. *J Cardiovas Pharmocol.* 1987;9 (suppl 4):S49-S53.

127. Nahas G, Trouve R, Demus JR, von Sitbon M. A calcium-channel blocker as antidote to the cardiac effects of cocaine intoxication. *N Engl J Med.* 1985;313:519-520.

128. Billman GE, Hoskins RS. Cocaine-induced ventricular fibrillation: protection afforded by the calcium antagonist verapamil. *FASEB J.* 1988;2:2990-2995.

129. Derlet RW, Albertson TE. Potentiation of cocaine toxicity with calcium channel blockers. *Am J Emerg Med.* 1989;7:464-468.

130. Hale SL, Alker KJ, Rezkalla SH, Eisenhauer AC, Kloner RA. Nifedipine protects the heart from the acute deleterious effects of cocaine if administered before but not after cocaine. *Circulation.* 1991;83:1437-1443.

131. Smith M, Garner D, Niemann JT. Pharmacologic interventions after an LD50 cocaine insult in a chronically instrumented rat model: are beta-blockers contraindicated? *Ann Emerg Med.* 1991;20:768-771.

132. Hollander JE, Hoffman RS, Burstein JL, Shih RD, Thode HC Jr Cocaine-associated myocardial infarction. Mortality and complications. Cocaine-Associated Myocardial Infarction Study Group. *Arch Intern Med.* 1995;155:1081-1086.

133. Vargas R, Gillis RA, Ramwell PW. Propranolol promotes cocaine-induced spasm of porcine coronary artery. *J Pharmacol Exp Ther.* 1991;257:644-646.

134. Karch S. Managing cocaine crisis. *Ann Emerg Med.* 1988;18:228-229.

135. Kerr GW, McGuffie AC, Wilkie S. Tricyclic antidepressant overdose: a review. *Emerg Med J.* 2001;18:236-241.

136. Glauser J. Tricyclic antidepressant poisoning. *Cleve Clin J Med.* 2000;67:704-706, 709-713, 717-709.

137. Frommer DA, Kulig KW, Marx JA, Rumack B. Tricyclic antidepressant overdose. A review. *JAMA.* 1987;257:521-526.

138. Braden NJ, Jackson JE, Walson PD. Tricyclic antidepressant overdose. *Pediatr Clin North Am.* 1986;33:287-297.

139. Foulke GE, Albertson TE, Walby WF. Tricyclic antidepressant overdose: emergency department findings as predictors of clinical course. *Am J Emerg Med.* 1986;4:496-500.

140. Glassman AH. Cardiovascular effects of tricyclic antidepressants. *Annu Rev Med.* 1984; 35:503-511.

141. Marshall JB, Forker AD. Cardiovascular effects of tricyclic antidepressant drugs: therapeutic usage, overdose, and management of complications. *Am Heart J.* 1982;103: 401-414.

142. Callaham M, Kassel D. Epidemiology of fatal tricyclic antidepressant ingestion: implications for management. *Ann Emerg Med.* 1985;14:1-9.

143. Wedin GP, Oderda GM, Klein-Schwartz W, Gorman RL. Relative toxicity of cyclic antidepressants. *Ann Emerg Med.* 1986;15:797-804.

144. Litovitz TL, Holm KC, Bailey KM, Schmitz BF. 1991 annual report of the American Association of Poison Control Centers National Data Collection System. *Am J Emerg Med.* 1992;10:452-505.

145. Wolfe TR, Caravati EM, Rollins DE. Terminal 40-ms frontal plane QRS axis as a marker for tricyclic antidepressant overdose. *Ann Emerg Med.* 1989;18:348-351.

146. Liebelt EL, Francis PD, Woolf AD. ECG lead aVR versus QRS interval in predicting seizures and arrhythmias in acute tricyclic antidepressant toxicity. *Ann Emerg Med.* 1995;26:195-201.

147. Liebelt EL, Ulrich A, Francis PD, Woolf A. Serial electrocardiogram changes in acute tricyclic antidepressant overdoses. *Crit Care Med.* 1997;25:1721-1726.

148. Harrigan RA, Brady WJ. ECG abnormalities in tricyclic antidepressant ingestion. *Am J Emerg Med.* 1999;17:387-393.

149. Shannon M, Merola J, Lovejoy FH Jr. Hypotension in severe tricyclic antidepressant overdose. *Am J Emerg Med.* 1988;6:439-442.

150. Blackman K, Brown SG, Wilkes GJ. Plasma alkalinization for tricyclic antidepressant toxicity: a systematic review. *Emerg Med (Fremantle).* 2001;13:204-210.

151. Mackway-Jones K. Towards evidence based emergency medicine: best BETs from the Manchester Royal Infirmary. Alkalinisation in the management of tricyclic antidepressant overdose. *J Accid Emerg Med.* 1999; 16:139-140.

152. McCabe JL, Cobaugh DJ, Menegazzi JJ, Fata J. Experimental tricyclic antidepressant toxicity: a randomized, controlled comparison of hypertonic saline solution, sodium bicarbonate, and hyperventilation. *Ann Emerg Med.* 1998;32:329-333.

153. Liebelt EL. Targeted management strategies for cardiovascular toxicity from tricyclic antidepressant overdose: the pivotal role for alkalinization and sodium loading. *Pediatr Emerg Care.* 1998;14:293-298.

154. Bessen HA, Niemann JT. Improvement of cardiac conduction after hyperventilation in tricyclic antidepressant overdose. *J Toxicol Clin Toxicol.* 1985;23:537-546.

155. Hoffman JR, McElroy CR. Bicarbonate therapy for dysrhythmia and hypotension in tricyclic antidepressant overdose. *West J Med.* 1981;134:60-64.

156. Brown TC. Sodium bicarbonate treatment for tricyclic antidepressant arrhythmias in children. *Med J Aust.* 1976;2:380-382.

157. Brown TC, Barker GA, Dunlop ME, Loughnan PM. The use of sodium bicarbonate in the treatment of tricyclic antidepressant-induced arrhythmias. *Anaesth Intensive Care.* 1973;1:203-210.

158. Sasyniuk BI, Jhamandas V, Valois M. Experimental amitriptyline intoxication: treatment of cardiac toxicity with sodium bicarbonate. *Ann Emerg Med.* 1986;15: 1052-1059.

159. Nattel S, Mittleman M. Treatment of ventricular tachyarrhythmias resulting from amitriptyline toxicity in dogs. *J Pharmacol Exp Ther.* 1984;231:430-435.

160. Bou-Abboud E, Nattel S. Relative role of alkalosis and sodium ions in reversal of class I antiarrhythmic drug-induced sodium channel blockade by sodium bicarbonate. *Circulation.* 1996;94:1954-1961.

161. Liberatore MA, Robinson DS. Torsade de pointes: a mechanism for sudden death associated with neuroleptic drug therapy? *J Clin Psychopharmacol.* 1984;4:143-146.

162. Tzivoni D, Banai S, Schuger C, Benhorin J, Keren A, Gottlieb S, Stern S. Treatment of torsade de pointes with magnesium sulfate. *Circulation.* 1988;77:392-397.

163. Perticone F, Adinolfi L, Bonaduce D. Efficacy of magnesium sulfate in the treatment of torsade de pointes. *Am Heart J.* 1986;112: 847-849.

164. Iseri LT, Chung P, Tobis J. Magnesium therapy for intractable ventricular tachyarrhythmias in normomagnesemic patients. *West J Med.* 1983;138:823-828.

165. Keren A, Tzivoni D, Gavish D, Levi J, Gottlieb S, Benhorin J, Stern S. Etiology, warning signs and therapy of torsade de pointes. A study of 10 patients. *Circulation.* 1981;64: 1167-1174.

166. Goldberg RJ, Capone RJ, Hunt JD. Cardiac complications following tricyclic antidepressant overdose. Issues for monitoring policy. *JAMA.* 1985;254:1772-1775.

167. Ellison DW, Pentel PR. Clinical features and consequences of seizures due to cyclic anti-depressant overdose. *Am J Emerg Med.* 1989;7:5-10.

168. Teba L, Schiebel F, Dedhia HV, Lazzell VA. Beneficial effect of norepinephrine in the treatment of circulatory shock caused by tricyclic antidepressant overdose. *Am J Emerg Med.* 1988;6:566-568.

169. Tran TP, Panacek EA, Rhee KJ, Foulke GE. Response to dopamine vs norepinephrine in tricyclic antidepressant-induced hypotension. *Acad Emerg Med.* 1997;4:864-868.

170. Knudsen K, Abrahamsson J. Epinephrine and sodium bicarbonate independently and additively increase survival in experimental amitriptyline poisoning. *Crit Care Med.* 1997;25:669-674.

171. Vernon DD, Banner W, Dean M. Dopamine and norepinephrine are equally effective for treatment of shock in amitriptyline intoxication. *Crit Care Med.* 1990;18:S239.

172. Dick M, Curwin J, Tepper D. Digitalis intoxication recognition and management. *J Clin Pharmacol.* 1991;31:444-447.

173. Antman EM, Smith TW. Digitalis toxicity. *Annu Rev Med.* 1985;36:357-367.

174. Moorman JR, Pritchett EL. The arrhythmias of digitalis intoxication. *Arch Intern Med.* 1985;145:1289-1292.

175. Antman EM, Wenger TL, Butler VP Jr, Haber E, Smith TW. Treatment of 150 cases of life-threatening digitalis intoxication with digoxin-specific Fab antibody fragments. Final report of a multicenter study. *Circulation.* 1990;81:1744-1752.

176. Martiny SS, Phelps SJ, Massey KL. Treatment of severe digitalis intoxication with digoxin-specific antibody fragments: a clinical review. *Crit Care Med.* 1988;16:629-635.

177. Ordog GJ, Benaron S, Bhasin V, Wasserberger J, Balasubramanium S. Serum digoxin levels and mortality in 5,100 patients. *Ann Emerg Med.* 1987;16:32-39.

178. Sonnenblick M, Abraham AS, Meshulam Z, Eylath U. Correlation between manifestations of digoxin toxicity and serum digoxin, calcium, potassium, and magnesium concentrations and arterial pH. *Br Med J (Clin Res Ed).* 1983;286:1089-1091.

179. Whang R, Oei TO, Watanabe A. Frequency of hypomagnesemia in hospitalized patients receiving digitalis. *Arch Intern Med.* 1985; 145:655-656.

180. Davey M, Caldicott D. Calcium salts in management of hyperkalemia. *Emerg Med J.* 2002;19:92-93.

181. Sharff JA, Bayer MJ. Acute and chronic digitalis toxicity: presentation and treatment. *Ann Emerg Med.* 1982;11:327-331.

182. Smith TW, Butler VP Jr, Haber E, Fozzard H, Marcus FI, Bremner WF, Schulman IC, Phillips A. Treatment of life-threatening digitalis intoxication with digoxin-specific Fab antibody fragments: experience in 26 cases. *N Engl J Med.* 1982;307:1357-1362.

183. Woolf AD, Wenger T, Smith TW, Lovejoy FH Jr. The use of digoxin-specific Fab fragments for severe digitalis intoxication in children. *N Engl J Med.* 1992;326:1739-1744.

184. Reisdorff EJ, Clark MR, Walters BL. Acute digitalis poisoning: the role of intravenous magnesium sulfate. *J Emerg Med.* 1986; 4:463-469.

185. Cohen L, Kitzes R. Magnesium sulfate and digitalis-toxic arrhythmias. *JAMA.* 1983; 249:2808-2810.

Special Resuscitation Situations Part 1: Hypothermia

Epidemiology

Unintentional hypothermia is defined as a decrease in core body temperature below 35°C or 36°C (95°F or 96.8°F). ACLS providers will most often encounter patients in cardiac arrest associated with unintentional hypothermia in 1 of 3 clinical settings:

- Cold stress or exposure (often subacute) in persons with thermoregulatory impairment

- Cold weather exposure

- Cold water immersion (with or without submersion)

Cold exposure in persons with impaired thermoregulatory function is surprisingly the most frequent cause of death from hypothermia.[1-13] *Impaired thermoregulatory function* may develop in many patient groups: the elderly, insulin-dependent diabetics, the malnourished, the alcohol- or drug-intoxicated, the chronically ill, and the multiply medicated, medically disabled. These patients have decreased basal metabolism, dysfunctional shivering thermogenesis, and impaired vasoconstriction.

- Patients with impaired thermoregulatory function who are impoverished, semistarved, or homeless and disabled, are particularly at risk for cold exposure from lack of shelter, inadequate clothing, or improper residential heating.[4,12,13] Authors have applied the phrase "accidental urban hypothermia" to many of these patients.[14]

- This "at risk" population may develop hypothermia at ambient temperatures not usually considered "cold weather." Hypothermia is most likely to develop when these patients suffer cold exposure over long periods of time.[4,12,13]

Cold weather exposure can produce hypothermia in healthy people with normal thermogenesis when they experience long periods of adverse weather conditions. A number of predisposing factors play a role in the development of significant hypothermia in healthy people: severity of the cold weather, insulation properties of clothing or shelter, wind chill in a windy or exposed setting, exhaustion after heavy outdoor exercise, wet clothing, inadequate caloric intake, and associated injuries (such as frostbite or fractures) that interfere with self-protective actions.

Cold water immersion can also lead to significant hypothermia in healthy people. Sudden immersion in cold water (usually defined as water temperature <21°C or <70°F) most often occurs in association with boating or recreational aquatic mishaps.[15]

- Cooling occurs rapidly during cold water immersion because conductive heat loss is 25 to 35 times faster in water than in air. In water at 4.44°C (40°F), mortality approaches 50% after 1 hour. For perspective on water temperatures, note that the mean January water temperature is 21°C (70°F) off Miami, 24°C (75°F) off Honolulu, 11°C (52°F) off San Francisco, 14°C (57°F) off San Diego, and 3°C (37°F) off New York City.[15]

- Victims of cold water immersion also face a high risk of *cold water submersion* with resultant aspiration, asphyxia, hypoxia, and even death (see Part 2 of this chapter).

- The protective value of hypothermia in cold water immersion with subsequent submersion is probably exaggerated. Recent experiments suggest that cold water immersion produces exhaustion (and subsequent submersion) faster than it produces a neurologically protective degree of core hypothermia.[16-18] Nearly all reports of successful resuscitation with full neurologic recovery describe prolonged cold water submersion in icy water (< 5°C or 41°F).

Therapeutic hypothermia is intentional lowering of the patient's body temperature to reduce oxygen demand and metabolic rate. This therapy is undertaken to reduce complications of inadequate perfusion or reperfusion injury. New recommendations developed by the International Liaison Committee on Resuscitation (ILCOR) advocate the use of therapeutic hypothermia as follows:

- When the initial rhythm was ventricular fibrillation (VF), unconscious adult patients with spontaneous circulation after out-of-hospital cardiac arrest should be cooled to 32°C to 34°C for 12 to 24 hours.

- For any other rhythm or for cardiac arrest in hospital, such cooling may also be beneficial.

Pathophysiology

Severe hypothermia (body temperature <30°C or <86°F) is associated with marked depression of cerebral blood flow and oxygen consumption, reduced cardiac output, and decreased arterial pressure.[19] Victims can appear to be clinically dead because of marked depression of brain function.[19-21]

Hypothermia may exert a protective effect on the brain and organs during cardiac arrest if the victim cools rapidly with no hypoxia before the cardiac arrest.[22,23] If the victim cools rapidly, oxygen consumption decreases and metabolism slows before the arrest, and this reduces organ ischemia during the arrest.[24]

- This protective effect appears to account for the rare occurrence of resuscitation with intact neurologic recovery after hypothermic cardiac arrest.[25]

- The effects of hypothermia on cerebral oxygen consumption and metabolism are thought to be the mechanism for the therapeutic effects of induced hypothermia. Induced hypothermia for comatose survivors of out-of-hospital ventricular fibrillation cardiac arrest has produced marked improvements in survival to hospital discharge,[26] 6-month mortality rate,[27] and neurologic outcomes.[27]

Severe unintentional hypothermia is a preventable health problem associated with significant morbidity and mortality, especially in urban areas. In inner cities hypothermia has a high association with mental illness, poverty, and use of drugs and alcohol.[28,29] In some rural areas more than 90% of deaths from hypothermia are associated with elevated blood alcohol levels.[30]

Hypothermia: Definitions, Signs, and Symptoms

The severity of hypothermia is determined from the victim's core body temperature. The Table presents the most commonly used definitions of hypothermia severity, based on a range of core body temperatures:

- **Mild hypothermia** (34°C to 36°C or 93.2°F to 96.8°F): The clinical hallmark of mild hypothermia is the onset of shivering, which can become severe. Shivering represents a centrally mediated attempt at thermogenesis.[19] The onset of mental confusion and disorientation marks the symptomatic transition from mild to moderate hypothermia.

- **Moderate hypothermia** (30°C to <34°C or 86°F to <93.2°F): The hallmark of moderate hypothermia is progressive loss of higher cognitive functions with onset of marked confusion, disorientation, stupor, and loss of consciousness. With moderate hypothermia shivering diminishes and eventually disappears completely.

- **Severe hypothermia** (<30°C or <86°F): The hallmark of severe hypothermia is unconsciousness with immobility and the progressive loss of all signs of life. The vital functions disappear completely in roughly the following order as hypothermia becomes more and more severe:

  — Loss of consciousness and all voluntary movement

  — Loss of papillary light reflexes

  — Loss of deep tendon reflexes

  — Loss of spontaneous respirations

  — Loss of organized cardiac rhythm (onset of VF)

- **Profound hypothermia** (<20°C or <68°F): Profound hypothermia may be considered as a subcategory of severe hypothermia.[20,21] This category, however, has little clinical utility because it has no therapeutic implications. Profound hypothermia is managed the same way as severe hypothermia.

  — The hallmark of profound hypothermia is the total loss of any sign of life. Cardiac activity is completely lost, and the monitor displays only asystole. The EEG is totally silent with no detectable brain activity. No distinction can be made from death.

  — There have been rare case reports of successful resuscitation of victims with profound hypothermia using internal rewarming. Few of these patients have demonstrated complete neurologic recovery.[25]

General Care of All Hypothermia Victims

The answers to 2 clinical questions shape the treatment of unintentional hypothermia:

- First, is the victim in cardiopulmonary arrest?

- Second, what is the core temperature?

The Hypothermia Algorithm (Figure) shows how the answers to these 2 questions determine the recommended actions for victims of unintentional hypothermia.

Box 1: Initial Therapy for All Patients

Remove wet garments

Protect against heat loss and wind chill

- In the prehospital setting, if the victim maintains a perfusing rhythm, rescuers focus on prevention of cardiac arrest. To prevent cardiac arrest:

  — Prevent further heat loss.

  — Begin passive rewarming.

  — Begin clinical monitoring, particularly measurement of core temperature and monitoring of cardiac rhythm.

  — Provide rapid transport to definitive care.

- Prevent further conductive, convective, evaporative, and radiant heat losses by shielding the victim from wind, removing wet garments, and insulating the victim with blankets (especially reflective metallic-foil wraps), insulated sleeping bags and pads, dry clothing, or even newspapers or cardboard.

FIGURE. Hypothermia Algorithm.

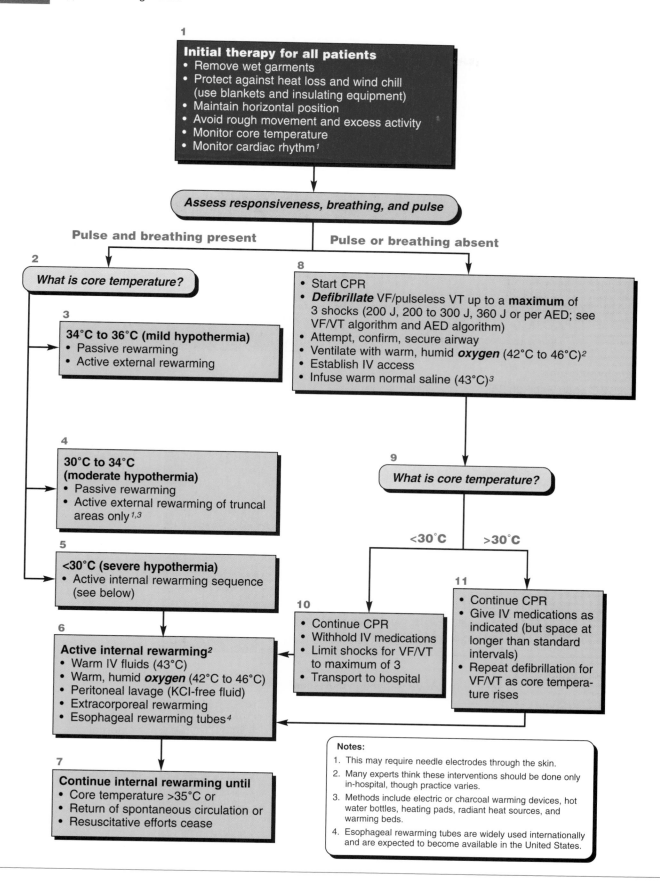

1

Initial therapy for all patients
- Remove wet garments
- Protect against heat loss and wind chill (use blankets and insulating equipment)
- Maintain horizontal position
- Avoid rough movement and excess activity
- Monitor core temperature
- Monitor cardiac rhythm[1]

Assess responsiveness, breathing, and pulse

Pulse and breathing present | **Pulse or breathing absent**

2

What is core temperature?

3

34°C to 36°C (mild hypothermia)
- Passive rewarming
- Active external rewarming

8
- Start CPR
- **Defibrillate** VF/pulseless VT up to a **maximum** of 3 shocks (200 J, 200 to 300 J, 360 J or per AED; see VF/VT algorithm and AED algorithm)
- Attempt, confirm, secure airway
- Ventilate with warm, humid *oxygen* (42°C to 46°C)[2]
- Establish IV access
- Infuse warm normal saline (43°C)[3]

4

30°C to 34°C (moderate hypothermia)
- Passive rewarming
- Active external rewarming of truncal areas only[1,3]

9

What is core temperature?

5

<30°C (severe hypothermia)
- Active internal rewarming sequence (see below)

<30°C   **>30°C**

10
- Continue CPR
- Withhold IV medications
- Limit shocks for VF/VT to maximum of 3
- Transport to hospital

11
- Continue CPR
- Give IV medications as indicated (but space at longer than standard intervals)
- Repeat defibrillation for VF/VT as core temperature rises

6

Active internal rewarming[2]
- Warm IV fluids (43°C)
- Warm, humid *oxygen* (42°C to 46°C)
- Peritoneal lavage (KCl-free fluid)
- Extracorporeal rewarming
- Esophageal rewarming tubes[4]

7

Continue internal rewarming until
- Core temperature >35°C or
- Return of spontaneous circulation or
- Resuscitative efforts cease

Notes:
1. This may require needle electrodes through the skin.
2. Many experts think these interventions should be done only in-hospital, though practice varies.
3. Methods include electric or charcoal warming devices, hot water bottles, heating pads, radiant heat sources, and warming beds.
4. Esophageal rewarming tubes are widely used internationally and are expected to become available in the United States.

TABLE. Hypothermia: Definitions, Signs and Symptoms, and Recommended Therapy*

Core Temperature*		Signs and Symptoms	Recommended Therapy		
°C	°F				
Mild hypothermia[31] 34°C to 36°C or 93.2°F to 96.8°F					
36°	96.8°	Muscle tone increases ("preshivering"). Metabolic rate and blood pressure increase to adjust for heat loss. Shivering begins.	Passive external rewarming	Active external rewarming: all areas	
35°	95°	Shivering continues and reaches maximum thermogenesis level. Victim is still mentally responsive.			
34°	93.2°	Extreme subjective coldness; some amnesia and dysarthria. Poor judgment and maladaptive behavior begin. Blood pressure is adequate; tachycardia and then progressive bradycardia occur.			
Moderate hypothermia 30°C to <34°C or 86°F to <93.2°F					
33°	91.4°	Mental confusion increases; ataxia; apathy; shivering decreases. Maximum respiratory stimulation with tachypnea, then progressive drop in minute volume.	Passive external rewarming	Active external rewarming: truncal areas only	
32°	89.6°	Consciousness is much more clouded; victim may become stuporous. Shivering almost stopped. Oxygen consumption <75% normal. Pupils may be dilated.			
31°	87.8°	Thermogenesis through shivering stops. Severe peripheral vasoconstriction; blood pressure is difficult to obtain.			
30°	86°	Muscles increasingly rigid; more loss of consciousness; risk of atrial fibrillation and other arrhythmias. Cardiac output drops to <67% of normal.			
Severe hypothermia <30°C or <86°F (purple shading = risk of VF with rough movements)					
29°	82.4°	Pulse and respirations slow perceptibly; cardiac arrhythmias become more frequent. Pupils usually dilated. Paradoxical undressing observed.	Passive external rewarming	Active external rewarming: truncal areas only	Active internal rewarming
28°	82.4°	**High risk of VF if heart is irritated from rough movements. Oxygen consumption <50% normal.**			
27°	80.6°	**Consciousness usually lost; all voluntary motion stops.**			

Core Temperature*		Signs and Symptoms	Recommended Therapy		
°C	°F		Passive external rewarming	Active external rewarming: truncal areas only	Active internal rewarming
26°	78.8°	Deep tendon and pupillary light reflexes usually absent. Victim can appear dead.			
25°	77°	VF can occur spontaneously even without irritation.			
24°	75.2°	Pulmonary edema, severe hypotension, and severe bradycardia may develop.			
23°	73.4°	VF risk very high; deathlike appearance; no corneal or oculocephalic reflexes.			
22°	71.6°	VF occurs spontaneously in majority of victims. Oxygen consumption <25% normal.			
21°	69.8°	VF amplitude diminishes.			
20°	68°	VF becomes very fine, more like "coarse asystole"; EEG signals flatten.			
Profound hypothermia (<20°C or <68°F)					
19°	66.2°	Either PEA or asystole; EEG almost flat.			
18°	64.4°	Almost invariably asystole.			
17°	62.6°	EEG totally silent.			
16°	60.8°	Total irreversible cardiac and brain death (except in rare cases).			
15°	59°	Lowest recorded infant core temperature with intact neurologic recovery from accidental hypothermia.[32]			
13.7°	56.6°	Lowest recorded adult core temperature with full neurologic recovery from accidental hypothermia.[25]			
10°	50°	Oxygen consumption <8% normal.			
9°	48.2°	Lowest recorded core temperature for survival from therapeutic hypothermia.[21]			

*Adapted with permission from *ACLS Scenarios: Core Concepts for Case-Based Learning* by R.O. Cummins (Copyright 1996 Mosby, Inc.) with additional data from References 19-21.

- Begin the process of passive rewarming with the insulating and shielding actions noted above.

Maintain horizontal position

- Try to keep hypothermic victims in a horizontal position from the time of initial rescue and extrication (as feasible).

- Hypothermic victims are often volume depleted from "cold diuresis" with dysfunctional cardiovascular regulatory mechanisms.[33,34]

Avoid rough movement and excess activity

- Try to avoid rough movement and excess activity. But do not delay urgently needed procedures such as rescue breathing, intubation, insertion of a vascular catheter, or even CPR chest compressions. Perform procedures gently, and monitor cardiac rhythm closely.

- An exaggerated fear of "precipitating VF" and other arrhythmias in hypothermic victims should not cause prehospital personnel to withhold essential interventions. But as the Table shows, spontaneous VF or VF secondary to jarring movements becomes a realistic risk only at severe levels of hypothermia (<30°C or <86°F).

Monitor core temperature

See Box 2, below.

Monitor cardiac rhythm

- Monitor the cardiac rhythm. If the victim's skin is extremely cold, it may be impossible to record the cardiac rhythm using adhesive electrodes. In such cases you may use a sterile needle (1.5 inch, 22 gauge works well) to attach the electrodes to the skin. Use the needle as you would use a safety pin. Insert the needle through the electrode, through a small piece of skin, and back through the electrode.

Box 2. Determine Core Body Temperature

The victim's core body temperature will determine subsequent treatment decisions.

- Measure core temperature using a rectal or tympanic membrane thermometer. Standard mercury-filled glass thermometers are useful only for mild hypothermia because they do not register temperatures below 34°C (93.2°F).

- Lower-reading rectal probe thermometers with electronic-digital circuitry are readily available. They should be standard equipment in all EMS vehicles, Emergency Departments, and first aid stations where hypothermic victims might require care.

Box 3. Mild Hypothermia: 34°C to 36°C (93.2°F to 96.8°F)

- Two methods are used to rewarm patients with mild hypothermia:

  — Passive rewarming (always)

  — Active external rewarming (when indicated)

Passive rewarming

- As a general rule passive rewarming is the treatment of choice for hypothermia victims who can shiver (shivering thermogenesis stops at core temperatures below 32°C or 89.6°F). A wide variety of insulating materials are effective for *passive rewarming*. Blankets and reflective metallic-foil wraps are the most common. Passive rewarming occurs through internal heat generation by the patient. Rewarming rates are relatively slow, in the range of only 0.25°C to 0.5°C (0.45°F to 0.9°F) per hour.[35] In some studies, however, passive rewarming during out-of-hospital care was associated with a *fall* in core temperature.[36]

  — Providers should also initiate and maintain passive rewarming for victims with moderate or severe hypothermia (see the Table). But passive rewarming alone will not effectively raise core body temperature for these patients or patients in cardiac arrest with any level of hypothermia.[24]

Active external rewarming

- *Active external rewarming: all areas* can be accomplished with a variety of *heating* and *heated* devices. Examples of heating devices are radiant heat, forced hot air, or warm bath water. Heated devices include warmed plastic bags of IV solutions, heated blankets, or chemical-reaction warm packs. In general, do not place heated devices directly on the patient's skin.

  — When you use these devices, you must monitor both the patient and the device; use them with care and caution.

  — With all active external devices, especially chemical warm packs, verify that the temperature of the warming pack does not increase enough to cause skin burns. This is a particular risk for insensate victims of hypothermia. There are reports of chemical heating packs reaching hazardous temperatures.

- In this form of passive rewarming, the entire body, including all 4 extremities and fingers and toes are warmed. There is risk in external rewarming.

  — As the arms and legs are rewarmed externally, rapid dilation of peripheral blood vessels occurs. As this cold blood returns to the central circulation, core body temperature may continue to fall—a phenomenon informally termed *afterdrop*.

  — Topical application of heated devices—especially to the fingers and toes—may result in tissue injury because peripheral tissues are often severely vasoconstricted. If heated devices like warm packs are used, apply them to truncal areas only (neck, armpits, or groin).

Box 4. Moderate Hypothermia: 30°C to <34°C (86°F to <93.2°F)

The approach to patients with moderate hypothermia is also rewarming using 2 methods:

■ Passive rewarming

■ Active external rewarming: *truncal areas only*

Active external rewarming: truncal areas only

■ Active external rewarming for moderate and severe hypothermia should specifically *exclude* rewarming of the arms and legs.

   — The afterdrop phenomenon occurs much more frequently with moderate and severe hypothermia.

In addition, an *afterdrop acidosis* is more of a risk if the arms and legs are included in active external rewarming efforts.

■ Active external rewarming of truncal areas can be accomplished in several ways.

   — Many of the innovative commercial rewarming techniques, such as forced hot air and warm water baths, cannot be used because these methods will not exclude the extremities.

   — In wilderness medicine, body-to-body contact inside an insulated bag has been used to increase core temperature at rates similar to spontaneous shivering.[37]

   — The most convenient and least expensive device for truncal rewarming is the classic hot water bottle, disguised in most Emergency Departments as warmed plastic bags of IV fluids. (*Note:* Microwave warming of crystalloid fluids has been shown to be thermally safe.[38])

   — The addition of 1 or 2 standard electric heating pads under the patient's back and waist provides frugal yet respectable core temperature rewarming rates of about 1°C (1.8°F) per hour.[35]

   — Forced-air warming blankets, with or without canopies,[39] are effective devices widely used for postoperative hypothermia.[40] They can produce rewarming rates of 1°C to 3°C (1.8°F to 5.4°F) per hour.[41] These devices have successfully rewarmed victims in hypothermic cardiac arrest; thus they may be useful in areas where cardiopulmonary bypass facilities are unavailable.[42]

   — More elaborate and expensive techniques are available. These techniques include electric-powered warming vests; combustible-fueled warming belts and vests using charcoal, butane gas, or flammable liquids; and sophisticated truncal-centric heating mattresses.

■ Most heating devices should be applied first to the groin and axillary regions. Placement at these locations allows healthcare personnel unrestricted access to the patient's chest, neck, and arms for monitoring, diagnostic testing, and intravenous access.

   — Active external rewarming of truncal areas can rewarm at a rate of about 1°C (1.8°F) per hour.[35]

   — The number (and temperature) of heated devices applied to truncal areas determines the rewarming rate. Rewarming devices arrayed in the groin and axillae, around the neck, and next over the abdomen and then the chest can achieve even faster rewarming rates.

Box 5. Severe Hypothermia: <30°C (<86°F)

Active internal rewarming

■ The unique treatment for severe hypothermia is the addition of *active internal rewarming*. Note that during active internal rewarming both passive rewarming and active external rewarming of truncal areas should continue (see the Table).

■ Healthcare personnel can accomplish active internal rewarming with several techniques. No randomized, controlled clinical trials comparing the efficacy of these methods have been reported.[24]

   — Active internal rewarming should start with simple, inexpensive, and minimally invasive techniques, such as warm IV fluids and warm, humid oxygen.

   — Active internal rewarming techniques also include more complex and invasive interventions. *Peritoneal lavage* is one example of "run-in/run-out heated lavage." These moderately invasive techniques include lavage of the stomach, colon, bladder, pleural cavity, and mediastinum.

   — *Extracorporeal rewarming* includes full aortic-caval cannulation cardiopulmonary bypass[43] and a variety of femoral artery-vein (arterial-venous) and femoral vein-vein (veno-venous) bypass[44] methods.

   — *Esophageal rewarming tubes* can be inserted.

■ During active internal rewarming of hypothermic patients in cardiac arrest, rescuers should remember the following:

   — Use as many rewarming techniques simultaneously as possible while continuing CPR chest compressions and maintaining access to the patient.

   — Start with the simple and minimally invasive techniques. Progress to the more complex approaches as more resources and personnel become available. The following sequence may be used:

      • When the patient arrives in the ED, active external rewarming of truncal areas has already begun. The patient should be receiving warm, humid oxygen by tracheal tube and warm saline IV infusion.

      • ED staff place an electric heating pad under the trunk and abdomen and apply warmed plastic bags of IV solution to the axillae and groin.

      • The emergency physician opens a dialysis tray before inserting a peritoneal dialysis catheter to begin peritoneal lavage. In the nearby operating room, technicians are preparing a cardiac bypass device to initiate extracorporeal rewarming as soon as the surgical team arrives to start the procedure.

Box 6. Active Internal Rewarming

It is difficult to initiate an effective active internal rewarming strategy outside the hospital.[45] In fact, some experts think that active internal rewarming should be done only in hospital, though practice varies.[20,21]

Warm, humid oxygen (administered temperature: 42°C to 46°C or 108°F to 115°F)

■ Most experts recommend administration of warm, humid oxygen as a mainstay of active internal rewarming for victims with severe hypothermia but no cardiac arrest.[19-21,46,47] This method is particularly useful when other methods of internal rewarming are unavailable or delayed.[46]

■ With the aerosol heated to 40°C (104°F), this technique rewarms at a rate of 1°C to 1.5°C (1.8°F to 2.7°F) per hour. Heated to 45°C (113°F), rewarming rates increase to 1.5°C to 2°C (2.7°F to 3.6°F) per hour.[14,29,48]

Warm IV fluids (42°C to 44°C or 108°F to 111°F)

■ Infuse warm saline centrally at rates of approximately 150 to 200 mL/h IV.

■ Avoid excessive fluid administration; aim to provide sufficient fluid intake to maintain urinary output of 0.5 to 1 mL/kg per hour.

Peritoneal lavage (KCl-free fluid, warmed to 43°C or 109°F)

■ For peritoneal lavage use warm, potassium-free fluid. Administer 2 L at a time and then remove it, with zero dwell time, using Y-connector tubing.

■ Many experienced clinicians consider peritoneal lavage the preferred run-in/run-out heated lavage technique.[49]

Peritoneal lavage has several advantages for emergency active internal rewarming:

— Ready availability in most hospitals and Emergency Departments

— Simple equipment requirements

— No requirement for special training or technical skills

— Other anatomic sites may be used for heated lavage, including the stomach, colon, bladder, chest (closed thoracic cavity lavage),[14,29] and heart (direct cardiac lavage can be performed after open thoracotomy and cardiac massage).[50]

Extracorporeal rewarming (cardiac bypass)

■ Extracorporeal rewarming is the most effective technique for core rewarming of hypothermic patients in cardiac arrest.[51] When available this is the treatment of choice for these victims.

■ Extracorporeal rewarming techniques have considerable advantages:

— They provide adequate support of oxygenation, ventilation, and perfusion.

— They enable rapid rates of core rewarming (up to 1°C or 1.8°F every 5 minutes).[51]

■ Extracorporeal rewarming techniques have serious drawbacks:

— A requirement for special equipment that is unavailable in many hospitals

— A requirement for highly trained personnel

— Long delays imposed by the need to assemble the equipment and the specialized team and by the time needed to perform the procedures

■ Note that several other active internal rewarming techniques have resulted in neurologically intact survival from hypothermic cardiac arrest. These techniques include

— Peritoneal lavage[52]

— Peritoneal lavage combined with warm water bags, warm IV fluids, and continuous CPR[53]

— Continuous, closed thoracostomy lavage using 2 chest tubes[54,55]

— Forced, heated air[42,56] (an active external rewarming technique)

Esophageal rewarming tubes

■ Use of esophageal rewarming tubes in the United States has not been reported, but these tubes have been used extensively and successfully in Europe.[57]

Box 7. Continue Internal Rewarming

Continue internal rewarming until:

■ **Core temperature >35°C (95°F)** *or*

■ **Return of spontaneous circulation** *or*

■ **Resuscitative efforts cease**

■ During rewarming, patients who have been hypothermic for more than 45 to 60 minutes are likely to require volume administration because their vascular space expands with vasodilation. Healthcare providers must closely monitor heart rate and perfusion and hemodynamics at this time. Routine administration of steroids, barbiturates, or antibiotics has not been documented to help increase survival or decrease postresuscitation damage.[58,59]

■ Significant hyperkalemia may develop during rewarming.

— Extreme hyperkalemia has been reported in avalanche victims who sustain crushing injuries and hypothermia.[24]

— Severe hyperkalemia has also been reported among hypothermic patients who did not sustain crushing injuries.[29] In fact the severity of hyperkalemia has been linked with mortality.

— Management of hyperkalemia should follow the currently recommended ACLS guidelines. The recommendations include administration of calcium chloride, sodium bicarbonate, glucose plus insulin, and nebulized albuterol (see Chapter 5, Table 5, in this volume and the *ECC Handbook,* "Hyperkalemia, Sympathomimetic and Inotropic Drugs"). More aggressive measures to reduce extremely high serum potassium levels may include dialysis or exchange transfusion.

- Because severe hypothermia is frequently preceded by problems such as drug overdose, alcohol intoxication, or trauma, the clinician must look for and address these underlying conditions while treating the hypothermia. If the victim appears malnourished or has chronic alcoholism, administer thiamine (100 mg IV) early during rewarming. If submersion with asphyxiation preceded the victim's hypothermia, successful resuscitation will be unlikely.

- In the field rescuers may withhold resuscitation if the victim has obvious lethal injuries or if the body is frozen so completely that chest compressions are impossible and the nose and mouth are blocked with ice.[29]

- Many experienced clinicians subscribe to the aphorism that "hypothermic cardiac arrest patients are not dead until they're warm and dead."

  — The underlying principle here is that patients who appear dead after prolonged exposure to cold temperatures should be rewarmed to near-normal core temperatures while CPR and other resuscitative interventions are provided. If the victim remains in cardiac arrest, then cardiovascular unresponsiveness is confirmed and resuscitative efforts can be withdrawn.

  — Complete rewarming is not indicated for all victims. Physicians should use their clinical judgment to decide when resuscitative efforts should cease for a hypothermic arrest victim. Providers should act in the best interest of the patient and should not be guided by an aphorism.

Box 8. Hypothermic Cardiac Arrest

It is important to note that for cardiac arrest victims, rescuers should initiate BLS interventions without reference to core temperature. Temperature assessment and core-temperature-based decisions come later.

Start CPR

- The general BLS approach still targets airway, breathing, circulation, and AED-based defibrillation. The BLS provider, however, must modify some aspects of this treatment for hypothermic victims in cardiac arrest.

  — Pulse and respiratory rates will be slow, breathing will be shallow, and peripheral vasoconstriction will make pulses difficult to feel. For these reasons the BLS rescuer should first assess for breathing (for 30 to 45 seconds) and then for pulse (for 30 to 45 seconds) to confirm respiratory arrest, pulseless cardiac arrest, or bradycardia profound enough to require CPR.

  — If the victim is not breathing, initiate rescue breathing immediately. If possible and practical, administer warm, humid oxygen (42°C to 46°C or 108°F to 115°F) during bag-mask ventilation.

  — If the victim is also pulseless with no detectable signs of circulation, start chest compressions immediately. Do *not* withhold BLS until the temperature is measured or the victim is rewarmed.

Defibrillate VF/pulseless VT

- Clinical studies have not established the core body temperature at which defibrillation should first be attempted in hypothermic VF patients and how often it should be repeated. In general, rescuers should attempt defibrillation (up to 3 shocks) without regard to core body temperature. It is unacceptable to delay defibrillation attempts to assess core temperature.

- By giving 3 shocks the rescuer can document the presence of shock-refractory VF before it is necessary to determine core body temperature.

- If the victim has severe hypothermia (core temperature <30°C or <86°F), successful conversion to normal sinus rhythm may be impossible until rewarming is accomplished.[60]

Attempt, confirm, secure airway

- Rescuers should first attempt to provide ventilation with 100% oxygen by bag-mask after placement of an oropharyngeal airway.

- Tracheal intubation is required if the hypothermic victim is unconscious or if bag-mask ventilation is inadequate. Intubation will serve 2 purposes:

  — It will enable provision of effective ventilation with warm, humid oxygen.

  — It will isolate the airway to reduce the likelihood of aspiration.

- There have been some reports that physical manipulations (including tracheal or nasogastric intubation, temporary pacing, or insertion of a pulmonary artery catheter) can precipitate VF in victims of severe hypothermia.[61,62] But when procedures such as tracheal intubation or chest compressions are specifically and urgently indicated, do not withhold them.

  — In a prospective multicenter study of hypothermia victims, careful tracheal intubation did not result in a single incident of VF.[55] In fact the fear of precipitating VF during tracheal intubation may be exaggerated,[24] and it should not prevent or delay careful intubation.

Ventilate with warm, humid oxygen (42°C to 46°C or 108°F to 115°F)

Establish IV access

Infuse warm normal saline (43°C or 109°F)

Box 9. What Is Core Temperature?

- For the victim of hypothermia in cardiac arrest, rescuers should initiate CPR, attempt defibrillation with up to 3 shocks, and establish a secure airway without reference to the core temperature.

- Further care, in particular the administration of medications and additional defibrillation, is determined by the core temperature, specifically whether that core temperature is less than or greater than 30°C (86°F).

Box 10. Hypothermic Cardiac Arrest: Core Temperature <30°C (<86°F)

Continue CPR

Withhold IV medications

- Administration of epinephrine and vasopressin has been shown to improve coronary artery perfusion pressure in pigs during severe hypothermia with cardiac arrest.[63] But the human hypothermic heart may be unresponsive to cardioactive drugs, pacemaker stimulation, and defibrillation.[62] With markedly reduced drug metabolism, medications such as vasopressors and antiarrhythmics may accumulate to toxic levels if given repeatedly.

- For these reasons providers should *withhold IV medications* if the victim's core body temperature is <30°C (<86°F).

Defibrillation

- Clinical studies have not established the core body temperature at which defibrillation should first be attempted in hypothermic VF patients and how often it should be repeated. In general, rescuers should attempt defibrillation (up to 3 shocks) without regard to core body temperature. It is unacceptable to

delay defibrillation attempts to assess core temperature.

- The major modification in the guidelines for defibrillation is recommended when the hypothermia victim fails to respond to 3 shocks. Rescuers should defer subsequent defibrillation attempts until an accurate core temperature is obtained.

  — If the core temperature is <30°C (<86°F), continue to withhold defibrillation attempts (shocks). The fibrillating myocardium at that temperature is unlikely to respond.[62]

  — Shocks can resume whenever the core temperature is >30°C (86°F).

- Bradycardia may be a physiologic consequence of severe hypothermia, but cardiac pacing is unlikely to be effective. Cardiac pacing is not indicated unless bradycardia persists after rewarming to >30°C (>86°F).

Transport to hospital

- At this point in the algorithm, emergency responders should transport the hypothermic patient in persistent cardiac arrest to the nearest appropriate emergency facility. In-hospital personnel can initiate or continue active internal rewarming (see Box 6).

Box 11. Hypothermic Cardiac Arrest: Core Temperature >30°C (>86°F)

Continue CPR

Give IV medications as indicated

- With markedly reduced drug metabolism, medications such as vasopressors and antiarrhythmics may accumulate to toxic levels if given repeatedly.

- If the victim's core body temperature is >30°C (>86°F), *give IV medications* as indicated, but space them at longer than standard intervals. A commonly used, but non–evidence-based guide

for this interval is to double or triple the normal interval.

Defibrillation

- Clinical studies have not established the core body temperature at which defibrillation should first be attempted in hypothermic VF patients and how often it should be repeated. In general, rescuers should attempt defibrillation (up to 3 shocks) without regard to core body temperature. It is unacceptable to delay defibrillation attempts to assess core temperature.

- Shocks can resume whenever the core temperature is >30°C (86°F). Rescuers should use the recommended drug-shock, drug-shock pattern. Because resuscitation medications are being spaced at longer intervals, the shocks will also be farther apart.

Transport to hospital

- At this point in the algorithm emergency responders should transport the hypothermic patient in persistent cardiac arrest to the nearest appropriate emergency facility.

- In-hospital personnel can initiate or continue active internal rewarming (see Box 6). Note that active internal rewarming is indicated when the patient with hypothermia develops cardiac arrest even if the victim's core temperature is >30°C. Because the patient has suffered cardiac arrest, the hypothermia is severe, and the more rapid and consistent rewarming method (see Box 8) is indicated.

Therapeutic Hypothermia

In 2002 the results of 2 prospective randomized trials comparing mild hypothermia with normothermia in comatose survivors of out-of-hospital cardiac arrest were published.[26] One of these studies was undertaken in 9 centers in 5 European countries[19]; the other took place in 4 hospitals in Melbourne, Australia.[26] Both of these studies involved a highly select group of patients, excluding up to 92% of out-of-hospital cardiac arrest patients assessed initially for eligibility.[27] Exclusions included

■ Persistent hypotension (systolic blood pressure less than 90 mm Hg despite inotropes)

■ Causes of coma other than cardiac arrest (eg, head injury, drug overdose, cerebrovascular accident)

There seems good evidence to recommend the use of induced mild hypothermia in the comatose survivors of out-of-hospital cardiac arrest due to VF.[64] Many in-hospital cardiac arrests are of non-cardiac etiology, and as therapeutic hypothermia has not been studied to any significant extent in this population, the relative risks and benefits of the intervention are unknown. It is quite possible that patients remaining comatose after in-hospital arrest of cardiac etiology will also benefit from thera-peutic hypothermia. Until further data is available, therapeutic hypothermia should not be used for patients with severe cardio-genic shock or life-threatening arrhythmias, those who are pregnant, or those who have a primary coagulopathy.[64]

For further information about this state-ment, see the AHA ECC website **www.americanheart.org/cpr.**

Critical Concepts: Differentiating Cardiac Arrest Due to Hypothermia From Normothermic Cardiac Arrest in a Cold Environment

■ Hypothermia may exert a protective effect on the brain and organs if core body temperature drops rapidly while the victim is still breathing and has a pulse. But when emergency person-nel discover a victim of hypothermia in cardiac arrest, they may find it im-possible to resolve a critical question: Did the patient suffer a normothermic cardiac arrest in a cold environment, or did the patient have spontaneous circulation but suffer progressive hypothermia ending in apnea and cardiac asystole? This question is important because the answer has important prognostic implications.

— If the victim cools rapidly before arrest, a decrease in oxygen con-sumption and metabolism can precede the arrest and reduce organ ischemia.

— If the arrest occurs while the vic-tim is normothermic and then the victim later develops hypothermia, the hypothermia cannot exert any protective effect.

■ Emergency personnel and hospital providers are often unable to deter-mine the precise sequence of events, but they may be able to speculate based on the circumstances of the arrest.

— For example, a normothermic person experiencing VF arrest while shoveling snow will develop core body hypothermia only *after* the arrest.

— A lone cross-country skier with a compound tibia-fibula fracture may experience a drop in core temperature over many hours before cardiac arrest occurs.

■ The hypothermic victim also may have sustained additional organ insults before the arrest, such as asphyxiation from submersion. In cold water immersion, for example, significant hypothermia will occur rapidly. But it may be hypothermia-induced exhaustion followed by sub-mersion, aspiration, and hypoxia, with eventual cardiac arrest. Success-ful resuscitation may be very unlike-ly in such circumstances.

■ The recommended "default deci-sion" is for rescuers to initiate full BLS and ACLS interventions when it is clinically impossible to deter-mine whether the arrest or the hypo-thermia occurred first. Emergency care providers should modify these interventions as described in this chapter if significant hypothermia is documented.

References

1. Exposure-related hypothermia deaths—District of Columbia, 1972-1982. *MMWR Morb Mortal Wkly Rep.* 1982;31:669-671.

2. Hypothermia—United States. *MMWR Morb Mortal Wkly Rep.* 1983;32:46-48.

3. Hypothermia-associated deaths—United States, 1968-1980. *MMWR Morb Mortal Wkly Rep.* 1985;34:753-754.

4. Hypothermia prevention. *MMWR Morb Mortal Wkly Rep.* 1988;37:780-782.

5. Hypothermia-related deaths—Cook County, Illinois, November 1992-March 1993. *MMWR Morb Mortal Wkly Rep.* 1993;42:917-919.

6. Hypothermia-related deaths—North Carolina, November 1993-March 1994. *MMWR Morb Mortal Wkly Rep.* 1994;43:849, 855-846.

7. Hypothermia-related deaths—New Mexico, October 1993-March 1994. *MMWR Morb Mortal Wkly Rep.* 1995;44:933-935.

8. Hypothermia-related deaths—Vermont, Oc-tober 1994-February 1996. *MMWR Morb Mortal Wkly Rep.* 1996;45:1093-1095.

9. Hypothermia-related deaths—Virginia, No-vember 1996-April 1997. *MMWR Morb Mortal Wkly Rep.* 1997;46:1157-1159.

10. Hypothermia-related deaths—Georgia, January 1996-December 1997, and United States, 1979-1995. *MMWR Morb Mortal Wkly Rep.* 1998;47:1037-1040.

11. Hypothermia-related deaths—Alaska, Octo-ber 1998-April 1999, and trends in the United States, 1979-1996. *MMWR Morb Mortal Wkly Rep.* 2000;49:11-14.

12. Hypothermia-related deaths—Suffolk County, New York, January 1999-March 2000, and United States, 1979-1998. *MMWR Morb Mortal Wkly Rep.* 2001;50:53-57.

13. Hypothermia-related deaths—Utah, 2000, and United States, 1979-1998. *MMWR Morb Mortal Wkly Rep.* 2002;51:76-78.

14. Miller JW, Danzl DF, Thomas DM. Urban accidental hypothermia: 135 cases. *Ann Emerg Med.* 1980;9:456-461.

15. Steinman AM, Giesbrecht G. Immersion into cold water. In: Auerbach PS, ed. *Wilderness Medicine: Management of Wilderness and Environmental Emergencies.* 4th ed. St Louis, Mo: Mosby; 2002:197-225.

16. Tipton M, Eglin C, Gennser M, Golden F. Immersion deaths and deterioration in swimming performance in cold water. *Lancet.* 1999; 354:626-629.

17. Ryan JM. Immersion deaths and swim failure—implications for resuscitation and prevention [editorial]. *Lancet.* 1999;354:613.

18. Teramoto S, Ouchi Y. Swimming in cold water. *Lancet.* 1999;354:1733.

19. Delaney K. Hypothermic sudden death. In: Paradis NA, Halperin HR, Nowak R, eds. *Cardiac Arrest: The Science and Practice of Resuscitation Medicine.* Baltimore, Md: Williams & Wilkins; 1996:745-760.

20. Danzl DF. Accidental hypothermia. In: Rosen P, Barkin R, eds. *Emergency Medicine: Concepts and Clinical Practice.* St Louis, Mo: Mosby; 1998:963-986.

21. Danzl DF. Accidental hypothermia. In: Auerbach PS, ed. *Wilderness Medicine: Management of Wilderness and Environmental Emergencies.* 4th ed. St Louis, Mo: Mosby; 2002: 135-177.

22. Holzer M, Behringer W, Schorkhuber W, Zeiner A, Sterz F, Laggner AN, Frass M, Siostrozonek P, Ratheiser K, Kaff A. Mild hypothermia and outcome after CPR. Hypothermia for Cardiac Arrest (HACA) Study Group. *Acta Anaesthesiol Scand Suppl.* 1997; 111:55-58.

23. Sterz F, Safar P, Tisherman S, Radovsky A, Kuboyama K, Oku K. Mild hypothermic cardiopulmonary resuscitation improves outcome after prolonged cardiac arrest in dogs. *Crit Care Med.* 1991;19:379-389.

24. Larach MG. Accidental hypothermia. *Lancet.* 1995;345:493-498.

25. Gilbert M, Busund R, Skagseth A, Nilsen PÅ, Solbø JP. Resuscitation from accidental hypothermia of 13.7°C with circulatory arrest. *Lancet.* 2000;355:375-376.

26. Bernard SA, Gray TW, Buist MD, Jones BM, Silvester W, Gutteridge G, Smith K. Treatment of comatose survivors of out-of-hospital cardiac arrest with induced hypothermia. *N Engl J Med.* 2002;346:557-563.

27. Hypothermia After Cardiac Arrest Study Group. Mild therapeutic hypothermia to improve the neurologic outcome after cardiac arrest. *N Engl J Med.* 2002;346:549-556.

28. Woodhouse P, Keatinge WR, Coleshaw SR. Factors associated with hypothermia in patients admitted to a group of inner city hospitals. *Lancet.* 1989;2:1201-1205.

29. Danzl DF, Pozos RS, Auerbach PS, Glazer S, Goetz W, Johnson E, Jui J, Lilja P, Marx JA, Miller J, Mills W Jr, Nowak R, Shields R, Vicario S, Wayne M. Multicenter hypothermia survey. *Ann Emerg Med.* 1987;16:1042-1055.

30. Gallaher MM, Fleming DW, Berger LR, Sewell CM. Pedestrian and hypothermia deaths among Native Americans in New Mexico: between bar and home. *JAMA.* 1992;267:1345-1348.

31. Hayward JS, Eckerson JD. Physiological responses and survival time prediction for humans in ice-water. *Aviat Space Environ Med.* 1984;55:206-211.

32. Nozaki R, Ishibashi K, Adachi N, Nishihara S, Adachi S. Accidental profound hypothermia [letter]. *N Engl J Med.* 1986;315:1680.

33. Reed HL, Shakir KM. Diuresis related to cold exposure. *JAMA.* 1985;253:776-777.

34. Allen DE, Gellai M. Mechanisms for the diuresis of acute cold exposure: role for vasopressin? *Am J Physiol.* 1993;264(3 pt 2): R524-R532.

35. Greif R, Rajek A, Laciny S, Bastanmehr H, Sessler DI. Resistive heating is more effective than metallic-foil insulation in an experimental model of accidental hypothermia: a randomized controlled trial. *Ann Emerg Med.* 2000;35:337-345.

36. Kober A, Scheck T, Fulesdi B, Lieba F, Vlach W, Friedman A, Sessler DI. Effectiveness of resistive heating compared with passive warming in treating hypothermia associated with minor trauma: a randomized trial. *Mayo Clin Proc.* 2001;76:369-375.

37. Giesbrecht GG, Sessler DI, Mekjavic IB, Schroeder M, Bristow GK. Treatment of mild immersion hypothermia by direct body-to-body contact. *J Appl Physiol.* 1994;76:2373-2379.

38. Lindhoff GA, MacG Palmer JH. An assessment of the thermal safety of microwave warming of crystalloid fluids. *Anaesthesia.* 2000;55:251-254.

39. Giesbrecht GG, Pachu P, Xu X. Design and evaluation of a portable rigid forced-air warming cover for prehospital transport of cold patients. *Aviat Space Environ Med.* 1998;69: 1200-1203.

40. Giesbrecht GG, Ducharme MB, McGuire JP. Comparison of forced-air patient warming systems for perioperative use. *Anesthesiology.* 1994;80:671-679.

41. Giesbrecht GG, Schroeder M, Bristow GK. Treatment of mild immersion hypothermia by forced-air warming. *Aviat Space Environ Med.* 1994;65:803-808.

42. Koller R, Schnider TW, Neidhart P. Deep accidental hypothermia and cardiac arrest—rewarming with forced air. *Acta Anaesthesiol Scand.* 1997;41:1359-1364.

43. Dobson JA, Burgess JJ. Resuscitation of severe hypothermia by extracorporeal rewarming in a child. *J Trauma.* 1996;40:483-485.

44. Waters DJ, Belz M, Lawse D, Ulstad D. Portable cardiopulmonary bypass: resuscitation from prolonged ice-water submersion and asystole. *Ann Thorac Surg.* 1994;57: 1018-1019.

45. Sterba JA. Efficacy and safety of prehospital rewarming techniques to treat accidental hypothermia. *Ann Emerg Med.* 1991;20:896-901.

46. Weinberg AD. The role of inhalation rewarming in the early management of hypothermia. *Resuscitation.* 1998;36:101-104.

47. Giesbrecht GG, Paton B. Review article on inhalation rewarming. *Resuscitation.* 1998; 38:59-60.

48. Hayward JS, Eckerson JD, Kemna D. Thermal and cardiovascular changes during three methods of resuscitation from mild hypothermia. *Resuscitation.* 1984;11:21-33.

49. Otto RJ, Metzler MH. Rewarming from experimental hypothermia: comparison of heated aerosol inhalation, peritoneal lavage, and pleural lavage. *Crit Care Med.* 1988;16: 869-875.

50. Brunette DD, McVaney K. Hypothermic cardiac arrest: an 11 year review of ED management and outcome. *Am J Emerg Med.* 2000; 18:418-422.

51. Walpoth BH, Walpoth-Aslan BN, Mattle HP, Radanov BP, Schroth G, Schaeffler L, Fischer AP, von Segesser L, Althaus U. Outcome of survivors of accidental deep hypothermia and circulatory arrest treated with extracorporeal blood warming. *N Engl J Med.* 1997;337: 1500-1505.

52. Pickering BG, Bristow GK, Craig DB. Case history number 97: core rewarming by peritoneal irrigation in accidental hypothermia with cardiac arrest. *Anesth Analg.* 1977;56: 574-577.

53. Lexow K. Severe accidental hypothermia: survival after 6 hours 30 minutes of cardiopulmonary resuscitation. *Arctic Med Res.* 1991;50(suppl 6):112-114.

54. Iversen RJ, Atkin SH, Jaker MA, Quadrel MA, Tortella BJ, Odom JW. Successful CPR in a severely hypothermic patient using continuous thoracostomy lavage. *Ann Emerg Med.* 1990;19:1335-1337.

55. Hall KN, Syverud SA. Closed thoracic cavity lavage in the treatment of severe hypothermia in human beings. *Ann Emerg Med.* 1990;19: 204-206.

56. Kornberger E, Schwarz B, Lindner KH, Mair P. Forced air surface rewarming in patients with severe accidental hypothermia. *Resuscitation.* 1999;41:105-111.

57. Kristensen G, Drenck NE, Jordening H. Simple system for central rewarming of hypothermic patients. *Lancet.* 1986;2:1467-1468.

58. Moss J. Accidental severe hypothermia. *Surg Gynecol Obstet.* 1986;162:501-513.

59. Safar P. Cerebral resuscitation after cardiac arrest: research initiatives and future directions [published erratum appears in *Ann Emerg Med.* 1993;22:759]. *Ann Emerg Med.* 1993; 22:324-349.

60. Southwick FS, Dalglish PH Jr. Recovery after prolonged asystolic cardiac arrest in profound hypothermia: a case report and literature review. *JAMA*. 1980;243:1250-1253.

61. Schneider SM. Hypothermia: from recognition to rewarming. *Emerg Med Rep*. 1992;13:1-20.

62. Reuler JB. Hypothermia: pathophysiology, clinical settings, and management. *Ann Intern Med*. 1978;89:519-527.

63. Krismer AC, Lindner KH, Kornberger R, Wenzel V, Mueller G, Hund W, Oroszy S, Lurie KG, Mair P. Cardiopulmonary resuscitation during severe hypothermia in pigs: does epinephrine or vasopressin increase coronary perfusion pressure? *Anesth Analg*. 2000;90:69-73.

64. Therapeutic hypothermia after cardiac arrest. An advisory statement by the Advanced Life Support Task Force of the International Liaison Committee on Resuscitation (ILCOR). *Circulation*. In press.

Special Resuscitation Situations
Part 2: Submersion

Submersion: Overview

■ Submersion events, imprecisely referred to as *drowning* or *near-drowning* (see "Submersion Definitions" below), are most common in the pediatric and young adult age groups.[1-3] These events can be traumatic for the relatives and loved ones of victims and for emergency providers.

— Parents, baby-sitters, or guardians may experience grief and guilt for failing to protect the victim. They may also feel intense anger toward others who did not provide adequate supervision.

— Neighbors, friends, bystanders, and emergency personnel may feel guilty for participating in a rescue attempt that resulted in death or neurologic impairment.

■ Many issues surrounding prevention of submersion events are complex and controversial:

— Appropriate targets for injury prevention efforts.[4]

— Siblings bathing together without adult supervision.[5] In one study from Utah every bathtub drowning occurred when siblings were bathing together without adult supervision.[5] Submersions occurred when one sibling reportedly stood or sat on another or held a sibling under the water.[5]

— Pediatric "drowning proofing" is an unproven concept[6] that is specifically discouraged by the American Academy of Pediatrics.[7]

— Legal ordinances for swimming supervision[8] and pool fencing vary widely.[9-12]

— Legal ordinances regulating water sports, personal watercraft,[13,14] boating,[15] life vests,[16] and flotation devices[17] vary widely.[18]

— Some submersion episodes that involve homicide,[19] manslaughter,[20] and suicide[21-23] are euphemistically termed "nonaccidental" or "intentional" drownings.

■ Many fatal submersion events or those that result in neurologic impairment are preventable tragedies. Many are the result of poor judgment, alcohol consumption,[24-27] or inadequate supervision of children.[5,26]

■ Despite the ACLS emphasis on immediate treatment, the definitive therapy for submersion events is *prevention*. As in cardiac arrests associated with hypothermia (see Part 1 of this chapter) or trauma (see Part 5 of this chapter), the most effective way to reduce the number of deaths due to submersion is to prevent the initiating event or provide immediate treatment to prevent a cardiac arrest. Once a victim of submersion, hypothermia, or trauma deteriorates to a state of cardiac arrest, the chances for a successful outcome are minimal.

■ Rescue of submersion victims occurs on or near the water, exposing rescue teams to danger. Never forget the principle of rescuer safety: rescuers should make sure the area is safe and should avoid becoming second victims.

Pathophysiology

Submersion leads to hypoxia that can ultimately cause cardiac arrest.

■ Submersion hypoxia can produce other complications, including hypoxic encephalopathy and acute respiratory distress syndrome (ARDS). These complications of submersion events are beyond the scope of this chapter.

■ The duration of hypoxia is the critical determinant of submersion outcome. The duration of hypoxia can be reduced first by early rescue from the water, then by immediate provision of basic and advanced life support. Rapid **A**irway and **B**reathing support play the major role in resuscitation from submersion. This emphasis contrasts with emphasis on rapid initiation of **C**hest compressions and **D**efibrillation, appropriate for most adult victims of sudden cardiac arrests.

Rescuers should be prepared to treat trauma (see Part 5 of this chapter) or hypothermia (see Part 1) that may be associated with submersion.

■ Submersion victims may require cervical spine precautions. C-spine immobilization is recommended for victims of submersion associated with trauma, such as a dive or fall into water.[28] If you are unsure if trauma occurred, assume that C-spine immobilization is needed.

- Submersion victims may develop primary or secondary hypothermia:

  — *Primary hypothermia* can develop when a submersion occurs in icy water (<5°C, <41°F). In icy water core body hypothermia may develop before the submersion causes significant hypoxia. It is possible that such cold-water submersion may provide some protection from hypoxia and organ ischemia. The published studies reporting good outcome from prolonged submersion describe young, small victims submerged in icy water.

  — *Secondary hypothermia* occurs as a consequence of heat loss through evaporation after rescue from the water and during attempted resuscitation. Hypothermia in these victims offers no protective effects.

Submersion Definitions

Unsatisfactory Nomenclature

A number of experts have noted that there are almost as many terms for drowning and submersion events as there are authors.[1-3]

- People often incorrectly apply the term *drowning* to victims who die within 24 hours of a submersion episode. But the term should apply only to submersion victims who fail to regain or maintain a pulse and respirations after initial resuscitative efforts.

- The term *near-drowning* is applied to submersion victims who survive more than 24 hours, but only if active interventions were needed for one or more submersion complications. Such complications can include pneumonia, ARDS, sepsis, or neurologic sequelae.

- Rescuers and emergency personnel find these definitions irrelevant because 24 hours must pass before the distinction can be made between drowning and near-drowning.

Table 1 presents many of the terms used in discussions about submersion, the conventional definitions, and some shortcomings of the terms. It is obvious that these terms and definitions lack many of the essential criteria for a successful nomenclature:

- The definitions are not based on consensus; the terms have different meanings for different users. In published articles the terms are defined by individual assertion rather than by international, multispecialty consensus.

- The terms do not adequately discriminate among mutually exclusive sets of patients.

- The terms fail to reflect different levels of severity and lack any relationship to outcomes.

- The terms fail to reflect clinical reality because many victims cannot be classified until hours, even days, pass.

- The terms fail to guide clinical care because they are unrelated to prognosis or outcome.

- The classification of victims is not based on simple or readily applied assessments.

The Need for Uniform Definitions and Reporting

As suggested above, researchers, EMS managers, and clinicians need a uniform approach for international reporting of submersion outcomes. Researchers in the area of out-of-hospital resuscitation faced a similar problem in the 1970s and 1980s.[32,33] In the early 1990s international efforts led to the development of the "Utstein Style for Uniform Reporting of Outcomes From Cardiac Arrest" for out-of-hospital events,[34] in-hospital events,[35] and pediatric cardiopulmonary emergencies.[36]

Critical Concepts: Prevention of Submersion Episodes

- Keep only a few inches of water in the bathtub when bathing young children. Never leave young children unsupervised in bathtubs.

- Never leave children alone in or near the pool even for a moment.

- Be sure adults and adolescents are trained in CPR so that they can rescue a child if necessary.

- Surround your pool on all 4 sides with a sturdy 5-foot fence. The house should not form one of the barriers to the pool if there is a doorway from the home to the pool area. Be sure that the gates self-close and self-latch at a height that children cannot reach.

- Keep rescue equipment—a shepherd's hook (a long pole with a hook on the end) and a life preserver—and a portable telephone near the pool.

- Avoid inflatable swimming aids such as "floaties." They are *not* a substitute for approved life vests and can give children a false sense of security.

- Generally children are not developmentally ready for swim lessons until after their fourth birthday.[7] Swim programs for children under 4 should *not* be seen as a way to decrease the risk of drowning.

- Whenever infants or toddlers are in or around water, an adult should be within arm's length, providing "touch supervision."

Proposed Approach to Defining and Grading Submersion Events

To stimulate international discussion of the shortcomings of submersion nomenclature and initiate preliminary solutions,

TABLE 1. Submersion-Related Nomenclature: Conventional Definitions and Shortcomings

Term	Conventional Definition	Shortcomings
Submersion event *(Also may be referred to as "drowning event")*	■ A person's head (or airway openings) becomes covered or stays covered with liquid (usually water) ■ Duration is sufficient to pose a risk of hypoxia ■ Aspiration into the hypopharynx, trachea, or bronchioles occurs to a degree that induces repeated coughing	■ Covers such a wide range of events that some grading of pathophysiologic severity must be used[29]: — Grade 0: Submersion does not induce coughing — Grade 1: Small aspiration results in coughing but normal lung auscultation — Grade 2: Small aspiration produces coughing and rales in one lung — Grade 3: Acute pulmonary edema (rales in both lungs), normal cardiac function (no hypotension) — Grade 4: Acute pulmonary edema (rales in both lungs), impaired cardiac function and hypotension — Grade 5: No spontaneous respirations, pulse present — Grade 6: No spontaneous respirations, no pulse
Drowning	■ Death from suffocation after a submersion event in liquid (usually water) ■ Death <24 hours after a submersion event	■ A postmortem term that should be applied only to people who have died from a submersion event. ■ A more precise definition would be failure to regain a pulse after initial resuscitative efforts.
Near-drowning	■ Survival for >24 hours after a submersion event ■ Event must be severe enough to require some medical intervention for submersion-related complications	■ An ambiguous term because it implies that all near-drowning victims survive. But it includes deaths from complications >24 hours after submersion.
Submersion syndrome	■ A term proposed to cover both drowning and near-drowning after a submersion episode (head goes below water)	■ More precision cannot be gained by lumping together 2 imprecisely defined terms. ■ People seldom are aware of or make the important distinctions between *immersion* and *submersion*.
Immersion syndrome	■ Sudden death after immersion (not submersion) in very cold water ■ Probably due to an arrhythmia induced by vagal stimulation	■ Often confused with *cold water immersion* (<25°C or <77°F),[30] which poses risks of hypothermia and submersion secondary to hypothermia (ie, swim failure).
Secondary drowning	■ Death occurring minutes to days after a near-drowning episode from a complication of the submersion	■ A problem term because it classifies death by initial event, not by complications (eg, ARDS). ■ Overlaps in some patients with near-drowning.
Postimmersion syndrome	■ Deterioration (not death) of an apparently well victim after a submersion event	■ Can be confused with immersion syndrome. ■ *Immersion* has a different meaning than *submersion*.

(Continued on next page)

TABLE 1. Submersion-Related Nomenclature: Conventional Definitions and Shortcomings (Continued)

Term	Conventional Definition	Shortcomings
"Wet" drowning or near-drowning	■ A drowning or near-drowning that occurs *with* significant aspiration ■ Occurs when a large amount of water enters the lungs	■ Unclear whether water entered because of respiratory efforts or passively after death. ■ A distinction between "wet" and "dry" has little or no clinical significance.
"Dry" drowning or near-drowning	■ A drowning or near-drowning that occurs *without* significant aspiration ■ Occurs when laryngospasm blocks entrance of water into the lungs	■ Found in <10% of drowning victims who go to autopsy. ■ Disputed by some experts. If no water is in lungs at autopsy, victim may have died before the submersion.[31] ■ If coughing is universally accepted as a critical finding, this term would disappear.

participants in the Guidelines 2000 Conference developed an approach to grading submersion episodes (Figure 1). This algorithm can be used by epidemiologists to support a prospective database of submersion cases.

The algorithm is largely derived from the work of Szpilman and his Brazilian collaborators.[29] It has been validated retrospectively, demonstrating a relationship to outcomes (Table 2). In the summer of 2002 the AHA cosponsored an international symposium on defining and grading submersion events. Participants expressed agreement with the general principles of this algorithm and reviewed early drafts of the Figure. The final version (Figure) reflects a number of modifications derived from this symposium. Continued use and evaluation of this algorithm, as well as final recommendations from the 2002 and subsequent symposia, could lead to future revisions and increased effectiveness.

The Proposed Submersion Episode Grading Algorithm: Underlying Concepts

■ Definitions of submersion events should reflect the pathophysiology of submersion.

— The pathophysiology of submersion represents a continuum from the moment of involuntary *submersion*

(head slips under the water), followed by some degree of aspiration, ineffective and then absent breathing, and then progressive hypoxia leading to irreversible apnea and then asystole (*drowning death*).

■ An effective grading system needs to reflect clinical signs demonstrated in

victims rescued during the stages in the submersion continuum.

— **Submersion:** The initial stage is an actual *submersion*. The head slips under water (or other liquid), there is no access to air, and some hypoxia develops, with some aspiration of fluid into the hypopharynx,

TABLE 2. Severity Grades for Submersion Events Based on Clinical Findings With Associated Mortality Rates

Severity Grade	Clinical Findings	Mortality (%)[29]
1	Some coughing, normal auscultation	0
2	Coughing; with abnormal auscultation: rales in some lung fields on one side	0.6
3	Coughing; abnormal auscultation with acute pulmonary edema (bilateral rales); good cardiac function (no hypotension)	5.2
4	Coughing; abnormal auscultation with acute pulmonary edema (bilateral rales) with poor cardiac function (hypotension)	19.4
5	No spontaneous respirations, pulse is present	44
6	Cardiopulmonary arrest: no spontaneous breathing, no pulse	93

trachea, and lungs. "Submersion" is not really a problem until either hypoxia or aspiration occurs. Otherwise a person is simply swimming under water or voluntarily holding his/her breath.

— **Aspiration:** Experienced observers consider entrance of water into the respiratory passages with resultant stimulation of gag and cough reflexes as an essential stage in submersion events. *Coughing* is a critical dichotomous assessment point (Box 6). Coughing is an obvious physical sign with prognostic significance. If the victim is not coughing and has normal lung auscultation, the victim is classified as a *water rescue*. Although aspiration is assumed to occur during the stereotypical "struggle to keep the head above water," observers report many different scenarios. Modell eloquently presents the range of submersion events that observers describe.[37]

— **Apnea or breathlessness:** Absence of spontaneous breathing is an unambiguous physical sign that also relates to outcomes. Many submersion definitions fail to mention presence or absence of spontaneous breathing when rescuers get the victim to shore or to a location where they can initiate resuscitative efforts.

— **Spontaneous circulation:** If the period of hypoxia is prolonged, the heart stops beating. Hypoxia produces a well-established sequence of cardiac deterioration with tachycardia, then bradycardia, then a pulseless phase of ineffective cardiac contractions (PEA or VF/pulseless VT phase), followed by complete loss of cardiac rhythm and electrical activity (asystole). For this reason the absence of a pulse and other signs of circulation are easily assessed by rescuers, and their absence suggests that significant hypoxia has developed.

Outcome of Submersion

The Challenges

Emergency care providers face a number of difficult questions when attempting resuscitation of submersion victims:

■ Should rescuers attempt resuscitation for a 60-year-old victim pulled from a tropical vacation swimming pool cyanotic, cold, breathless, and pulseless after 10 minutes of submersion?

■ What is the prognosis for a 5-year-old child who is cyanotic, cold, breathless, and pulseless when he is pulled from a frozen pond 30 minutes after falling through the ice and slipping underwater?

■ Should Emergency Department personnel continue CPR and ACLS interventions for submersion victims who remain breathless and pulseless after 40 minutes of resuscitative efforts in the field? What if a family member or emergency responder risked his/her life in recovering the victim from the water?

■ What is the value of restoring a heartbeat and spontaneous respirations to a child whose chance of meaningful neurologic recovery is virtually zero?

Such clinical and ethical challenges have stimulated considerable interest in outcome prediction for submersion victims. Accurate outcome prediction would assist rescuers in recognizing

■ Fatal submersion events for which resuscitative efforts should not be started

■ Submersion events for which resuscitative efforts should be stopped in the field without "lights and siren" transport

Accurate outcome prediction would also help prevent the tragedy of successful restoration of a beating heart and breathing lungs for victims with devastating and irreversible hypoxic neurologic insult.

Research in Outcome Prediction

Predictors of outcome have been generated on the basis of retrospective surveys and epidemiologic analyses rather than prospective studies. Retrospective analyses of a large observational database of submersions in children and adolescents (up to 20 years of age) from King County and Seattle, Washington, have contributed valuable insight into submersion outcome.[27,38-40] This work confirmed duration of submersion as the most powerful predictor of outcome.[40] With increasing duration of submersion, the following associations with death or severe neurologic impairment were observed:

■ 0 to <5 minutes: 10%

■ 5 to <10 minutes: 56%

■ 10 to <25 minutes: 88%

■ 25 minutes: 100%

Note how 5 more minutes of submersion in the 5 to <10 minutes group increases mortality almost 6 times compared with the 0 to <5 minutes group.

In a further analysis of 77 pediatric submersion victims for whom EMS personnel attempted resuscitation, 100% mortality was associated with the following factors[39]:

■ Submersion duration >25 minutes

■ Resuscitation duration >25 minutes

■ Pulseless cardiac arrest on arrival in the ED

Slightly lower mortality rates were also associated with the following factors[39]:

■ VT/VF was observed on the initial field ECG: 93% mortality

■ Pupils were dilated and unresponsive to light on arrival in the ED: 89% mortality

■ Severe acidosis was documented in the ED: 89% mortality

■ Respiratory arrest occurred after arrival in the ED: 87% mortality

FIGURE. Proposed Algorithm for Grading of Submersion Episodes to Facilitate Uniform International Reporting

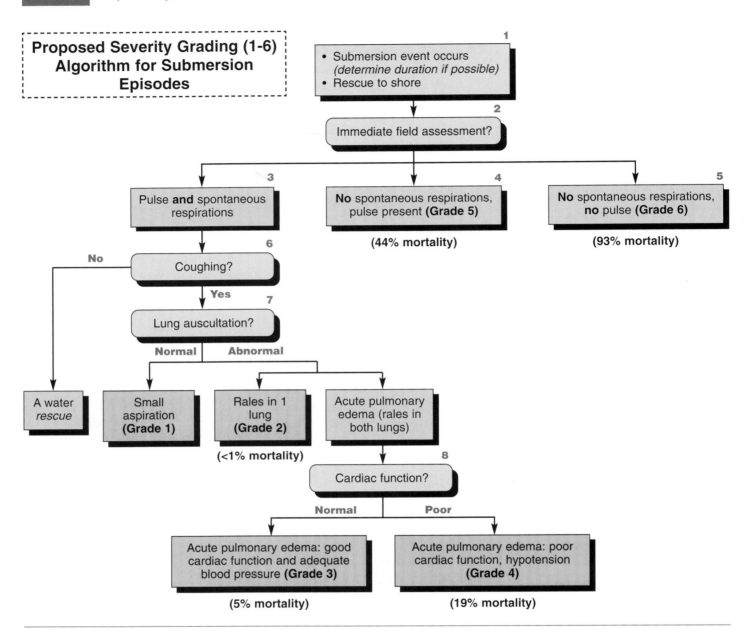

- Victims never regained consciousness, remaining comatose at the scene and on arrival at the hospital: 100% mortality

Submersion victims who have spontaneous circulation and breathing in the field, before arrival at the ED, usually recover with good neurologic outcomes. In the King County database, no deaths occurred among victims who were responsive at the scene or in the ED.[27]

Several classification systems have attempted to use clinical findings as predictors of outcome for submersion victims.[29,37] The most coherent and logical approach derives from a long-term analysis of 1831 submersion episodes from the beaches of Brazil.[29]

Unlike other researchers in this area, Szpilman and colleagues[29] did not start with an implicitly derived classification scheme and force each case into the

scheme. Instead they derived the classification grades empirically after recognizing that the worse the cardiopulmonary compromise, the worse the mortality rate (see Table 2). The Szpilman classification system is based on identification of cardiopulmonary compromise that is easily assessed by an on-scene physician using only 4 variables: coughing (yes or no), auscultation of the lungs, blood pressure, and heart rate.[29]

Critical Concepts: Application of Proposed Grading Algorithm for Submersion Episodes

Box 1

- A submersion event occurs. If possible determine the duration of submersion.

- If the rescuer can do so safely, the rescuer should open the victim's airway and check breathing and provide rescue breaths in the water if needed.

- Proceed with rescue to shore. Pay close attention to safety of both rescuer and victim. Take C-spine precautions (maintain cervical spine immobilization) as indicated.

Box 2

- After the victim is rescued to shore (or another firm surface), immediately assess the ABCs of BLS: airway, breathing, and circulation.

- Immediately initiate all indicated BLS, ACLS, and pediatric resuscitation interventions based on the presence or absence of a patent airway, spontaneous respirations, and spontaneous pulse. These interventions include the following:

  — Send a second rescuer to phone 911. The lone rescuer should remain with the victim and provide 1 minute of rescue support (whatever steps of CPR are needed) before leaving the victim to phone 911.

  — Provide basic life support, including all elements of the primary ABCs. When indicated provide ventilations and chest compressions. Continue until a defibrillator is available.

  — Once an AED is available, check for the presence of VF/VT ("shockable rhythm") and deliver defibrillatory shocks if indicated.

  — Provide advanced adult and pediatric life support, including insertion of airway devices, establishment of IV access, and administration of IV medications.

Box 3

- Submersion victims with spontaneous respirations and a sustained pulse are classified on the basis of 3 criteria:

  — Coughing (Box 6)

  — Lung auscultation (Box 7)

  — Cardiac function, eg, blood pressure (Box 8)

Box 4

- Submersion victims who have no spontaneous respirations but have a detectable pulse are classified as *Grade 5*. On the warm-water beaches of Brazil with rapid BLS- and ACLS-level response teams, 56% of submersion victims with a severity of Grade 5 survive to hospital discharge.[29]

- If spontaneous respirations cannot be restored during resuscitative efforts and spontaneous cardiac activity ceases (asystole), treat as a *Grade 6* (Box 5).

Box 5

- Submersion victims who have no spontaneous respirations and no pulse on initial field assessment are classified as *Grade 6*. In Brazil only 7% of these nonbreathing, pulseless submersion victims survive to hospital discharge.[29]

- Victims are classified as *drowning deaths* if they fail to respond to initial resuscitative efforts and fail to regain or sustain spontaneous respirations and pulse.

Box 6

- Auscultate the lungs. Assess whether victim is coughing.

- Coughing in submersion victims implies water aspiration.

- Submersion victims who are not coughing, have clear lungs on auscultation, and have maintained spontaneous circulation and respirations since rescue to shore are classified as *water rescues*.

- Submersion victims who are coughing repeatedly are further classified by the findings on lung auscultation.

Box 7

- The auscultation findings are used to further classify submersion victims with coughing:

  — Grade 1: Normal lung auscultation. Because these victims have been coughing, they are considered to have aspirated only a small amount of water.

  — Grade 2: Lung auscultation reveals some rales, but in only one lung.

  — Grades 3 and 4: Lung auscultation reveals *acute pulmonary edema* (rales in both lungs). See Box 8 to separate Grade 3 from Grade 4.

Box 8

- In victims with acute pulmonary edema (rales in both lungs), cardiac function and blood pressure distinguish between Grades 3 and 4:

  — Grade 3: Good cardiac function and adequate blood pressure (5% mortality reported in Brazil[29])

  — Grade 4: Impaired cardiac function and hypotension (19% mortality reported in Brazil[29])

Outcome Prediction for Submersion Victims: Conclusions

Fate Factors but No System Factors for Submersion Victims

Adult Out-of-Hospital Cardiac Arrest

The landmark work of Eisenberg et al[41] on out-of-hospital cardiac arrest identified what he termed *fate factors* and *system factors*.

- *Fate factors* are age, gender, initial arrest rhythm, location of arrest, and whether the arrest was witnessed. Although probability of survival is related to these factors, they cannot be changed or modified by rescuers.

- *System factors* include time to CPR, time to defibrillation, and time to and quality of early advanced care. These factors are amenable to effective organization and implementation of prehospital care. Community-based efforts to improve system factors and establish a strong Chain of Survival have revolutionized the approach to emergency medical services worldwide.[42]

Submersion Events

The epidemiologic studies of submersion events paint a pessimistic picture for improving submersion outcomes. Multiple studies have established that outcome is determined largely by a single fate factor—

duration of submersion.[29,39,40,43,44] The longer it takes to identify and rescue a submersion victim, the worse the outcome.

The duration of hypoxia during submersion cannot be changed despite the best BLS and ALS efforts. Immediate bystander CPR, however, can limit the duration of hypoxia to the time of submersion only. Delayed CPR results in a longer period of hypoxia.

Immediate provision of BLS and early ALS contribute to the best outcome possible, given the duration of submersion. Nonetheless the relative contributions of these interventions are modest at best. Table 3 illustrates this problem. (Note that these are not published figures but rather data extrapolated from published sources.[29,39,40,43,44])

Table 3 shows that early BLS and ACLS significantly improve the chances of survival. But this data also shows the greater power that duration of submersion exerts over outcome. For example, victims rescued from the water within 5 minutes of submersion have a 70% chance of survival with late BLS and ACLS care and a 90% chance with immediate care. A person rescued from the water several minutes later, after 5 to <10 minutes of submersion, has markedly lower chances of survival regardless of whether BLS and ACLS care is immediate (44%), early (35%), or late (30%).

Although survival from submersion episodes has increased in recent years, this increase does not appear to be attributable to improvements in medical treatment.[27]

"Do-Not-Start" and "When-to-Stop" Guidelines for Submersion Events

With the duration of submersion such a powerful determinant of outcome, one obvious guideline for emergency personnel would be not to initiate resuscitative efforts for a submersion victim with no respirations, no pulse, and a duration of submersion >25 minutes. But there are 2 critical problems with this guideline:

- It is often impossible to determine the precise duration of submersion.

- There are well-publicized anecdotes of successful resuscitations after prolonged submersions. The survivors in these cases are almost exclusively young children submerged in icy cold water, and many of these "survivors" have severe neurologic impairment. It is impossible to derive valid information from lay press reports of submersions or rescues. It is difficult for EMS systems to adopt specific do-not-start guidelines in the face of public perception that "miracle survivors" are commonplace.[45]

It seems reasonable to develop do-not-start and when-to-stop guidelines, based on objective information on the duration of submersion, for submersion victims who

TABLE 3. Probability of Neurologically Intact Survival to Hospital Discharge Based on Duration of Submersion and Time to Basic and Advanced Life Support* (Extrapolated on Published Data[29,39,40,43,44])

Duration of Submersion (minutes)	Probability of Survival With Late BLS and Late ACLS	Probability of Survival With Early BLS and Late ACLS	Probability of Survival With Immediate BLS and ACLS
0 to <5	70%	80%	90%
5 to <10	30%	35%	44%
10 to <25	3%	5%	12%
≥25	0%	0%	0%

*Late is defined as BLS and ACLS personnel arriving >10 minutes after water rescue; early, BLS personnel arrive <10 minutes after water rescue; and immediate, BLS and ACLS personnel are present when victim is recovered from the water.

are in cardiopulmonary arrest upon rescue from the water (submersion severity grade 6). Very few of these victims are going to survive. For example, even in an excellent system like the one on Brazilian beaches, where physicians respond to submersion events, the survival rate for victims in cardiopulmonary arrest is only 7%, regardless of the duration of submersion.[29]

- As a rule of thumb, about half of victims submerged for 5 to <10 minutes are pulseless upon water rescue.[29,39,40]

- Virtually all victims who ultimately survive from severity grade 6 (not breathing, no pulse) will demonstrate a pulse in the field after a period of full BLS and ACLS interventions.

- King County data confirm this observation, noting that survival is unlikely if cardiac arrest persists despite resuscitation attempts for 25 minutes.[39,40] In studies from this EMS system, no one, not even pediatric victims, survived to hospital discharge if spontaneous circulation did not return within 25 minutes of the start of resuscitative efforts.

  — Informal clinical guidelines in many EMS systems have evolved along the lines of "In normothermic victims, if pulse and respirations have not returned after 25 to 35 minutes of BLS and ALS support, they never will."

If the victim fails to respond to initial BLS, rescuers should evaluate the core temperature as soon as possible to rule out hypothermia. The rescuer should consider prolonging resuscitation attempts for a grade 6 submersion victim if the victim's core temperature is <30°C (86°F). A core temperature at this level is an indication for active internal rewarming.

- If the core temperature is >34°C (93.2°F), the hypothermia is insignificant and should not alter the duration of the resuscitation attempt.

- Between a core temperature of 30°C (86°F) and 34°C (93.2°F), clinical practice varies. Conservative protocols prolong the resuscitative effort until

active external rewarming of truncal areas brings the core temperature up to >34°C (93.2°F). Little evidence supports this approach.

Resuscitation Guidelines for Cardiac Arrest Associated With Submersion

BLS Guidelines for Submersion Victims

Rescuer Safety

A cardinal rule of emergency medicine holds that the rescuer's primary obligation is to his/her personal safety. The rescuer must avoid creating "a second victim." The rescuer must always minimize danger to himself/herself. Rescuers should never attempt risky actions that are beyond the scope of their training and experience.

Associated Trauma

Submersion events may be associated with trauma, and the issue of cervical spine immobilization is a difficult one. If the likelihood of head, neck, or spinal cord injury is significant, the rescuer should immobilize the head and neck and open the airway with a jaw thrust. But these maneuvers take time and may delay the effective provision of rescue breathing.

- Rescuers should suspect spinal injuries in all submersions associated with diving; body, wind, or board surfing; falls from motorboats or sailboats; hang gliding; parasailing; or submersions associated with falls from or crashes of personal watercraft. Rescuers should immobilize the cervical spine for these victims.

- *Routine* cervical spine immobilization of *all* submersion victims is not recommended.[28] In a retrospective survey of more than 2244 submersion victims, only 11 (<0.5%) had a C-spine injury, and all 11 had obvious trauma from diving, falling from height, or a motor vehicle crash.[28]

First-responding rescuers who suspect a spinal cord injury should

- Use their hands to stabilize the victim's neck in a neutral position (without flexion or extension).

- Open the airway using a jaw thrust without head tilt or chin lift. This method of airway opening is very difficult to perform in water, so the rescuer must weigh the likelihood of cervical spine injury against the need for immediate rescue breathing in the water.

- Provide rescue breathing while maintaining the head in a neutral position. This method of rescue breathing is very difficult during in-water rescue.

- Float the victim, supine, onto a horizontal back-support device before removing the victim from the water.

- Align and support the head, neck, chest, and body if the victim must be turned.

- If you must move the victim, use a log-roll.

Associated Hypothermia

Consider the potential for hypothermia in all *submersion* events, especially when the initial *immersion* occurs in cold water. It is important to recognize that immersion in cold water is more likely to result in submersion with hypoxia than in development of protective central hypothermia.[46-48] This occurs because swimming in cold water typically produces a sequence of exhaustion, "swim-failure" (inability to maintain horizontal swimming angle with body becoming more vertical relative to water surface), increasingly severe submersions, and finally hypoxia.

This potentially terminal hypoxia occurs at relatively modest levels of central hypothermia. These levels of hypothermia are insufficient to prevent organ ischemia.[48] For example, in the Tipton et al study,[48] competitive swimmers became exhausted after 60 to 90 minutes of swimming in 10°C (50°F) water. At that time of "swim failure" their rectal temperatures had only dropped to 35°C (94.5°F), a temperature that was still too high to exert any protective effect.[48]

To treat associated hypothermia, remove wet garments, dry the victim as soon as possible, and provide active rewarming when indicated (see Part 1: "Hypothermia").

- Cover the victim with blankets or other materials to provide passive rewarming and to prevent further heat loss.

- Obtain rectal or tympanic (core body) temperature as soon as practical, and initiate hypothermia protocols as indicated in the Hypothermia Algorithm (Figure 1 in Part 1 of this chapter).

- If significant hypothermia is thought to be present, resuscitative efforts should continue until core temperature is measured to ensure that hypothermia is not contributing to ineffective resuscitative efforts.

Airway and Breathing

Airway and **B**reathing are the first and most important treatment steps for the submersion victim, and they should begin as soon as they can safely be provided. Rescue breathing should begin in the water if possible.[49]

- Flotation devices and some appliances can facilitate support of airway and breathing in the water if rescuers are trained in their use. Untrained rescuers should not attempt to use such adjuncts. Rescuers should not delay rescue breathing for lack of such equipment if they can otherwise provide it safely.

No Need to Drain Water From the Lungs

Do not attempt to drain water from the lungs. Lay rescuers may think that draining the lungs of water after submersion makes intuitive sense.[2] But the total volume of water aspirated by submersion victims is modest, is distributed widely throughout the lungs, and is absorbed rapidly into the central circulation.[50] There is no need to drain the lungs after submersion, and no evidence that attempts will remove fluid from the lungs. Attempts

to drain lungs after fluid aspiration in research settings showed that most fluid obtained comes from the stomach and not from the lungs.[51]

Reviews of this topic by the Institute of Medicine,[51] by the American Heart Association,[52] and in recognized textbooks in resuscitation[3] and emergency medicine[1,2] all conclude that there is no evidence to justify routine attempts to drain water from the lungs after submersion.

Attempts to remove water from the breathing passages by any means other than suction can be harmful.[53-63] Abdominal thrusts, for example, have been reported to cause regurgitation of gastric contents and subsequent aspiration,[54,55,57] spinal cord injuries,[51] pharyngeal obstruction,[63] and rupture of the stomach.[53,56,58-61]

Most important, provision of the Heimlich maneuver delays the initiation of ventilation that is critical to reverse hypoxia. Although proposals for routine use of the Heimlich maneuver for submersion victims occasionally surface in the lay press,[64] this maneuver should be reserved for victims of choking and foreign-body airway obstruction.[65,66] *It should not be used routinely for submersion victims.*

Recent evidence suggests that chest compressions are superior to the Heimlich maneuver for generating intrathoracic pressures sufficient to expel foreign material.[67] The international *ECC Guidelines 2000* recommend that healthcare providers provide the Heimlich maneuver only if submersion victims have evidence of foreign-body airway obstruction.[68]

Vomiting During Resuscitation

Vomiting often occurs during chest compressions or rescue breathing, complicating efforts to maintain a patent airway. In a 10-year study in Australia vomiting occurred in more than 65% of victims who needed rescue breathing and in 86% of those who required both rescue breathing and chest compressions.[43] Even in victims who required no interventions after water rescue, vomiting occurred in 50% once they reached shore.

If vomiting occurs, turn the victim's mouth to the side and remove the vomitus with a finger sweep, a cloth, or suction. If head, neck, or spinal cord injury may be present, remove the vomitus by log-rolling the victim with the head, neck, and torso aligned and turned as a unit.

Chest Compressions

As soon as the victim is removed from the water and 2 rescue breaths are delivered, check for signs of circulation:

- The lay rescuer will check for general signs of circulation (breathing, coughing, or movement in response to rescue breaths).

- The healthcare provider will check for general signs of circulation plus the presence of a central pulse. The pulse may be difficult to detect in a submersion victim, particularly if the victim is cold.

If signs of circulation are absent, start chest compressions at once. In general, rescuers should attempt chest compressions only on shore or on board a stable vessel or floating surface. External chest compressions can be performed in the water if rigid flotation devices are used or if the victim is extremely small and can be supported on the rescuer's forearm. Proper use of in-water resuscitation flotation devices requires device-specific training.

Defibrillation for BLS Providers

If there are no signs of circulation, rescuers should attach an AED to evaluate the rhythm and deliver a shock if prompted by the AED. Although most submersion victims demonstrate asystole, some victims may demonstrate VF/pulseless VT. You cannot safely attempt defibrillation in standing water. Victims will need to be moved out of standing water. Dry the patient's chest before attaching electrodes for monitoring or for defibrillation.

Deliver up to 3 shocks. Then if hypothermia is present, evaluate the victim's core body temperature. If the victim's core body temperature is <30°C (<86°F) and VF persists, do not give further shocks until the victim's core body temperature rises above 30°C (86°F). Resume BLS and ACLS care until that time (see Part 1: "Hypothermia" in this chapter).

ACLS Guidelines for Submersion Victims

Airway and Breathing

The submersion victim in cardiac arrest requires ACLS, including tracheal intubation. Early tracheal intubation is valuable for

- Improved oxygenation and ventilation

- Direct removal of foreign material from the tracheobronchial tree

- Application of continuous positive airway pressure (CPAP) or positive end-expiratory pressure (PEEP)

Circulation and Defibrillation

Victims in cardiac arrest may present with asystole (most common), pulseless electrical activity, or pulseless VT/VF. Rescuers should follow PALS and ACLS guidelines for treatment of these rhythms. Treat submersion victims with severe hypothermia (core body temperature <30°C or <86°F) according to the recommendations for hypothermia:

- Limit defibrillation attempts to 3 if hypothermia is severe, and withhold further shocks and intravenous medications until the core body temperature rises above 30°C or 86°F.

- If moderate hypothermia is present (core body temperature 30°C to 34°C or 86°F to 93.2°F), space intravenous medications at longer than standard intervals (see Part 1: "Hypothermia" in this chapter). Attempt defibrillation with each drug administered in a drug-shock, drug-shock pattern.

- In children and adolescents VT/VF on the initial ECG is an extremely poor prognostic sign.[39]

Summary

- Prevention remains the most powerful therapeutic intervention for submersion events.

- Limiting the duration of submersion remains the second most powerful therapeutic intervention.

- Resuscitation-focused organizations must develop an international consensus approach to uniform reporting of submersion events and their outcomes. The lack of an agreed-upon nomenclature is a major obstacle to effective research in the epidemiology and treatment of submersion events.

- Submersion events must be graded by severity. This grading is based on the clinical signs, ranging from simple aspiration with coughing to apnea with a beating heart to cardiopulmonary arrest (no breathing, no pulse).

- Do-not-start and when-to-stop guidelines are urgently needed to reduce danger to rescue personnel, poor use of resources, and the number of survivors with profound neurologic impairment.

  — Evidence now exists that supports the following "do-not-start resuscitation" guideline: *Do not start resuscitative efforts for victims of submersion who were submerged for >25 minutes if there are no respirations and no heartbeat upon rescue from the water and if the victim is normothermic (core body temperature >34°C). No* international consensus group has yet made such a recommendation.

  — Evidence now exists that supports the following "when-to-stop resuscitation" guideline: *Stop resuscitative efforts if there has been no response (no respirations, no heartbeat) after >25 minutes of full BLS and ACLS interventions.* No international consensus group has yet made such a recommendation.

  — Isolated reports of neurologically intact survivors after >25 minutes of submersion or >25 minutes of attempted resuscitation pose the major obstacle to definitive do-not-start and when-to-stop guidelines. An inspirational anecdote will always trump good science in this regard.

- When treating submersion victims, rescuers should consider the possibility of associated trauma and associated hypothermia.

  — A history or strong suspicion of trauma associated with a submersion event is the major indication for C-spine immobilization.

  — Routine C-spine immobilization for all submersion victims is not recommended at this time because it may compromise the delivery of rescue breathing.

  — The neuroprotective value of hypothermia for submersion victims in cardiac arrest is probably exaggerated. This effect is possible only when the hypothermia is severe (core body temperature <30°C or <86°F) and the body cooling preceded the submersion hypoxia.

- ACLS personnel should strongly support effective prevention activities, which may at times require legislative and regulatory initiatives. Important prevention activities include

  — Safe pool design with self-closing, self-locking gates and fencing that encloses the pool on all sides

  — Trained lifeguards at public pools and beaches

  — Public swim areas fully equipped with rigid backboards, cervical collars, and BLS supplies, including AEDs

  — Swimming and lifesaving classes

  — Lay rescuer CPR-AED training

— Widespread availability and appropriate use of personal flotation devices

— Unremitting, responsible, and mature adult supervision for all infants and children when near any source of the 1 to 2 inches of water necessary for a submersion death

References

1. Feldhaus KM, Knopp RK. Near-drowning. In: Rosen P, Barkin R, eds. *Emergency Medicine: Concepts and Clinical Practice*. 4th ed. St. Louis, Mo: Mosby; 1998:1061-1066.

2. Newman AB, Stewart RD. Submersion incidents. In: Auerbach PS, ed. *Wilderness Medicine: Managment of Wilderness and Environmental Emergencies*. 4th ed. St. Louis, Mo: Mosby; 2001.

3. Shaw KN, Lavelle JM. Drowned and near-drowned patients. In: Paradis NA, Halperin HR, Nowak RM, eds. *Cardiac Arrest: The Science and Practice of Resuscitation Medicine*. Baltimore, Md: Williams and Wilkins; 1997:820-829.

4. Quan L, Bennett E, Cummings P, Henderson P, Del Beccaro MA. Do parents value drowning prevention information at discharge from the emergency department? *Ann Emerg Med*. 2001;37:382-385.

5. Jensen LR, Williams SD, Thurman DJ, Keller PA. Submersion injuries in children younger than 5 years in urban Utah. *West J Med*. 1992; 157:641-644.

6. Pitt WR, Cass DT. Preventing children drowning in Australia. *Med J Aust*. 2001;175:603-604.

7. Swimming programs for infants and toddlers. Committee on Sports Medicine and Fitness and Committee on Injury and Poison Prevention. American Academy of Pediatrics. *Pediatrics*. 2000;105:868-870.

8. Blum C, Shield J. Toddler drowning in domestic swimming pools. *Inj Prev*. 2000;6:288-290.

9. Morgenstern H, Bingham T, Reza A. Effects of pool-fencing ordinances and other factors on childhood drowning in Los Angeles County, 1990-1995. *Am J Public Health*. 2000; 90:595-601.

10. Wirtz SJ, Barrett-Miller J, Barrow S, Bates R, Baxter L, Huddart-Wolfe L, Kerr M, Lawrence D, Rose D, Trent R, Weiss B, Woo S, Woods R, Yuwiler J, Zenzola J. Prevention of toddler drowning in pools: isolation vs perimeter fencing. *Am J Public Health*. 2001;91:468-470.

11. Thompson DC, Rivara FP. Pool fencing for preventing drowning in children. *Cochrane Database Syst Rev*. 2000:CD001047.

12. Logan P, Branche CM, Sacks JJ, Ryan G, Peddicord J. Childhood drownings and fencing of outdoor pools in the United States, 1994. *Pediatrics*. 1998;101:E3.

13. Jones CS. Drowning among personal watercraft passengers: the ability of personal flotation devices to preserve life on Arkansas waterways, 1994-1997. *J Ark Med Soc*. 1999;96:97-98.

14. Shatz DV, Kirton OC, McKenney MG, Ginzburg E, Byers PM, Augenstein JS, Sleeman D, Aguila Z. Personal watercraft crash injuries: an emerging problem. *J Trauma*. 1998;44: 198-201.

15. Chochinov A. Alcohol "on board," man overboard—boating fatalities in Canada. *CMAJ*. 1998;159:259-260.

16. Quan L, Bennett E, Cummings P, Trusty MN, Treser CD. Are life vests worn? A multiregional observational study of personal flotation device use in small boats. *Inj Prev*. 1998;4:203-205.

17. Bennett E, Cummings P, Quan L, Lewis FM. Evaluation of a drowning prevention campaign in King County, Washington. *Inj Prev*. 1999;5:109-113.

18. Langley JD, Warner M, Smith GS, Wright C. Drowning-related deaths in New Zealand, 1980-94. *Aust N Z J Public Health*. 2001;25: 451-457.

19. Lau G. Did he drown or was he murdered? *Med Sci Law*. 2002;42:172-180.

20. Charatan F, Eaton F, Eaton L. Woman may face death penalty in postnatal depression case. *BMJ*. 2002;324:634.

21. Nowers MP. Suicide by drowning in the bath. *Med Sci Law*. 1999;39:349-353.

22. Byard RW, Houldsworth G, James RA, Gilbert JD. Characteristic features of suicidal drownings: a 20-year study. *Am J Forensic Med Pathol*. 2001;22:134-138.

23. Wirthwein DP, Barnard JJ, Prahlow JA. Suicide by drowning: a 20-year review. *J Forensic Sci*. 2002;47:131-136.

24. Howland J, Birckmayer J, Hemenway D, Cote J. Did changes in minimum age drinking laws affect adolescent drowning (1970-90)? *Inj Prev*. 1998;4:288-291.

25. Bell NS, Amoroso PJ, Yore MM, Senier L, Williams JO, Smith GS, Theriault A. Alcohol and other risk factors for drowning among male active duty U.S. army soldiers. *Aviat Space Environ Med*. 2001;72:1086-1095.

26. Warner M, Smith GS, Langley JD. Drowning and alcohol in New Zealand: what do the coroner's files tell us? *Aust N Z J Public Health*. 2000;24:387-390.

27. Cummings P, Quan L. Trends in unintentional drowning: the role of alcohol and medical care. *JAMA*. 1999;281:2198-2202.

28. Watson RS, Cummings P, Quan L, Bratton S, Weiss NS. Cervical spine injuries among submersion victims. *J Trauma*. 2001;51:658-662.

29. Szpilman D. Near-drowning and drowning classification: a proposal to stratify mortality based on the analysis of 1,831 cases. *Chest*. 1997;112:660-665.

30. Steinman AM, Hayward JS. Cold water immersion. In: Auerbach PS, ed. *Wilderness Medicine: Management of Wilderness and Environmental Emergencies*. 3rd ed. St Louis, Mo: Mosby; 1995:104-128.

31. Orlowski JP, Szpilman D. Drowning: rescue, resuscitation, and reanimation. *Pediatr Clin North Am*. 2001;48:627-646.

32. Eisenberg MS, Cummins RO, Larsen MP. Numerators, denominators, and survival rates: reporting survival from out-of-hospital cardiac arrest. *Am J Emerg Med*. 1991;9:544-546.

33. Eisenberg MS, Cummins RO, Damon S, Larsen MP, Hearne TR. Survival rates from out-of-hospital cardiac arrest: recommendations for uniform definitions and data to report. *Ann Emerg Med*. 1990;19:1249-1259.

34. Cummins RO, Chamberlain DA, Abramson NS, Allen M, Baskett PJ, Becker L, Bossaert L, Delooz HH, Dick WF, Eisenberg MS, et al. Recommended guidelines for uniform reporting of data from out-of- hospital cardiac arrest: the Utstein Style. A statement for health professionals from a task force of the American Heart Association, the European Resuscitation Council, the Heart and Stroke Foundation of Canada, and the Australian Resuscitation Council. *Circulation*. 1991;84:960-975.

35. Cummins RO, Chamberlain D, Hazinski MF, Nadkarni V, Kloeck W, Kramer E, Becker L, Robertson C, Koster R, Zaritsky A, et al. Recommended guidelines for reviewing, reporting, and conducting research on in-hospital resuscitation: the in-hospital 'Utstein style'. American Heart Association. *Circulation*. 1997;95:2213-2239.

36. Zaritsky A, Nadkarni V, Hazinski M, Foltin G, Quan L, Wright J, Fiser D, Zideman D, O'Malley P, Chameides L, Cummins R. Recommended guidelines for uniform reporting of pediatric advanced life support: the pediatric Utstein style. *Circulation*. 1995;92:2006-2020.

37. Modell JH. Drowning. *N Engl J Med*. 1993; 328:253-256.

38. Quan L. Near-drowning. *Pediatr Rev*. 1999; 20:255-259.

39. Quan L, Kinder D. Pediatric submersions: prehospital predictors of outcome. *Pediatrics*. 1992;90:909-913.

40. Quan L, Wentz KR, Gore EJ, Copass MK. Outcome and predictors of outcome in pediatric submersion victims receiving prehospital care in King County, Washington. *Pediatrics*. 1990;86:586-593.

41. Eisenberg MS. Who shall live? Who shall die? In: Eisenberg MS, Bergner L, E.P. H, eds. *Sudden Cardiac Death in the Community*. Philadelphia, Pa: Praeger Scientific; 1984:44-58.

42. Cummins RO, Ornato JP, Thies WH, Pepe PE. Improving survival from sudden cardiac arrest: the "chain of survival" concept. A statement for health professionals from the Advanced Cardiac Life Support Subcommittee and the Emergency Cardiac Care Committee, American Heart Association. *Circulation*. 1991;83:1832-1847.

43. Manolios N, Mackie I. Drowning and near-drowning on Australian beaches patrolled by life-savers: a 10-year study, 1973-1983. *Med J Aust*. 1988;148:165-167, 170-171.

44. Suominen P, Baillie C, Korpela R, Rautanen S, Ranta S, Olkkola KT. Impact of age, submersion time and water temperature on outcome in near-drowning. *Resuscitation*. 2002; 52:247-254.

45. Cummins R. Personal communications regarding confidential medical reviews and consultations to medical-legal professionals. Seattle, Wash; 2002.

46. Ryan JM. Immersion deaths and swim failure—implications for resuscitation and prevention. *Lancet*. 1999;354:613.

47. Teramoto S, Ouchi Y. Swimming in cold water. *Lancet*. 1999;354:1733.

48. Tipton M, Eglin C, Gennser M, Golden F. Immersion deaths and deterioration in swimming performance in cold water. *Lancet*. 1999;354:626-629.

49. Kyriacou DN, Arcinue EL, Peek C, Kraus JF. Effect of immediate resuscitation on children with submersion injury. *Pediatrics*. 1994;94: 137-142.

50. Modell JH, Davis JH. Electrolyte changes in human drowning victims. *Anesthesiology*. 1969;30:414-420.

51. Rosen P, Stoto M, Harley J. The use of the Heimlich maneuver in near drowning: Institute of Medicine report. *J Emerg Med*. 1995;13: 397-405.

52. Quan L. Drowning issues in resuscitation. *Ann Emerg Med*. 1993;22:366-369.

53. Visintine RE, Baick CH. Ruptured stomach after Heimlich maneuver. *JAMA*. 1975;234:415.

54. Redding JS. The choking controversy: critique of evidence on the Heimlich maneuver. *Crit Care Med*. 1979;7:475-479.

55. Orlowski JP. Vomiting as a complication of the Heimlich maneuver. *JAMA*. 1987;258: 512-513.

56. Cowan M, Bardole J, Dlesk A. Perforated stomach following the Heimlich maneuver. *Am J Emerg Med*. 1987;5:121-122.

57. Fink JA, Klein RL. Complications of the Heimlich maneuver. *J Pediatr Surg*. 1989;24: 486-487.

58. van der Ham AC, Lange JF. Traumatic rupture of the stomach after Heimlich maneuver. *J Emerg Med*. 1990;8:713-715.

59. Dupre MW, Silva E, Brotman S. Traumatic rupture of the stomach secondary to Heimlich maneuver. *Am J Emerg Med*. 1993;11:611-612.

60. Bintz M, Cogbill TH. Gastric rupture after the Heimlich maneuver. *J Trauma*. 1996;40: 159-160.

61. Majumdar A, Sedman PC. Gastric rupture secondary to successful Heimlich manoeuvre. *Postgrad Med J*. 1998;74:609-610.

62. Nowitz A, Lewer BM, Galletly DC. An interesting complication of the Heimlich manoeuvre. *Resuscitation*. 1998;39:129-131.

63. Anderson S, Buggy D. Prolonged pharyngeal obstruction after the Heimlich manoeuvre [letter]. *Anaesthesia*. 1999;54:308-309.

64. Associated Press. Mom says 'thank you' to Heimlich; doctor's technique saved her son's life. In: *Cincinnati Post*. Cincinnati, Ohio 1999.

65. Heimlich HJ. A life-saving maneuver to prevent food-choking. *JAMA*. 1975;234:398-401.

66. Patrick E. A case report: the Heimlich maneuver. *Emergency*. 1981;13:45-47.

67. Langhelle A, Sunde K, Wik L, Steen PA. Airway pressure with chest compressions versus Heimlich manoeuvre in recently dead adults with complete airway obstruction. *Resuscitation*. 2000;44:105-108.

68. American Heart Association in collaboration with the International Liaison Committee on Resuscitation. Guidelines 2000 for Cardiopulmonary Resuscitation and Emergency Cardiovascular Care: International Consensus on Science, Part 8: Advanced Challenges in Resuscitation: Section 3: Special Challenges in ECC. *Circulation*. 2000;102:I229-I252.

Special Resuscitation Situations
Part 3: Severe, Life-Threatening Asthma

Overview

Severe, life-threatening asthma is a special resuscitation situation because effective therapy requires modification of ACLS approaches to assessment and therapy. Asthma is caused by bronchial hyperreactivity and chronic airway inflammation. Exposure to environmental allergens provokes a small number of asthma-related fatalities.[1] Most are related to severe underlying disease, inadequate baseline management, and acute exacerbations of inflammation. These potentially preventable deaths often strike the young, and they can be very painful for families, friends, and healthcare providers.

Several consensus groups have developed excellent practice guidelines for the diagnosis and treatment of asthma. These groups include the National Asthma Education and Prevention Program of the National Institutes of Health,[2,3] the Global Initiative for Asthma,[4] and the Canadian Association of Emergency Physicians and the Canadian Thoracic Society.[5] The following websites are useful:

- National Asthma Education and Prevention Program: **www.nhlbi.nih.gov**

- Global Initiative for Asthma: **www. cooke.gsf.de/gina/practical/prac.html**

The international ECC guidelines 2000 do not address care for chronic asthma or typical exacerbations.[6,7] The ACLS recommendations focus on the management of *acute severe life-threatening asthma attacks*. These attacks have several labels and definitions:

- **Near-fatal[8] severe life-threatening asthma[9]:** severe attacks that may be fatal; the patient should be admitted to the ICU.

- **Status asthmaticus:** attacks that fail to respond to continuous, aggressive treatment after a specified amount of time (eg, 4 hours).

A 3-item asthma severity scale has been developed for the Global Initiative for Asthma.[10] This scale is based on history, current medication use, and forced expiratory volume in 1 second (FEV_1):

- **Severe hypoxemia:** for example, Pao_2 <65 mm Hg with 40% inspired oxygen, often with hypercarbia ($Paco_2$ >40 mm Hg)

- **Severe airway obstruction:** defined by objective measures such as an FEV_1 or peak expiratory flow rate (PEFR) <50% of the predicted value

- **Speed of onset:** *rapid-onset asthma* develops in <2.5 hours; *slow-onset asthma* develops over several days[11]

- Severe, life-threatening asthma (see Table 1) will present to ACLS providers in 1 of 2 ways:

  - As a patient with clinical deterioration despite hours of therapy

  - In periarrest: the patient may have stopped breathing or appears likely to stop within minutes

Epidemiology

- More than 14 million people reported having asthma in 1995.[12] The incidence of asthma is increasing.

- In the decade of the 1990s asthmatics in the United States made more than 2 million visits each year to Emergency Departments.

  - Approximately 1 of 4 (500 000) of these visits resulted in an admission.

  - Of every 100 admissions, 1 person died (5000 deaths).[13]

- This figure of 5000 deaths underestimates the total number of fatal asthma episodes. Experts think that more than 50% of such deaths will not be recognized as asthma related because the patients die either at home or during transport to the hospital.

Life-Threatening and Fatal Asthma

Pathophysiology

Severe exacerbations of asthma can lead rapidly to death. Cardiac arrest in patients with bronchial asthma has been linked to a variety of pathophysiologic mechanisms:

- Severe bronchospasm and mucous plugging can cause asphyxia.[14] Experts think that bronchospasm with subsequent plugging of the narrowed airways by mucus causes the vast majority of asthma-related deaths. At autopsy these patients display marked mucous plugging, airway edema, exudation of plasma proteins, hypertrophy of airway smooth muscle, and cellular activation with increased production and activation of inflammatory mediators.[15-17]

- Bronchoconstriction and airway obstruction from mucous plugging lead to hyperinflation and increasing airway resistance. As a consequence the work of breathing increases dramatically. For example, at an FEV_1 of 50% of predicted, the work of breathing increases to 10 times normal. At an FEV_1 of <25% of predicted, severe respiratory muscle fatigue can contribute to the development of respiratory arrest and death unless urgent treatment is provided.

- Some patients experience a sudden severe onset of bronchospasm that responds rapidly to inhaled β_2-agonists.[18] This observation suggests that marked bronchiolar smooth muscle spasm is the major component in some cases of fatal asthma.

- Some patients who receive mechanical ventilation develop *auto-PEEP* (positive end-expiratory pressure). A simple explanation is that the inspiratory tidal volume is greater than the expiratory tidal volume. This net increase in volume leads to an increase in intrathoracic pressure (the auto-PEEP), which decreases venous return to the heart. Hemodynamic compromise rapidly follows, largely as a result of inadequate cardiac output.

- Severe asthma attacks can be fatal, particularly when combined with 1 or more asthma-related complications. These complications include tension pneumothorax (often bilateral), pneumomediastinum, pneumonia, lobar atelectasis (from mucous plugging, often of larger airways), cardiac dysfunction, and pulmonary edema.

- Experts have long suspected that fatal cardiac arrhythmias occur from the use (or misuse) of β-adrenergic agonists.[19,20] In reviews of asthma-related deaths,

however, several authors were unable to document an association between these drugs and fatal arrhythmias.[18,21,22] Recently registries of long QT pedigrees have confirmed that long QT syndrome patients with asthma have more cardiac events than cohort members without asthma.[23] In these patients the β-adrenergic agonists cause increased prolongation of the QT interval.[23]

Patterns, Signs, and Symptoms

Patterns

Fatal, near-fatal,[8] or life-threatening asthma[9] occurs more frequently in the following patient groups with asthma:

- Black men

- Inner-city residents

- Patients recently hospitalized for asthma[22]

- Patients who are steroid-dependent

- Patients recently intubated for asthma[22]

- Patients who delay seeking care for attacks and deteriorate at home

    Most deaths from asthma occur at home or during transport to an Emergency Department. Of interest for prehospital and ED providers, the number of patients with severe attacks of asthma who present to the ED at night is 10 times greater than the number presenting during the day; 2% of patients with acute asthma who present at night require intubation.

- Patients who fail to recognize the severity of their attack[24]

- Patients who attempt to treat themselves during attacks without notifying their primary provider about exacerbations

- Patients with a high level of denial on psychological evaluation[25]

- Patients who receive suboptimal treatment from their primary care provider

- Patients who are depressed or anxious[9]

- Patients whose asthma was diagnosed when they were <5 years of age[8]

A somewhat stereotypical picture emerges of noncompliance, inadequate medication regimens, and denial. But a case-control study of fatal and near-fatal asthma events based on the experiences of more than 400 specialists noted that the stereotype was inaccurate for about half of life-threatening asthma events.[26] Nearly half of near-fatal and fatal attacks occurred suddenly and unexpectedly, outside the hospital, in stable, younger, atopic patients who were reportedly compliant with their medical plan of care, using inhaled corticosteroids on a daily basis.[26]

Signs and Symptoms: Assessing Severity

The patient's report of subjective symptoms is an inaccurate gauge of asthma severity.

- Reported severity correlates poorly with objective severity scoring systems.

- Some patients with severe, life-threatening asthma have an impaired response to hypercapnia and hypoxia. Their perception of dyspnea appears to be blunted. These patients may present with severe abnormalities of oxygenation and respiratory acidosis.[27]

In severe asthma the severity of wheezing provides a poor indicator of airflow or adequacy of gas exchange. A patient with severe bronchospasm and obstruction may not move air and may not wheeze at all.[28,29] The silent asthmatic chest is an ominous sign. Treatment that results in the return of wheezes on auscultation is effective treatment.

An asthmatic who is sitting upright to breathe, using accessory inspiratory muscles in the neck and chest, is at risk for sudden respiratory failure. Somnolence, mental confusion, and a moribund or exhausted appearance are ominous signs that respiratory arrest is imminent.

The key to assessing severity is the use of asthma severity scores (Table 1). These include objective evaluation of clinical signs, airway obstruction and work of breathing, oxygenation (with oximetry) and ventilation, and either FEV_1 or PEFR.[28,29] Clinical severity scores are much more reliable than observations of healthcare providers.[29]

TABLE 1. Asthma Severity Score: Classification of Mild, Moderate, and Severe Asthma*

Parameter†	Mild	Moderate	Severe	Respiratory Arrest Imminent
Breathless	Walking Can lie down	Talking (Infant will have softer, shorter cry; difficulty feeding) Prefers sitting	At rest (Infant will stop feeding) Hunched forward	
Talks in	Sentences	Phrases	Words	
Alertness	May be agitated	Usually agitated	Usually agitated	Drowsy or confused
Respiratory rate	Increased	Increased	Often >30/min	
	Guide to rates of breathing associated with respiratory distress in awake children: Age Normal rate <2 months <60/min 2-12 months <50/min 1-5 years <40/min 6-8 years <30/min			
Accessory muscles and suprasternal retractions	Usually not	Usually	Usually	Paradoxical thoraco-abdominal movement
Wheeze	Moderate, often only end-expiration	Loud	Usually loud	Absence of wheeze
Pulse/minute	<100	100-120	>120	Bradycardia
	Guide to limits of normal pulse rate in children: Age Normal rate Infants (2-12 months) <160/min Toddler (1-2 years <120/min Preschool/school age (2-8 years) <110/min			
Pulsus paradoxus	Absent <10 mm Hg	May be present 10-25 mm Hg	Often present >25 mm Hg (adult) 25-40 mm Hg (child)	Absence suggests respiratory muscle fatigue
PEF after initial bronchodilator % predicted or % personal best	>80%	Approximately 60%-80%	<60% predicted or personal best (<100 L/min adults) or response lasts <2 hours	
Pao₂ (on air)‡ and/or Paco₂‡	Normal, test usually not necessary <45 mm Hg§	>60 mm Hg <45 mm Hg§	<60 mm Hg Possible cyanosis >45 mm Hg; possible respiratory failure	
SaO₂ %	>95%	91%-95%	<90%	

*Reproduced from National Heart, Lung, and Blood Institute and World Health Organization: Global Strategy for Asthma Management and Prevention NHLBI/WHO Workshop Report, US Department of Health and Human Services, Revised September 1997. Publication no. 97-2339.

†The presence of several parameters, but not necessarily all, indicate the general classification of the attack.

‡Kilopescals are used internationally; conversion would be appropriate in this regard.

§Hypercapnia (hypoventilation) develops more readily in young children than in adults and adolescents.

A peak flow meter provides a quick, accurate, and reproducible measure of PEFR in cooperative adults that is not influenced by the person supervising the test.[30-32] Emergency Departments should consider PEFR as a vital sign for an asthmatic. A peak flow meter should be used in offices and Emergency Departments that might treat patients with acute asthma. The device should be kept with a small box of the disposable mouthpieces and a copy of the expected normal flow rates for men and women. Table 2 presents the predicted average PEFRs for men and women based on age and height. The PEFR correlates well with the FEV_1 and is much easier to obtain.[28]

Differential Diagnosis

"All that wheezes is not asthma."

—Chevalier Jackson,
pioneer bronchoscopist
from Temple University

- When a patient presents with wheezing, the ACLS provider must determine if the patient has acute asthma. When a patient presents with extreme dyspnea, you may not be able to obtain a confirmatory history of asthma.

- Other conditions may cause patients to wheeze and to be acutely short of breath. These conditions include
  — Cardiac disease (congestive heart failure or myocarditis)
  — Emphysema
  — Pneumonia
  — Upper airway obstruction (structural or psychogenic, due to vocal cord dysfunction)
  — Acute allergic bronchospasm or anaphylaxis (aspirin, foods, or idiopathic)
  — Pulmonary embolism
  — Vasculitis (Churg-Strauss syndrome)[37]

- Bronchospasm also may be caused by medications, such as β-blockers,[38] or by drugs such as cocaine and opiates.[39,40]

- Abrupt discontinuation of corticosteroids may lead to life-threatening asthma.

Long-term corticosteroid use may produce a relative adrenal insufficiency because endogenous cortisol secretion is suppressed. If steroids are stopped abruptly, endogenous cortisol production may initially be inadequate, and this temporary adrenal insufficiency may precipitate a severe attack in these patients.

Clinical Deterioration Despite Usually Effective Therapy

- ACLS providers will most often treat people with severe, life-threatening asthma attacks in 1 of 2 scenarios:

  — **Deterioration despite treatment:** The asthmatic who deteriorates despite therapy

  — **Imminent respiratory arrest:** The periarrest asthmatic who stops breathing or is likely to stop breathing within minutes

- The immediate goal is to prevent deterioration to full cardiopulmonary arrest.

- These patients are challenging for emergency providers. The provider must make difficult decisions about noninvasive ventilation, tracheal intubation, and mechanical ventilation. Note that with appropriate first-line asthma therapy, life-threatening asthma attacks should be infrequent.

- The following section describes consensus recommendations for first-line asthma interventions that have been proven effective.

First-Line Therapy
Summary Recommendations

- **Definitely effective:** For patients presenting with a severe, life-threatening asthma episode, excellent evidence supports immediate initiation of the following first-line treatments:

  — Oxygen at 4 L/min

  — Inhaled β₂-agonists such as albuterol

- **Probably effective:** Good evidence supports the conditional use of these agents:

  — Systemic corticosteroids (oral or intravenous)

  — Ipratropium bromide

  — Magnesium sulfate

- **Possibly effective:** Several agents fall into the category of agents to consider as possibly helpful in certain clinical circumstances:

  — Epinephrine or terbutaline

  — Methylxanthines (aminophylline)

Definitely Effective Recommendations

Oxygen

- Oxygen should be started at 4 L/min for all patients with acute severe asthma. The immediate treatment goal is to achieve an arterial partial pressure of oxygen (PaO_2) of ≥92 mm Hg or oxyhemoglobin saturation ≥95%.

- Start supplementary oxygen before or simultaneously with initial inhaled β₂-agonists. Give oxygen to all asthmatic patients, including those with normal oxygen saturation.

  — Without administration of supplementary oxygen, a paradoxical worsening of hypoxemia could follow administration of inhaled bronchodilators.

  — β-Agonists may induce both pulmonary vasodilation and bronchodilation. This condition may produce a right-to-left shunt (shunting of systemic venous blood through the lungs so that it is desaturated when it returns to the left atrium); this will contribute to worsening of hypoxemia.

- Some patients may require high-flow oxygen by mask.

Inhaled β₂-Selective β-Agonists

- **Albuterol or *salbutamol*** are equivalent β₂-selective β-agonists that act by relaxing bronchial smooth muscles. These

TABLE 2. Average* Predicted Peak Expiratory Flow Rates (in L/min) for Age and Height

Normal Men

Age (y)	Height				
	60 inches (5 ft)	65 inches (5 ft 5 in)	70 inches (5 ft 10 in)	75 inches (6 ft 3 in)	80 inches (6 ft 8 in)
20	555	600	650	695	740
25	545	590	635	680	725
30	530	575	620	665	710
35	520	565	610	650	695
40	510	550	595	635	680
45	500	540	585	620	665
50	485	525	570	605	650
55	475	515	555	595	635
60	465	500	540	580	620
65	450	490	530	565	605
70	440	475	515	550	585

Normal Women

Age (y)	Height				
	55 inches (4 ft 7 in)	60 inches (5 ft)	65 inches (5 ft 5 in)	70 inches (5 ft 10 in)	75 inches (6 ft 3 in)
20	390	425	460	495	530
25	385	420	455	490	525
30	380	415	450	485	515
35	375	410	440	475	510
40	370	400	435	470	500
45	365	400	430	465	495
50	360	390	425	460	490
55	355	385	420	450	480
60	350	380	410	445	475
65	345	375	405	440	470
70	340	370	400	430	460

Based on data from several sources.[33-36] These values differ from the original source values. They have been rounded to the nearest 5 L/min. Each color represents a rate range.

*These average values are based on multiple measurements of PEFR for a large number of people. A person's PEFR can vary over time and can be repeatedly higher or lower than the average value. Calculation: % of normal PEFR = (measured PEFR ÷ predicted PEFR) × 100. The preferred clinical practice is to use a patient's "personal best" PEFR instead of the predicted PEFR. The personal best value is established over time while the patient is receiving effective treatment.

drugs provide rapid, short-acting reduction in bronchospasm with minimal adverse effects. Albuterol has gained almost universal acceptance as the therapeutic cornerstone for acute asthma.[41,42] When first developed albuterol was given intravenously. Now, however, inhaled albuterol (0.5 mL diluted in 2 to 2.5 mL normal saline), delivered through a nebulizer or a metered-dose inhaler (MDI), has proven much more effective than intravenous albuterol.

— Other commonly used β-agonists, with less $β_2$ selectivity than albuterol, are *terbutaline* (0.5 to 1 mg nebulized every 20 minutes × 3) and *metaproterenol* (0.4% solution, 2.5 mL nebulized every 20 minutes × 3).

■ **Metered-dose inhalers versus nebulizers:** Delivery by nebulizer has become the most common ED treatment for acute asthma attacks. But a number of studies suggest that MDIs with spacers have several advantages over nebulizers,[43-46] although the technique of administration must be precise:

— Less expensive

— Starting treatment is faster and easier

— More efficient use of staff time

■ **Dose:** "Aggressive dosing" for more severe cases calls for higher amounts of agents at shorter intervals:

— **Metered-dose inhaler:** 4 to 8 puffs every 15 to 20 minutes for 1 hour.

— **Nebulizer:** In the United States 2.5-mg doses of nebulized albuterol are administered every 20 minutes for 3 doses (7.5 mg total) for acute episodes of asthma.[47]

— But in one randomized, controlled trial, a "high-dose" nebulization regimen of 5 mg initially with an additional 5 mg 40 minutes later (10 mg total) produced faster and greater bronchodilation at 60 minutes than the regimen of three 2.5-mg doses.[47]

— For the asthmatic in periarrest, giving three 5-mg doses (15 mg total) at 20-minute intervals is acceptable.

■ **Levalbuterol (R-isomer of albuterol):** Recent research suggests that the R-isomer form of albuterol (levalbuterol; available in the United States as Xopenex inhalation solution) may produce more effective bronchodilation than the racemic form.[48-50] The relative benefits of levalbuterol—more expensive than albuterol—have not been determined.[42]

Probably Effective Recommendations

Corticosteroids

■ **Pharmacology:** Despite persistent and repeated study, researchers have not yet established the benefit of corticosteroids specifically for acute life-threatening asthma. The reason is simple: corticosteroids are slow to act. Corticosteroids produce an objective effect only after 3 to 4 hours. Improved airflow due to corticosteroids can be demonstrated only after 6 to 12 hours.

■ **Issues:** A number of debates swirl around the use of corticosteroids for acute severe asthma[51]:

— Do corticosteroids improve airflow? One meta-analysis reached a generally negative conclusion.[52]

— Do corticosteroids keep severe asthmatics out of the hospital? The same meta-analysis concluded that they do not.[52]

— Do *inhaled* corticosteroids confer benefits not observed with the oral or intravenous route? One study found that higher doses of metered-dose steroids (with spacer and mixed with albuterol) measurably improved pulmonary function and reduced bronchial edema, but only after 3 hours.[53]

— Do corticosteroids convey *any* benefit for severe asthmatics? Corticosteroids convey no unequivocal benefits during the several hours

severe asthmatics spend in the ED. Reduction of inflammation and bronchial edema, however, does reduce length of hospital stay, in-hospital complications, readmissions, and return visits to the ED.[54-56]

■ **Indications:** It is essential that corticosteroids be administered immediately for any patient with severe, life-threatening asthma.[42,57] The delayed onset of action of these agents will not affect initial management or the clinical course of acute asthma. But steroids started in the ED will serve the patient well during hospitalization. Other commonly accepted criteria[57] for immediately starting corticosteroids include

— Slow response (>20 minutes) to inhaled $β_2$-agonists (moderate to severe attack)

— ED visit within the previous 7 days (the "bounce-backs")

— Current use of oral corticosteroids ("steroid-dependent" patient)

— Recent tapering off corticosteroids ("steroid-dependent" patient)

■ **Dose:**

— *Methylprednisolone* 125 mg IV is given as an empiric starting dose in cases of severe asthma.[51,55,56,58] The weight-based dose is 2 mg/kg IV; repeat every 6 hours.

— Other corticosteroid choices are *hydrocortisone* (5 to 7 mg/kg IV; repeat every 4 to 6 hours and *dexamethasone* (0.25 mg/kg IV; repeat every 8 to 12 hours).

— But even questions of dose provoke debates. Some clinicians prescribe as little as 40 mg of IV methylprednisolone in the ED. Others use doses as high as 250 mg IV or its equivalent.

Anticholinergics

■ **Pharmacology:** Ipratropium bromide (Atrovent) is an anticholinergic (parasympatholytic) bronchodilator that is pharmacologically related to atropine.

— Ipratropium inhibits vagally mediated constriction of bronchial smooth muscles. The result is local, site-specific bronchodilation. There are no systemic effects.

— Ipratropium bromide produces less bronchodilation than inhaled β$_2$-agonists,[59,60] and it has a slower onset (about 20 minutes longer).[61]

— Ipratropium is most effective for "maintenance treatment" of bronchospasm that accompanies chronic bronchiolitis. It is considered a secondary drug for the treatment of chronic asthma.

■ **Use for severe, life-threatening asthma:** There does appear to be a role for ipratropium bromide *in combination* with inhaled β-agonists for acute events.

— This beneficial effect appears to occur specifically in cases of severe, life-threatening asthma. Note that the only age groups with relevant studies are children and adolescents.[62]

— A systematic analysis of randomized, controlled trials in children and adolescents with moderately severe asthma (FEV$_1$ <55% of predicted) noted that multiple doses of ipratropium added to inhaled β$_2$-agonists improved pulmonary function and reduced the rate of hospitalization by 30%.[63,64] But this benefit was not observed when the asthma attacks were only mild or moderate.[63]

— A meta-analysis of randomized, controlled trials limited to adult asthmatics observed a modest benefit from ipratropium combined with β$_2$-agonists (7% improvement in FEV$_1$, 22% improvement in PEFR).[65]

— The National Institutes of Health Expert Panel on Asthma endorses the combination of β$_2$-agonists plus an inhaled anticholinergic agent[2,3] for asthma patients with a PEFR or FEV$_1$ <80% of the predicted normal value.[2,3]

— Several companies produce inhalation solutions that combine ipratropium bromide with albuterol sulfate (eg, Combivent or DuoNeb).

■ **Dose:** Mix ipratropium bromide 0.5 mg in 2.5 mL of normal saline in a nebulizer with the first dose of albuterol. Higher doses or dosing intervals less than 4 hours confer no added benefits.

Magnesium Sulfate

■ **Pharmacology:** A number of clinical trials have reported that magnesium sulfate improves bronchodilation in patients persistently symptomatic after inhaled adrenergic agents and corticosteroids.[66-70]

■ **Use in severe, life-threatening asthma:** A recent Cochrane Database meta-analysis identified 7 prospective clinical trials of magnesium sulfate in acute asthma.[67,68] The reviewers concluded that only the subset of patients experiencing a severe asthma attack derived significant benefit from magnesium infusion. Although clinicians find the benefits of magnesium inconsistent,[66] magnesium is widely available and can be administered with few side effects. It appears to be a growing practice to give 2 to 3 g of magnesium sulfate IV to patients experiencing a severe, life-threatening asthma attack, especially to patients unresponsive to early therapy with inhaled β$_2$-agonists.

■ **Dose:** Give magnesium sulfate 2 to 3 g IV at rates of 200 mg/min to 1 g/min (1 g of magnesium sulfate = 98 mg of elemental magnesium).[54,67,69,70]

Possibly Effective Recommendations

Epinephrine

■ **Pharmacology:** Epinephrine is a nonselective β-agonist that requires parenteral (subcutaneous or intravenous) administration. Epinephrine is an effective bronchial smooth muscle dilator with rapid onset of action.

— The nonselective properties of epinephrine also produce tachycardia, acute blood pressure elevation, and myocardial irritability.

— Epinephrine will increase myocardial oxygen demand.

■ **Indications:**

— Adverse properties and side effects cause many experts to limit the use of epinephrine in acute asthma to patients under the age of 35 who are unable to use inhalers.

— The exclusion of patients over age 35 is probably unjustified,[71] particularly for subcutaneous epinephrine. Older prospective studies and reviews documented that subcutaneous epinephrine is well tolerated and effective for the treatment of older adults with asthma.[72,73]

■ **Use in severe, life-threatening asthma:** Subcutaneous epinephrine is seldom given to patients with severe asthma. This practice is a regrettable omission in many cases. Patients who are "too tight to wheeze" are the ones most likely to benefit from epinephrine. They cannot effectively inhale β$_2$-agonists through a metered-dose inhaler or nebulizer. As the patient deteriorates, the inspiratory flow rate decreases and compromises delivery of inhaled medications.

— **Withhold epinephrine?** Do not withhold epinephrine (even if it must be given IV) from patients with severe, life-threatening asthma solely because of their age. Do not withhold epinephrine from patients simply because of its reputation for adverse effects. For these patients epinephrine may eliminate the need for tracheal intubation and mechanical ventilation.

— **An important perspective:** If you are hesitant to give epinephrine to a severely distressed asthmatic, you should consider the fact that if the patient deteriorates further and suffers a cardiorespiratory arrest, the first drug you will administer is epinephrine 1 mg IV. This dose is 3 times the recommended subcutaneous epinephrine dose of 0.3 mg. Most clinicians agree that these patients are much better off receiving a small dose of epinephrine before their arrest than larger doses of epinephrine after a cardiopulmonary arrest.

- **Dose:** The total epinephrine dose is 0.01 mg/kg, usually divided into 3 doses given at time zero, 20 minutes, and 40 minutes. A 70-kg patient would therefore receive a total of 0.7 mg, given as approximately 0.25 mg/dose for 3 doses. (Epinephrine, at a concentration of 1:1000, is supplied as 1 mg in 1 mL ampules.)

  — A non–weight-based dose of 0.3 mg is often given to adults at time zero; this dose is used for convenience and easy recall.

  — You can give a second epinephrine dose of 0.3 mg in 20 minutes. Assess for clinical improvement before giving a third 0.3 mg dose.

Terbutaline Sulphate

- **Pharmacology:** Terbutaline is a selective β_2-agonist with pharmacologic and adverse effects similar to those of albuterol. Common trade names for terbutaline are Brethine and Bricanyl. Asthmatics use terbutaline in metered-dose inhalers, nebulized solution, or oral tablets. In the ED terbutaline is given by subcutaneous injection or intravenous infusion.

- **Use in severe, life-threatening asthma?** Compared with epinephrine, terbutaline has a slower onset of action (5 to 30 minutes), a longer time to peak effects (1 to 2 hours), and a much longer duration of action (3 to 6 hours). As an alternative to epinephrine, terbutaline has little role to play in adults with severe, life-threatening asthma because of the slow onset of action and longer time to peak effects. But in children at least one ED study has found terbutaline to be more efficacious than epinephrine for reversal of wheezing.[74]

- **Dose:** The dose of terbutaline is 0.25 mg subcutaneously. You can repeat this dose once in 30 to 60 minutes, but the total dose should not exceed 0.5 mg every 4 hours.

Methylxanthines (Aminophylline IV)

- **Pharmacology:** As a bronchodilator aminophylline is less effective than albuterol. Aminophylline is now almost never used as *primary therapy* in adults. Some clinicians have considered aminophylline as secondary therapy to be added to β_2-agonists and corticosteroids. The rationale has been that aminophylline may enhance the effects of those agents. A recent meta-analysis of 13 clinical trials concluded that the addition of aminophylline produced no increase in bronchodilation but an increase in adverse effects.[75] This increase in side effects is most evident in patients already taking oral theophyllines.

- **Indications[57]:**

  — A patient who is already taking a methylxanthine at the time of presentation.

  — A patient experiencing a severe, life-threatening asthma exacerbation who has not responded to inhaled β_2-agonists, corticosteroids, ipratropium, or subcutaneous epinephrine or terbutaline.

  — Some experienced clinicians report their use of aminophylline in adults for severe attacks in people who have had a positive response to the drug during previous attacks.

- **Dose:** For those rare patients who report a childhood response to aminophylline, use a loading dose of 5 mg/kg, given over 30 to 45 minutes. Follow with an infusion of 0.5 to 0.7 mg/kg per hour.

- **Side effects:** Side effects include nausea, vomiting, seizures, and cardiac arrhythmias. Theophylline is a substrate for the cytochrome p450 enzyme pathway. Theophylline levels are *increased* with concomitant administration of many drugs, such as cimetidine and verapamil. Theophylline levels are *decreased* with concomitant administration of isoproterenol, phenobarbital, phenytoin, and rifampin.

Reevaluation After First-Line Treatment

Response to Initial Treatment?

Clinical decision making for severe, life-threatening asthma is determined by the patient's response to initial treatment. This fact underscores the importance of asthma scoring systems that include evaluation of clinical appearance, work of breathing, pulse oximetry, and measurement of PEFR or FEV_1. One study evaluated patients with severe asthma (pretreatment PEFR <100 L/min) and noted the degree of improvement with initial therapy. Failure to achieve a PEFR >300 L/min after first-line treatment was associated with a 92% admission rate.

To aid decision making, use the severity scoring system (Table 1). In addition, you can place patients into one of the following categories after first-line treatment:

- Clinical improvement and FEV_1 or PEFR >70% of predicted after 1 to 3 hours of treatment: consider discharge home

- Some clinical improvement and FEV_1 or PEFR 50% to 70% of predicted after 4 hours of intensive treatment: "incomplete responder"

- Inadequate clinical improvement and FEV_1 or PEFR 25% to 50% of predicted after 4 hours of intensive treatment: hospital admission + noninvasive assisted ventilation

- No clinical improvement and FEV_1 or PEFR <25% of predicted after 4 hours of intensive treatment: ICU admission + assisted ventilation

Clinical Improvement and FEV_1 or PEFR >70% of Predicted After 1 to 3 Hours of Treatment: Consider Discharge Home

Most patients who improve clinically and are breathing room air with adequate oxygenation (oxyhemoglobin saturation of ≥95%) and FEV_1 or PEFR >70% of predicted after 1 to 3 hours of inhaled β_2-agonists, anticholinergics, and corticosteroids can be discharged home.[2,3] You may need to modify this disposition on the basis of the risk factors noted above and below.

- Observe these patients for at least 1 hour after they reach >70% of predicted FEV_1 or PERF to ensure their stability.[2,3]

- Review the discharge medications closely. Studies confirm the value of continued inhaled or oral steroids and of inhaled β_2-agonists *after* an acute attack.[52,76,77] These medications significantly reduce the need for return ED visits and subsequent hospitalizations.

Some Clinical Improvement and FEV₁ or PEFR 50% to 70% of Predicted After 4 Hours of Intensive Treatment: Incomplete Responders

Risk stratification for incomplete responders: Patients who achieve some clinical improvement but have persistent signs of moderate to severe asthma with improved oxygenation (oxyhemoglobin saturation of 90% to 95%) and FEV_1 or PEFR 50% to 70% of predicted after 4 hours of intensive treatment are classified as *incomplete responders*. They require careful triage. To borrow from the nomenclature for acute coronary syndromes, the responsible clinician must "risk stratify" these patients. Concurrent comorbidity, such as insulin-dependent diabetes, coronary artery disease, cerebrovascular disease, chronic obstructive pulmonary disease, or acute pneumonia, adds to the risk.

Low-risk incomplete responders: Some incomplete responders are at low risk for continued deterioration and may be discharged conditionally. Appropriate discharge requires that patients have adequate discharge medications, home resources, access to follow-up care, and a detailed discharge care plan.[3,5]

High-risk incomplete responders: Incomplete responders with 1 or more of the following risk factors should be hospitalized (with occasional individual exceptions).[2,24]

- History of intubation and mechanical ventilation for acute, life-threatening asthma

- Recent (within 2 to 4 weeks) hospitalization for asthma

- Bounce-back ED visits (ie, patient was evaluated and treated in an ED in the previous 24 to 48 hours)

- Duration of attack is 1 week or longer

- Current use of oral steroids (steroid-dependent); studies have not yet established whether patients currently using inhaled steroids should be stratified as high risk

- Inadequate home care resources

- Known or suspected poor compliance

Inadequate Clinical Improvement and FEV₁ or PEFR 25% to 50% of Predicted After 4 Hours of Intensive Treatment: Hospital Admission + Noninvasive Assisted Ventilation

With rare exceptions, emergency physicians should admit these patients to the hospital.

Pulmonologists, emergency physicians, and other specialists are gaining considerable experience with noninvasive assisted ventilation techniques for these patients. Noninvasive positive-pressure ventilation (NPPV) is rapidly emerging as an effective ED technique. These techniques, discussed in more detail below, are not initiated to prevent hospital admission. Their major clinical purpose is to prevent tracheal intubation. These techniques are judged "effective" only if the patient avoids tracheal intubation.

No Clinical Improvement and FEV₁ or PEFR <25% of Predicted After 4 Hours of Intensive Treatment: ICU Admission + Assisted Ventilation

These patients need not only hospital admission but also intensive monitoring and care. They are seriously ill. Tracheal intubation and mechanical ventilation may be necessary if the patient continues to be unresponsive to therapy.

Indications for ICU admission: In addition to an FEV_1 or PEFR <25% of predicted, other objective signs and clinical symptoms indicate the need for ICU admission and probable intubation:

- PaO_2 <65 mm Hg with 40% inspired oxygen (oxyhemoglobin saturation <90%)

- $PaCO_2$ >40 mm Hg (especially if rising during treatment in the ED)

- Altered level of consciousness

- Breathlessness that makes talking difficult

- Inability to lie in the supine position

- Increasing fatigue and tiredness

Noninvasive Assisted Ventilation

"The greatest challenge in intubating and managing the patient with asthma . . . is that the patient's clinical condition may worsen after intubation, when the patient may prove extremely difficult to ventilate and may be hemodynamically unstable. Thus the decision to intubate must be made carefully and the technique must be chosen to facilitate the best possible outcome."

—R.E. Schneider[78]

Description

As the above quotation makes clear, the decision to intubate a patient with asthma is difficult. Noninvasive assisted ventilation techniques are emerging as an effective way for patients with severe, life-threatening asthma to avoid the need for intubation and mechanical ventilation.[79-81]

Noninvasive positive-pressure ventilation uses a mechanical ventilation device to deliver positive-pressure ventilation through a mask to assist the patient's spontaneous respiratory efforts. The mask may cover a patient's face or nose or both. It must fit against the nose or face with a relatively tight seal.

Benefits

These devices are intended for patients suffering from severe life-threatening asthma that is refractory to bronchodilators and steroids. In the past, such compromised patients required tracheal intubation and mechanical ventilation. By preventing intubation these techniques convey numerous benefits. Table 3 provides a partial list of the benefits of noninvasive assisted ventilation.

NPPV can enable support of ventilation without the need for and hazards of tracheal tube placement. The patient, however, must have effective spontaneous respiratory effort and adequate airway protective mechanisms.

Requirements and Contraindications

Experienced clinicians often recommend NPPV for patients who do not respond satisfactorily to aggressive first-line therapy.[78,81] But 3 critical requirements remain. The patients must be

- Alert and able to protect airway
- Cooperative
- Demonstrating effective spontaneous respirations

Contraindications: Noninvasive assisted ventilation techniques are contraindicated for patients who are

- Severely hypoxemic: PaO_2 <60 mm Hg or O_2 saturation <90% on rebreathing mask

TABLE 3. Benefits of Noninvasive Assisted Ventilation

- Unloads and rests respiratory muscles
- Reduces the work of breathing
- Improves oxygenation
- Improves carbon dioxide elimination
- Increases bronchodilation (a mechanical effect)
- Decreases airway resistance (a mechanical effect)
- Reexpands areas of atelectasis
- Increases ability to remove secretions
- Helps to avoid tracheal intubation and its complications
- Eliminates the need for sedation
- Decreases dyspnea and increases the patient's comfort
- Maintains alertness and the ability to speak
- Maintains ability to swallow, eat, and drink

- Deteriorating steadily or rapidly
- Confused, somnolent, moribund, or uncooperative
- Unable to protect the airway
- Hypotensive (BP <90 mm Hg)
- Known to have ischemic heart disease
- Having ventricular arrhythmias

Sample Settings

Table 4 lists the initial steps to follow for NPPV.[78,81]

Bilevel Positive Airway Pressure

Bilevel positive airway pressure (BiPAP) has proven to be the most effective type of NPPV for life-threatening asthma. Intermittent assisted ventilation with a BiPAP ventilator may help to delay or eliminate the need for tracheal intubation.

The BiPAP ventilator is a variable-flow device that offers separate control of the inspiratory positive airway pressure and the expiratory positive airway pressure. Carefully selected settings allow this type of ventilator to counteract the effects of auto-PEEP. BiPAP devices reduce the work of breathing more than any other noninvasive respiratory support technique. They reduce the work of breathing by reducing the force required for exhalation and increasing the work of inspiration.

Most experts begin with an inspiratory positive airway pressure of 8 to 10 cm H_2O and an expiratory positive airway pressure of 3 to 5 cm H_2O.[82]

Tracheal Intubation for Life-Threatening Asthma

"The patient's clinical condition may worsen after intubation . . . . The decision to intubate must be made carefully. . . ."[78]

Indications

The major indications for rapid tracheal intubation in life-threatening asthma are

TABLE 4. Initial Steps and Settings for NPPV: Patients With Status Asthmaticus Approaching Respiratory Failure[78,81]

1. Secure a full face mask with head straps over the nose and mouth. Avoid a tight fit.
2. Connect the ventilator to the face mask. Use either a conventional mechanical ventilator or a ventilator specially made for NPPV.
3. Start with continuous positive airway pressure (CPAP) set to 0 cm H_2O. Slowly increase CPAP to maintain positive end-expiratory pressure even during spontaneous inspiration.
4. Set positive-pressure support (inspiratory pressure) of ventilation at 10 cm H_2O. Adjust on the basis of arterial blood gases, but do not exceed 25 cm H_2O.
5. Set tidal volume at 500 mL (7 mL/kg).
6. Set ventilation rate at <25 breaths/min.
7. Continue to administer nebulized medications through the system.

- Failure to improve after 4 hours of NPPV.
- Continued deterioration despite aggressive first-line therapy.
- Association with anaphylaxis (see Part 4: "Anaphylaxis").
- Deterioration with fatigue and exhaustion. With complete exhaustion the victim is simply too tired to maintain effective ventilation, and apnea and respiratory arrest are likely to develop.
- Onset of altered level of consciousness, confusion, or somnolence.
- A rising $PaCO_2$ (>40 mm Hg) with a falling pH. These values are particularly worrisome when associated with clinical signs of obtundation, somnolence, and poor muscle tone. These signs suggest the presence of patient exhaustion and respiratory failure. Note that isolated hypercarbia does not require immediate

tracheal intubation. *Treat the patient, not the numbers.*

- PaO$_2$ <50 mm Hg on a nonrebreathing mask, especially when associated with clinical signs of hypoxemia. These signs include severe agitation, confusion, and fighting against the oxygen mask.[83]

Rapid Sequence Intubation

Precautions

- Rapid sequence intubation (RSI) is the technique of choice for tracheal intubation in patients with severe, life-threatening asthma.[42,78] Other techniques, especially nasotracheal intubation, have a high rate of failure in these patients.

- Select the most experienced laryngoscopist to perform the procedure. In asthmatic patients the smallest amount of airway stimulation with a laryngoscope blade can provoke severe laryngospasm and reflex bronchoconstriction.

- It may be impossible to provide effective bag-mask ventilation when status asthmaticus is present. In patients with severe, life-threatening asthma, most air delivered with a bag and mask will divert away from the high-resistance airways and into the stomach. This can produce gastric distention, further decrease in effective ventilation, regurgitation, and aspiration.

- Use the largest tracheal tube (8 to 9 mm) possible. The larger the tube diameter, the less the airway resistance. Suctioning the airway secretions can be handled better with large-diameter tubes.

Premedications

- The most critical of the *LOAD* premedications (lidocaine, opioids, atropine, defasciculating agent) is lidocaine (see Vol. 1, Chapter 8: "Airway, Airway Adjuncts, Oxygenation, and Ventilation").

- Give lidocaine 1.5 to 2 mg/kg IV 3 minutes before administration of opioids, sedatives, or paralytics. This dose will reduce bronchospasm induced by laryngoscopy and intubation.

Sedation and Anesthesia

- Several anesthetics are powerful bronchodilators, especially *halothane* (not generally available) and other inhalational anesthetics (eg, *isoflurane*), *ketamine,* and *propofol.*[84,85]

- **Ketamine** is an effective sedative, analgesic, and dissociative anesthetic. Many experts recommend ketamine as the IV anesthetic of choice for patients with status asthmaticus. Ketamine possesses strong bronchodilator properties.[86,87]

  — Ketamine potentiates catecholamines and relaxes bronchiolar smooth muscle. Ketamine does not cause vasodilatation, circulatory collapse, or myocardial depression.

  — A dose of 2 mg/kg IV (1 to 4 mg/kg pediatrics) induces anesthesia in 30 seconds and lasts 10 to 15 minutes.

  — Because ketamine increases bronchial secretions, many experts also premedicate with **atropine** (0.01 mg/kg; minimum dose of 0.1 mg).

- **Propofol** is another sedative with bronchodilator properties.[88,89] It is effective for both intubation and maintenance of sedation during mechanical ventilation.

  — A dose of 2 to 2.5 mg/kg induces anesthesia in approximately 40 seconds and lasts 3 to 5 minutes.

  — This drug may cause hypotension.

- **Etomidate** is an acceptable hypnotic to use, though it lacks bronchodilator properties.[90] Etomidate is ultra–short-acting and has a safer hemodynamic profile than both ketamine and propofol.

  — A dose of 0.2 to 0.6 mg/kg (0.2 to 0.4 mg/kg pediatrics) induces anesthesia in 60 seconds and lasts 3 to 5 minutes.

  — This drug has no analgesic properties.

- **Inhaled volatile anesthetics:** Physicians who care for patients with severe asthma should be aware of reports of the use of inhaled volatile anesthetics for patients with severe life-threatening asthma.

  — The volatile anesthetics are powerful bronchial smooth muscle relaxants.

Agents like halothane, isoflurane, enflurane, and ether have been successful in the treatment of status asthmaticus refractory to all other treatments.[91]

  — Use these agents with extreme caution because they are also vasodilators and myocardial depressants. Some of these anesthetics sensitize the myocardium to catecholamines, leading to life-threatening arrhythmias.

Paralysis

- **Succinylcholine,** at a dose of 1 to 2 mg/kg, is the clear paralytic agent of choice for RSI in patients with severe asthma and no contraindications to the drug (see Vol. 1, Chapter 8, Table 5).[78]

- **Rocuronium,** at a dose of 0.6 to 1.2 mg/kg, is the second paralytic of choice.[92] Its rapid onset of action is similar to that of succinylcholine, but it has a longer duration of action.

Immediately After Intubation

The persistent problem—airway obstruction: Tracheal intubation enables use of external mechanical power to assist the patient's failing ventilation efforts. It does not solve the problem of airway obstruction. Patients with severe, life-threatening asthma may be extremely difficult to oxygenate prior to intubation, even with bag-mask ventilation. In addition, hypercarbia may create a respiratory acidosis. These problems with oxygenation and ventilation may persist even once the tube is in place.

Continue inhaled β$_2$-agonists: Because breathing efforts may be inadequate, the patient may not have had adequate distribution of β$_2$-agonists prior to intubation. Immediately after intubation inject 2.5 to 5 mg of albuterol directly into the tracheal tube.

Ventilate the patient slowly with 100% oxygen: When severe asthma is present, significant obstruction to air flow persists even after intubation. In fact, if there is no significant obstruction to airflow immediately after intubation, you should reevaluate the diagnosis of acute asthma and consider the possibility that the resistance to airflow was present in the upper airway (eg, vocal cord dysfunction, tumor, or a foreign body).

Anyone performing manual ventilation for patients with severe asthma after intubation should *slowly* ventilate at a rate of only 8 to 10 breaths/min, allowing adequate time for exhalation between delivered breaths. This slow respiratory rate and adequate exhalation time can minimize the development of auto-PEEP and its serious consequence of severe hypotension and pneumothorax. Prevention of hyperventilation and auto-PEEP is preferable to treatment of the complications.

Acute asthma is occasionally confused with exacerbation of emphysema, especially in the elderly. Hyperventilation immediately after intubation can cause dire consequences in elderly patients with emphysema.

Table 5 summarizes the steps needed to insert a tracheal tube and begin mechanical ventilatory support for patients with severe, life-threatening asthma.

Mechanical Ventilation in Patients With Severe Asthma

Difficulties and Complications

Mechanical ventilation in patients with severe, life-threatening asthma is challenging and may produce several significant complications.

■ **Auto-PEEP:** Clinicians who provide mechanical ventilatory support for patients with severe asthma must understand the concept of auto-PEEP:

— Although asthmatics experience some obstruction of inspiration, they experience *marked* obstruction of expiration. As resistance to exhalation increases, the inevitable result will be air trapping and "breath stacking" (inspired air enters and then cannot exit).

— With severe airway obstruction the duration of spontaneous expiration increases. But during mechanical ventilation, expiratory time is set. If expiratory time is inadequate, this can lead to "self-produced" or "auto-produced" PEEP. In this case, end-expiratory pressure increases without addition of PEEP to the mechanical ventilatory circuit.

— Increased intrathoracic pressure from auto-PEEP can reduce venous return to the heart. This reduced venous return can lead to reduced cardiac output, hemodynamic compromise, and hypotension.

— Note that hyperinflation and increased intrathoracic pressure can also produce barotrauma such as a tension pneumothorax.

■ **Ventilation with "permissive hypercarbia":** Adequate oxygenation is relatively easy to achieve with mechanical ventilation in patients with severe asthma. The problem is getting rid of the carbon dioxide–ventilation. To prevent the development of significant levels of auto-PEEP, the mechanical ventilator must be set with low tidal volume and low respiratory rate and long expiratory time. These settings will lead to an increase in $PaCO_2$, but a modest degree of hypercarbia is acceptable. This concept of controlled hypoventilation, using ventilator settings that result in a mild elevation of $PaCO_2$, is referred to as *permissive hypercarbia*.[93]

— Ventilatory support is controlled so that there is gradual development (over 3 to 4 hours) of hypercarbia ($PaCO_2$ levels may rise to 70 to 90 mm Hg). Acidemia also develops, with pH values in the range of 7.2 to 7.3, but the level is controlled by controlling the rise in $PaCO_2$.

TABLE 5. Summary of Steps to Initiate Mechanical Ventilatory Support for Severe, Life-Threatening Asthma[78]

This sequence is one example. Variations are acceptable.

1. Place the patient in an upright position if comfortable.
2. Administer *lidocaine* 1.5 to 2 mg/kg three minutes before administration of anesthesia.
3. Administer *ketamine* 2 mg/kg.
4. *Immediately* follow with *succinylcholine* 1.5 mg/kg.
5. As the patient loses consciousness, apply *cricoid pressure*. Gently place the patient in the supine position.
6. Perform *laryngoscopy* and *tracheal intubation*. Use an 8- to 9-mm tube if possible.
7. Perform primary and secondary confirmation of tube placement and begin mechanical ventilation support. Note that when patients have severe asthma, the esophageal detector device may reinflate rapidly, falsely suggesting tracheal tube placement despite the presence of the tube in the esophagus. Providers should perform primary confirmation of tube placement and use exhaled CO_2 as a secondary confirmation device.
8. Begin maintenance sedation (*benzodiazepine* or *propofol*) and paralysis (*rocuronium*). Continue for 4 to 6 hours.
9. Adjust mechanical ventilation parameters as recommended in Table 6.
10. Provide additional *ketamine* as needed.
11. Administer inhalational agents via the tracheal tube.
12. Monitor airway pressures to evaluate patient response to therapy
13. Administer fluids (eg, normal saline) if needed to counteract the fall in blood pressure from auto-PEEP.

Within 24 to 48 hours the patient's serum pH will be restored to near-normal levels because the kidneys will reabsorb bicarbonate to compensate for the respiratory acidosis.

— In addition to setting the ventilator for reduced tidal volume and slower respiratory rates, you should increase the inspiratory flow rate to 80 to 120 L/min.

— To tolerate such settings patients usually require complete paralysis and heavy sedation.

— Closely monitor patient tolerance of the respiratory acidosis, particularly during the first 24 to 48 hours of therapy, before renal compensation has occurred. In some patients arrhythmias may develop when acidosis is present, and this may limit the level of permissive hypercarbia used. It may be necessary to allow the $Paco_2$ to rise in smaller increments over a longer period of time.

■ Table 6 provides an example of initial settings for mechanical ventilation after tracheal intubation.

Imminent Respiratory Arrest

Most people who die from fatal asthma do so at home or on the way to the Emergency Department. ACLS providers, especially prehospital EMS professionals, may face a patient for whom respiratory arrest is imminent. If respiratory arrest has occurred, proceed at once to the assessments and interventions of the Primary and Secondary ABCD Surveys of ACLS. This event constitutes a "crash airway" situation. Follow the recommendations in Vol. 1, Chapter 8: "Airway, Airway Adjuncts, Oxygenation, and Ventilation" (refer to the "crash airway" algorithm, Figure 19), in particular the use of succinylcholine for paralysis if needed.

■ **Critical Action:** Do not hyperventilate the patient during bag-mask ventilation. Hyperventilation could exacerbate the problem of auto-PEEP with compromise of cardiac output.

■ Start supplementary **oxygen** at once; use a nonrebreathing mask with high-flow oxygen or a bag and mask.

■ Administer **epinephrine** 0.3 mg subcutaneously as quickly as possible. You are trying to prevent a cardiopulmonary arrest. Potential side effects of epinephrine are small relative to the risk of cardiopulmonary failure.

■ **Critical Decision:** The responsible clinician must make an immediate yet key decision: *Is the patient making inspiratory efforts capable of moving inhaled β₂-agonists into the lungs?*

— If the answer is *no,* do not waste time administering inhaled agents and waiting to see the effects.

— If the answer is *yes* or *maybe,* immediately administer an **inhaled β₂-agonist.** Administer the first dose with a metered-dose inhaler (with spacer) or nebulizer, whichever can be assembled more quickly.

— If **NPPV** is available, start it simultaneously, without waiting for a response to the epinephrine and β₂-agonists. Experienced and properly equipped EDs can begin noninvasive positive-pressure ventilation within a few minutes of the arrival of a critically ill asthmatic. Again the focus is to avoid the need for tracheal intubation.

■ **Evaluate immediate response:** Evaluate how well the patient responds in the first 10 to 20 minutes to the oxygen, epinephrine, inhaled β₂-agonists, and possibly NPPV. There should be unequivocal and significant objective improvement (eg, improvement in oxygenation and clinical appearance, a change in PEFR from a severe degree of obstruction of <100 L/min to 150 to 200 L/min.)

— If significant improvement does not occur, proceed to RSI if resources and skilled personnel are available. If time and resources allow premedication and sedation, give lidocaine

---

TABLE 6. Example of Initial Settings for Mechanical Ventilation After Tracheal Intubation[78]

1. Calculate the patient's **ideal body weight.**

2. **Tidal volume:** Set to 6 to 8 mL/kg.

3. **Respiratory rate:** Set to 8 to 10 breaths/min.

4. **Inspiratory flow rate:** Set to 80 to 100 L/min. The objective is to achieve a ratio of inspired to expired air (I:E) of 1:4 to 1:5.

5. **Positive inspiratory pressure:** Start at 10 cm H_2O. Do not set at >25 cm H_2O. Keep the **peak inspiratory pressure (PIP)** under 40 cm H_2O. This level will reduce the occurrence of barotrauma and hemodynamic compromise. Sudden increases in the inspiratory pressures may indicate a pneumothorax, obstructed tracheal tube, or mucous plugging. Conversely a precipitous fall in PIP may indicate extubation. Investigate any sudden change in PIP.

6. **Permissive hypercarbia:** Titrate tidal volume and respiratory rate to allow the gradual development of hypercarbia. It often will occur if inspiratory pressure is maintained at <25 cm H_2O.

7. **Continue sedation:** Maintain continuous sedation with propofol or a benzodiazepine.

8. **Maintain paralysis:** Maintain continuous paralysis with a longer-acting, nondepolarizing muscle relaxant, such as *rocuronium.*

9. **Administer inhalational medications:** Continue to provide (as indicated) the first-line asthma therapies (inhaled β₂-agonists, anticholinergics, and corticosteroids) by nebulizer delivery of drugs through the ventilator and tracheal tube.

Critical Concepts:
Troubleshooting Problems in the Intubated, Ventilator-Dependent Asthmatic

Patient Is Difficult to Ventilate

If the patient is extremely "tight" (with airway constriction) and difficult to ventilate, perform the following procedures *in order* until ventilation is adequate:

1. Ensure that the patient is adequately sedated and paralyzed so that there is a passive patient-ventilator interaction.

2. Check the tracheal tube for patency. Look for obstruction from kinking, mucous plugging, or biting. Suction the tube.

3. Change to a *square-wave pattern* of airflow. You may need to increase the time for exhalation, shorten the time for inhalation, and markedly increase the limit of peak inspiratory pressure to ensure that the patient is receiving the set tidal volume.

4. Reduce the respiratory rate to 6 to 8 breaths/min to reduce auto-PEEP to ≤15 mm Hg.

5. Reduce the tidal volume to 3 to 5 mL/kg to reduce auto-PEEP to ≤15 mm Hg.

6. Increase peak flow to >60 L/min (90 to 120 L/min is commonly used) to further shorten inspiratory time and increase exhalation time.[94]

Hypoxia or Hypotension Occurs After Intubation

There are 4 common causes of significant hypoxia or hypotension immediately after intubation:

1. Incorrect placement of the tracheal tube

2. Obstruction of the tracheal tube

3. Massive auto-PEEP buildup

4. Tension pneumothorax

1. Incorrect Placement of the Tracheal Tube

■ With any drop in oxygen saturation or exhaled CO_2, reconfirm tube position immediately. Do this even if correct tube position was verified by primary and secondary confirmation.

■ Check that the tracheal tube has not been inserted too far. It may be in either the right (most likely) or left main bronchus. The tube should be inserted to 21 cm (measure at the incisors) in most men and to 20 cm in most women. Use lengths slightly shorter (eg, 19 to 20 cm) in smaller adults.

■ If you suspect incorrect placement of the tracheal tube, evaluate the tube placement *immediately using primary and secondary confirmation techniques*. Do not take time to obtain a chest radiograph. It is appropriate to obtain a chest radiograph after intubation, but it may not confirm tube misplacement. Spontaneous extubation or tube migration into a main bronchus is always a respiratory emergency. This is particularly true if the patient has severe life-threatening asthma. The patient cannot tolerate the delay that would occur with a confirmatory radiograph (see Vol. 1, Chapter 8).

■ Note that patients with status asthmaticus can demonstrate false-negative results with the esophageal detector device. When the tracheal tube is in the esophagus of the patient with severe asthma, the detector bulb may re-expand immediately, suggesting tracheal tube placement. Providers must be aware that severe asthma may cause erroneous results with the esophageal detector device; they should use exhaled CO_2 detectors as another secondary confirmation device.

2. Obstruction of the Tracheal Tube

■ If the patient is difficult to ventilate manually, check for patency of the tube.

■ Attempt to suction the tube.

■ Check for tube obstructions from kinking, mucous plugging, or biting.

■ A true diagnosis may be elusive in patients with severe refractory asthma. Auscultatory clues may be missing because the chest is often silent. This lack of audible breath sounds comes from poor airflow and hyperinflation of the chest wall.

3. Massive Auto-PEEP Buildup

■ The most common cause of profound hypotension after intubation is a massive buildup of auto-PEEP.

— First, stop ventilating the patient for a brief time (20 to 40 seconds).

— This pause allows the auto-PEEP to dissipate.

— At the same time someone must monitor the patient's oxygenation. Resume ventilation if auto-PEEP dissipates or if the patient develops significant hypoxemia or clinical signs of deterioration.

4. Tension Pneumothorax

■ Evidence of a tension pneumothorax includes decreased chest expansion and decreased breath sounds on the side of the pneumothorax, shifting of the trachea away from the side of the pneumothorax, or the development of subcutaneous emphysema. The immediate lifesaving treatment is *needle decompression* to release air from the pleural space. This procedure is often followed by placement of a chest tube.

— Slowly insert a 16-gauge cannula (over-the-needle catheter) in the second intercostal space along the midclavicular line. Be careful to avoid direct puncture of the lung. Hearing or feeling the venting of compressed air is diagnostic.

— Several commercial products, based on the 1-way valve principle, are available. You can use these devices after relief of a tension pneumothorax to prevent further buildup of pneumatic tension. Nonetheless patients often require a chest tube.

■ *Caution!* An attempt at needle decompression or insertion of a chest tube in a patient with severe, refractory asthma without a pneumothorax can be a life-threatening error.

— The visceral pleura of the hyperinflated lung can be punctured, producing an iatrogenic pneumothorax. The person inserting the tube would not realize that puncture of the lung has occurred.

— Air would be released through the needle catheter or thoracostomy tube, just as occurs with relief of a tension pneumothorax.

— The high pressures in the contralateral, mechanically ventilated lung plus the coexisting auto-PEEP could generate a contralateral tension pneumothorax.

1.5 to 2 mg/kg and ketamine 2 mg/kg or propofol 2 to 2.5 mg/kg.

— If both the patient and clinician concur that significant improvement is under way, initiate a modified first-line asthma regimen (see below).

■ **Modified first-line therapy after initial improvement:**

— Administer **methylprednisolone** 125 mg IV (or equivalent).

— Add **ipratropium bromide** (0.5 mg diluted in 2.5 mL of normal saline in nebulizer) to the second dose of β_2-agonist, and administer both 10 to 20 minutes after the initial dose.

— Administer **magnesium sulfate** 2 to 3 g IV.

— Consider **aminophylline** 5 mg/kg over 30 to 45 minutes, followed by an infusion of 0.5 to 0.7 mg/kg per hour *if* patient has a history of positive response to the drug. Monitor for arrhythmias.

— Consider **terbutaline** 0.25 mg subcutaneously.

Final Interventions to Consider

ACLS providers may encounter a patient with severe asthma and progressive hypoxia and hypercarbia refractory to the therapy described above. Certainly consultation with a pulmonologist or critical care specialist is always appropriate for refractory asthmatic patients. At that time, if at all possible, a pulmonologist or critical care specialist should be consulted. The following "interventions of desperation" have occasionally met with some success, at least as recounted in case reports and anecdotes.

■ **Empiric bilateral needle decompression for bilateral pneumothoraxes:** Evidence from anecdotal case reports[95,96] and surveys of chest radiographs suggest that unrecognized bilateral tension pneumothoraxes may underlie some cases of fatal asthma. There is insufficient published data to support a recommendation for empiric attempts at bilateral

needle decompression in all severely compromised asthma patients. The critical point is "to consider" whether unrecognized pneumothoraces may have precipitated an asthmatic cardiac arrest.

■ **Intravenous β-agonist (isoproterenol):** Isoproterenol given by IV infusion over 60 to 90 minutes has been effective for severely ill patients unable to tolerate inhalational therapy. Start with 0.1 µg/kg per minute; increase to a maximum of 6 µg/kg per minute. Titrate according to heart rate.

■ **Extracorporeal membrane oxygenation (ECMO).** There are increasing reports of success with this technique in mechanically ventilated patients who could not be adequately oxygenated.[97]

Additional therapies such as so-called "lung massage" have been reported to benefit some patients in status asthmaticus. But positive reports from animal studies[98] were not verified in humans,[99] and such techniques should not be attempted.

Table 7 lists interventions to consider for asthma patients facing imminent respiratory arrest.

TABLE 7. Imminent Respiratory Arrest in Severe, Life-Threatening Asthma: Interventions to Consider

■ Oxygen: high flow, nonrebreathing mask

■ Epinephrine: 0.1 to 0.3 mg IV

■ β_2-agonists: by MDI and spacer or nebulizer

■ Noninvasive positive-pressure ventilation: if immediately available

■ Magnesium sulfate IV

■ Inhaled ipratropium bromide

■ Corticosteroids IV

■ Methylxanthines (aminophylline) IV

■ For severe refractory respiratory failure:

— Empiric bilateral needle decompression

— Metaproterenol or isoproterenol IV

— ECMO

References

1. Wobig EK, Rosen P. Death from asthma: rare but real. *J Emerg Med.* 1996;14:233-240.

2. National Asthma Education and Prevention Program. Expert panel report: guidelines for the diagnosis and management of asthma update on selected topics—2002. *J Allergy Clin Immunol.* 2002;110(5 suppl):S141-S219.

3. Emond SD, Camargo CA Jr, Nowak RM. 1997 National Asthma Education and Prevention Program guidelines: a practical summary for emergency physicians. *Ann Emerg Med.* 1998; 31:579-589.

4. Alvey Smaha D. Asthma emergency care: national guidelines summary. *Heart Lung.* 2001; 30:472-474.

5. Beveridge RC, Grunfeld AF, Hodder RV, Verbeek PR. Guidelines for the emergency management of asthma in adults. CAEP/CTS Asthma Advisory Committee. Canadian Association of Emergency Physicians and the Canadian Thoracic Society. *CMAJ.* 1996;155:25-37.

6. Part 8: advanced challenges in resuscitation. Section 3: special challenges in ECC. 3B: submersion or near-drowning. European Resuscitation Council. *Resuscitation.* 2000;46:273-277.

7. American Heart Association in collaboration with International Liaison Committee on Resuscitation. Guidelines 2000 for Cardiopulmonary Resuscitation and Emergency Cardiovascular Care: International Consensus on Science, Part 8: Advanced Challenges in Resuscitation: Section 3: Advanced Challenges in ECC. *Circulation.* 2000;102(suppl I):I229-I252.

8. Mitchell I, Tough SC, Semple LK, Green FH, Hessel PA. Near-fatal asthma: a population-based study of risk factors. *Chest.* 2002;121: 1407-1413.

9. Kolbe J, Fergusson W, Vamos M, Garrett J. Case-control study of severe life threatening asthma (SLTA) in adults: psychological factors. *Thorax.* 2002;57:317-322.

10. Liard R, Leynaert B, Zureik M, Beguin FX, Neukirch F. Using Global Initiative for Asthma guidelines to assess asthma severity in populations. *Eur Respir J.* 2000;16:615-620.

11. Wasserfallen JB, Schaller MD, Feihl F, Perret CH. Sudden asphyxic asthma: a distinct entity? *Am Rev Respir Dis.* 1990;142:108-111.

12. Benson V, Marano MA. Current estimates from the National Health Interview Survey, 1995. *Vital Health Stat 10.* 1998:1-428.

13. Weiss KB, Gergen PJ, Hodgson TA. An economic evaluation of asthma in the United States. *N Engl J Med.* 1992;326:862-866.

14. Molfino NA, Nannini LJ, Martelli AN, Slutsky AS. Respiratory arrest in near-fatal asthma. *N Engl J Med.* 1991;324:285-288.

15. Reid LM. The presence or absence of bronchial mucus in fatal asthma. *J Allergy Clin Immunol.* 1987;80:415-416.

16. Bhaskar KR, O'Sullivan DD, Coles SJ, Kozakewich H, Vawter GP, Reid LM. Characterization of airway mucus from a fatal case of status asthmaticus. *Pediatr Pulmonol.* 1988; 5:176-182.

17. Sur S, Crotty TB, Kephart GM, Hyma BA, Colby TV, Reed CE, Hunt LW, Gleich GJ. Sudden-onset fatal asthma: a distinct entity with few eosinophils and relatively more neutrophils in the airway submucosa? *Am Rev Respir Dis.* 1993;148:713-719.

18. Kallenbach JM, Frankel AH, Lapinsky SE, Thornton AS, Blott JA, Smith C, Feldman C, Zwi S. Determinants of near fatality in acute severe asthma. *Am J Med.* 1993;95:265-272.

19. Robin ED, McCauley R. Sudden cardiac death in bronchial asthma, and inhaled β-adrenergic agonists. *Chest.* 1992;101:1699-1702.

20. Robin ED, Lewiston N. Unexpected, unexplained sudden death in young asthmatic subjects. *Chest.* 1989;96:790-793.

21. Abramson MJ, Bailey MJ, Couper FJ, Driver JS, Drummer OH, Forbes AB, McNeil JJ, Haydn Walters E. Are asthma medications and management related to deaths from asthma? *Am J Respir Crit Care Med.* 2001;163:12-18.

22. McFadden ER Jr, Warren EL. Observations on asthma mortality. *Ann Intern Med.* 1997; 127:142-147.

23. Rosero SZ, Zareba W, Moss AJ, Robinson JL, Hajj Ali RH, Locati EH, Benhorin J, Andrews ML. Asthma and the risk of cardiac events in the long QT syndrome. Long QT Syndrome Investigative Group. *Am J Cardiol.* 1999;84: 1406-1411.

24. Turner MO, Noertjojo K, Vedal S, Bai T, Crump S, Fitzgerald JM. Risk factors for near-fatal asthma: a case-control study in hospitalized patients with asthma. *Am J Respir Crit Care Med.* 1998;157:1804-1809.

25. Campbell DA, Yellowlees PM, McLennan G, Coates JR, Frith PA, Gluyas PA, Latimer KM, Luke CG, Martin AJ, Ruffin RE. Psychiatric and medical features of near fatal asthma. *Thorax.* 1995;50:254-259.

26. Hannaway PJ. Demographic characteristics of patients experiencing near-fatal and fatal asthma: results of a regional survey of 400 asthma specialists. *Ann Allergy Asthma Immunol.* 2000;84:587-593.

27. Kikuchi Y, Okabe S, Tamura G, Hida W, Homma M, Shirato K, Takishima T. Chemosensitivity and perception of dyspnea in patients with a history of near-fatal asthma. *N Engl J Med.* 1994;330:1329-1334.

28. Nowak RM, Pensler MI, Sarkar DD, Anderson JA, Kvale PA, Ortiz AE, Tomlanovich MC. Comparison of peak expiratory flow and FEV_1 admission criteria for acute bronchial asthma. *Ann Emerg Med.* 1982;11:64-69.

29. Shim CS, Williams MH Jr. Evaluation of the severity of asthma: patients versus physicians. *Am J Med.* 1980;68:11-13.

30. Levin E, Gold MI. The mini-Wright expiratory peak flow meter. *Can Anaesth Soc J.* 1981; 28:285-287.

31. Jones KP, Mullee MA. Measuring peak expiratory flow in general practice: comparison of mini Wright peak flow meter and turbine spirometer. *BMJ.* 1990;300:1629-1631.

32. Pedersen OF, Rasmussen TR, Omland O, Sigsgaard T, Quanjer PH, Miller MR. Peak expiratory flow and the resistance of the mini-Wright peak flow meter. *Eur Respir J.* 1996; 9:828-833.

33. Weng TR, Levison H. Standards of pulmonary function in children. *Am Rev Respir Dis.* 1969;99:879-894.

34. Nunn AJ, Gregg I. New regression equations for predicting peak expiratory flow in adults. *BMJ.* 1989;298:1068-1070.

35. Leiner GC, Abramowitz S, Small MJ, Stenby VB, Lewis WA. Expiratory peak flow rate. Standard values for normal subjects: use as a clinical test of ventilatory function. *Am Rev Respir Dis.* 1963;88:644-651.

36. Leiner GC, Abramowitz S, Lewis WA, Small MJ. Dyspnea and pulmonary function tests. *Am Rev Respir Dis.* 1965;92:822-823.

37. Brenner BE, Chavda K, Karakurum M, Camargo CA. Circadian differences among 4096 patients presenting to the emergency department with acute asthma. *Acad Emerg Med.* 1999;6:523.

38. Odeh M, Oliven A, Bassan H. Timolol eyedrop-induced fatal bronchospasm in an asthmatic patient. *J Fam Pract.* 1991;32:97-98.

39. Weitzman JB, Kanarek NF, Smialek JE. Medical examiner asthma death autopsies: a distinct subgroup of asthma deaths with implications for public health preventive strategies. *Arch Pathol Lab Med.* 1998;122:691-699.

40. Levenson T, Greenberger PA, Donoghue ER, Lifschultz BD. Asthma deaths confounded by substance abuse: an assessment of fatal asthma. *Chest.* 1996;110:604-610.

41. Delbridge T, Domeier R, Key CB. Prehospital asthma management. *Prehosp Emerg Care.* 2003;7:42-47.

42. Marik PE, Varon J, Fromm R Jr. The management of acute severe asthma. *J Emerg Med.* 2002;23:257-268.

43. Bowton DL, Goldsmith WM, Haponik EF. Substitution of metered-dose inhalers for hand-held nebulizers: success and cost savings in a large, acute-care hospital. *Chest.* 1992;101: 305-308.

44. Bowton DL. Metered-dose inhalers versus hand-held nebulizers: some answers and new questions. *Chest.* 1992;101:298-299.

45. Colacone A, Afilalo M, Wolkove N, Kreisman H. A comparison of albuterol administered by metered dose inhaler (and holding chamber) or wet nebulizer in acute asthma. *Chest.* 1993; 104:835-841.

46. Idris AH, McDermott MF, Raucci JC, Morrabel A, McGorray S, Hendeles L. Emergency department treatment of severe asthma: metered-dose inhaler plus holding chamber is equivalent in effectiveness to nebulizer. *Chest.* 1993; 103:665-672.

47. McFadden ER Jr, Strauss L, Hejal R, Galan G, Dixon L. Comparison of two dosage regimens of albuterol in acute asthma. *Am J Med.* 1998;105:12-17.

48. Gawchik SM, Saccar CL, Noonan M, Reasner DS, DeGraw SS. The safety and efficacy of nebulized levalbuterol compared with racemic albuterol and placebo in the treatment of asthma in pediatric patients. *J Allergy Clin Immunol.* 1999;103:615-621.

49. Nelson HS. Clinical experience with levalbuterol. *J Allergy Clin Immunol.* 1999;104(2 pt 2): S77-S84.

50. Nelson HS, Bensch G, Pleskow WW, DiSantostefano R, DeGraw S, Reasner DS, Rollins TE, Rubin PD. Improved bronchodilation with levalbuterol compared with racemic albuterol in patients with asthma. *J Allergy Clin Immunol.* 1998;102:943-952.

51. McFadden ER Jr. Inhaled glucocorticoids and acute asthma: therapeutic breakthrough or nonspecific effect? *Am J Respir Crit Care Med.* 1998;157:677-678.

52. Rodrigo G, Rodrigo C. Corticosteroids in the emergency department therapy of acute adult asthma: an evidence-based evaluation. *Chest.* 1999;116:285-295.

53. Rodrigo G, Rodrigo C. Inhaled flunisolide for acute severe asthma. *Am J Respir Crit Care Med.* 1998;157:698-703.

54. Rowe BH, Bretzlaff JA, Bourdon C, Bota GW, Camargo CA. Systematic review of magnesium sulfate in the treatment of acute asthma. *Cochrane Database Syst Rev.* 1998;(4).

55. Rowe BH, Keller JL, Oxman AD. Effectiveness of steroid therapy in acute exacerbations of asthma: a meta-analysis. *Am J Emerg Med.* 1992;10:301-310.

56. Rowe BH, Spooner CH, Ducharme FM, Bretzlaff JA, Bota GW. Early emergency department treatment of acute asthma with systemic corticosteroids. *Cochrane Database Syst Rev.* 2000: CD002178.

57. Mengert TJ. Asthma. In: Copass MK, ed. *Emergency Medical Therapy.* 4th ed. Philadelphia, Pa: WB Saunders; 1996:300-316.

58. McFadden ER Jr. Dosages of corticosteroids in asthma. *Am Rev Respir Dis.* 1993;147: 1306-1310.

59. Rodrigo G, Rodrigo C, Burschtin O. A metaanalysis of the effects of ipratropium bromide in adults with acute asthma. *Am J Med.* 1999; 107:363-370.

60. Rodrigo G, Rodrigo C. Ipratropium bromide in acute asthma: small beneficial effects? *Chest.* 1999;115:1482.

61. Karpel JP, Schacter EN, Fanta C, Levey D, Spiro P, Aldrich T, Menjoge SS, Witek TJ. A comparison of ipratropium and albuterol vs albuterol alone for the treatment of acute asthma. *Chest.* 1996;110:611-616.

62. Qureshi F, Zaritsky A, Lakkis H. Efficacy of nebulized ipratropium in severely asthmatic children. *Ann Emerg Med.* 1997;29:205-211.

63. Plotnick LH, Ducharme FM. Combined inhaled anticholinergics and β_2-agonists for initial treatment of acute asthma in children. *Cochrane Database Syst Rev.* 2000:CD000060.

64. Plotnick LH, Ducharme FM. Should inhaled anticholinergics be added to β_2 agonists for treating acute childhood and adolescent asthma? A systematic review. *BMJ.* 1998;317: 971-977.

65. Stoodley RG, Aaron SD, Dales RE. The role of ipratropium bromide in the emergency management of acute asthma exacerbation: a metaanalysis of randomized clinical trials. *Ann Emerg Med.* 1999;34:8-18.

66. Cydulka RK. Why magnesium for asthma? *Acad Emerg Med.* 1996;3:1084-1085.

67. Rowe BH, Bretzlaff JA, Bourdon C, Bota GW, Camargo CA Jr. Intravenous magnesium sulfate treatment for acute asthma in the emergency department: a systematic review of the literature. *Ann Emerg Med.* 2000;36: 181-190.

68. Rowe BH, Bretzlaff JA, Bourdon C, Bota GW, Camargo CA Jr. Magnesium sulfate for treating exacerbations of acute asthma in the emergency department. *Cochrane Database Syst Rev.* 2000:CD001490.

69. Schiermeyer RP, Finkelstein JA. Rapid infusion of magnesium sulfate obviates need for intubation in status asthmaticus. *Am J Emerg Med.* 1994;12:164-166.

70. Silverman RA, Osborn H, Runge J, Gallagher EJ, Chiang W, Feldman J, Gaeta T, Freeman K, Levin B, Mancherje N, Scharf S. IV magnesium sulfate in the treatment of acute severe asthma: a multicenter randomized controlled trial. *Chest.* 2002;122:489-497.

71. Safdar B, Cone DC, Pham KT. Subcutaneous epinephrine in the prehospital setting. *Prehosp Emerg Care.* 2001;5:200-207.

72. Cydulka R, Davison R, Grammer L, Parker M, Mathews J IV. The use of epinephrine in the treatment of older adult asthmatics. *Ann Emerg Med.* 1988;17:322-326.

73. Quadrel M, Lavery RF, Jaker M, Atkin S, Tortella BJ, Cody RP. Prospective, randomized trial of epinephrine, metaproterenol, and both in the prehospital treatment of asthma in the adult patient. *Ann Emerg Med.* 1995;26: 469-473.

74. Victoria MS, Battista CJ, Nangia BS. Comparison between epinephrine and terbutaline injections in the acute management of asthma. *J Asthma.* 1989;26:287-290.

75. Parameswaran K, Belda J, Rowe BH. Addition of intravenous aminophylline to β_2-agonists in adults with acute asthma. *Cochrane Database Syst Rev.* 2000:CD002742.

76. Rowe BH, Bota GW, Fabris L, Therrien SA, Milner RA, Jacono J. Inhaled budesonide in addition to oral corticosteroids to prevent asthma relapse following discharge from the emergency department: a randomized controlled trial. *JAMA.* 1999;281:2119-2126.

77. Edmonds ML, Camargo CA, Pollack CV, Rowe BH. Early use of inhaled corticosteroids in the emergency department treatment of acute asthma. *Cochrane Database Syst Rev.* 2001: CD002308.

78. Schneider RE. Asthma and COPD. In: Schneider RE, ed. *Manual of Emergency Airway Management.* Philadelphia, Pa: Lippincott Williams & Wilkins; 2000:164-168.

79. Hillberg RE, Johnson DC. Noninvasive ventilation. *N Engl J Med.* 1997;337:1746-1752.

80. Hotchkiss JR, Marini JJ. Noninvasive ventilation: an emerging supportive technique for the emergency department. *Ann Emerg Med.* 1998;32:470-479.

81. Meduri GU, Cook TR, Turner RE, Cohen M, Leeper KV. Noninvasive positive pressure ventilation in status asthmaticus. *Chest.* 1996; 110:767-774.

82. Panacek EA, Pollack C. Medical management of severe asthma. In: Brenner BE, ed. *Emergency Asthma.* New York, NY: Marcel-Dekker; 1999:395-417.

83. Brenner BE, Abraham E, Simon RR. Position and diaphoresis in acute asthma. *Am J Med.* 1983;74:1005-1009.

84. Maltais F, Sovilj M, Goldberg P, Gottfried SB. Respiratory mechanics in status asthmaticus: effects of inhalational anesthesia. *Chest.* 1994;106:1401-1406.

85. Rooke GA, Choi JH, Bishop MJ. The effect of isoflurane, halothane, sevoflurane, and thiopental/nitrous oxide on respiratory system resistance after tracheal intubation. *Anesthesiology.* 1997;86:1294-1299.

86. Howton JC, Rose J, Duffy S, Zoltanski T, Levitt MA. Randomized, double-blind, placebo-controlled trial of intravenous ketamine in acute asthma. *Ann Emerg Med.* 1996;27:170-175.

87. Hemmingsen C, Nielsen PK, Odorico J. Ketamine in the treatment of bronchospasm during mechanical ventilation. *Am J Emerg Med.* 1994;12:417-420.

88. Eames WO, Rooke GA, Wu RS, Bishop MJ. Comparison of the effects of etomidate, propofol, and thiopental on respiratory resistance after tracheal intubation. *Anesthesiology.* 1996; 84:1307-1311.

89. Kress JP, O'Connor MF, Pohlman AS, Olson D, Lavoie A, Toledano A, Hall JB. Sedation of critically ill patients during mechanical ventilation: a comparison of propofol and midazolam. *Am J Respir Crit Care Med.* 1996;153:1012-1018.

90. Bergen JM, Smith DC. A review of etomidate for rapid sequence intubation in the emergency department. *J Emerg Med.* 1997;15:221-230.

91. Saulnier FF, Durocher AV, Deturck RA, Lefebvre MC, Wattel FE. Respiratory and hemodynamic effects of halothane in status asthmaticus. *Intensive Care Med.* 1990;16: 104-107.

92. Hudson ME, Rothfield KP, Tullock WC, Firestone LL. Haemodynamic effects of rocuronium bromide in adult cardiac surgical patients. *Can J Anaesth.* 1998;45:139-143.

93. Tuxen DV. Permissive hypercapnic ventilation. *Am J Respir Crit Care Med.* 1994;150: 870-874.

94. Mayo P, Radeos MS. The severe asthmatic: intubated and difficult to ventilate. In: Brenner BE, ed. *Emergency Asthma.* New York, NY: Marcel-Dekker; 1999:469-487.

95. Josephson E, Goetting M. Asthmatic cardiac arrest: an indication for empiric bilateral tube thoracotomies. *Ann Emerg Med.* 1989;18:457.

96. D'Urzo AD, D'Urzo DK, Chapman KR. Case report: pneumothorax and asthma. *Can Fam Physician.* 1999;45:1524-1525.

97. Shapiro MB, Kleaveland AC, Bartlett RH. Extracorporeal life support for status asthmaticus. *Chest.* 1993;103:1651-1654.

98. Van der Touw T, Tully A, Amis TC, Brancatisano A, Rynn M, Mudaliar Y, Engel LA. Cardiorespiratory consequences of expiratory chest wall compression during mechanical ventilation and severe hyperinflation. *Crit Care Med.* 1993;21:1908-1914.

99. Van der Touw T, Mudaliar Y, Nayyar V. Cardiorespiratory effects of manually compressing the rib cage during tidal expiration in mechanically ventilated patients recovering from acute severe asthma. *Crit Care Med.* 1998;26:1361-1367.

Special Resuscitation Situations Part 4: Anaphylaxis

Definitions

Anaphylaxis is a multisystem syndrome of allergic reaction that can involve the cutaneous, cardiovascular, respiratory, and gastrointestinal systems. By definition two or more systems must be involved to make the diagnosis of anaphylaxis.[1] Clinical signs include urticaria (hives) or angioedema, vasodilation, bronchospasm, abdominal pain, and vomiting. Death from anaphylaxis is most frequently caused by cardiovascular collapse with severe hypotension.

■ **Immunologic definitions.** A hypersensitivity reaction, anaphylaxis is mediated by the antibody subclasses IgE and IgG4. The classic form of anaphylaxis involves prior sensitization with later reexposure, although reactions can occur without documented history of prior exposure.

— Some anaphylactic reactions may be mediated by complement (eg, allergic reactions to blood products). Generally signs of an anaphylactic reaction develop after reexposure to a sensitizing antigen.

— *Anaphylactoid reactions* are similar to anaphylactic reactions but they are triggered by materials such as radiocontrast material and certain parenteral medications and are not mediated by an IgE antibody response.

— The clinical presentation and management of anaphylactic and anaphylactoid reactions are similar, so it is not necessary to distinguish between them when determining treatment for an acute attack.

■ **Clinical definitions.** Some authors define *anaphylaxis* as a generalized, rapid-onset allergic reaction (including urticaria) with laryngeal edema, angioedema, or bronchospasm from increased bronchial smooth muscle tone, which causes shortness of breath.[2] Anaphylaxis is graded as severe if loss of consciousness (syncope) or hypotension occurs. These effects are produced by the release of mediators, including histamine, leukotriene C_4, prostaglandin D_2, and tryptase.

Incidence

Although prior exposure is essential for development of true anaphylaxis, reactions occur even when no documented prior exposure exists. Thus patients may appear to react to their initial exposure to an antibiotic or insect sting. As we age we all are exposed to potential allergens that can create sensitivity. For this reason children are at lowest risk and the elderly are at the greatest risk of developing anaphylaxis.

■ The annual incidence of anaphylaxis is unknown. Researchers do not use national or international standards for either *numerators* (case definitions) or *denominators* (source of cases).

— A population-based study from the state of Minnesota[3] estimated the annual rate of *occurrence* of anaphylaxis to be 30 per 100 000 person-years (95% CI).

— Because some people had more than one episode of anaphylaxis, the average annual rate of *incidence* of anaphylaxis was lower at 21 per 100 000 person-years (95% CI, 17 to 25).[3]

— Clinicians identified a suspect allergen in 68% of cases of anaphylaxis. The most commonly identified allergens were food, medication, and insect sting. Seven percent of persons with anaphylaxis required hospitalization.

■ In the United Kingdom investigators reported an annual incidence rate using the number of patients evaluated at the accident and emergency department (ED) of a single hospital as the denominator.[2]

— Anaphylaxis, defined as a generalized allergic reaction that caused shortness of breath, occurred in 1 of 2300 ED patients.

— Severe anaphylaxis, with loss of consciousness, occurred in 1 of 6000 ED patients.

■ The annual incidence of severe anaphylactic reactions in 3 European countries has been estimated at 154 per 1 million hospitalized patients, with 4 deaths per 1 million hospitalized patients.[4]

Etiology

■ Insect stings, drugs, contrast media, and some foods (eg, milk, eggs, and fish in children and shellfish in adults) are the most common causes of anaphylaxis.

— The issue of hypersensitivity to Hymenoptera (membrane-winged insects—bees, ants, and wasps) insect stings has become particularly complex and controversial because of medical, economic, and legal issues related to the poor performance of venom skin testing as a diagnostic test,[5,6] and the absence of appropriate indications for Hymenoptera desensitization.

— In one recent study of people who had been stung once *and* who had a reaction to that sting, subjects were given a challenge sting at rest. Of these subjects, 35% to 60% experienced anaphylaxis from the challenge sting.[7]

■ Peanut and tree nut (Brazil, almond, hazel, and macadamia nuts) allergies have recently been recognized as particularly dangerous.[8]

■ Aspirin, nonsteroidal anti-inflammatory agents, parenteral penicillins, radiologic contrast media, and many other drugs and toxins, vaccines, beer, and latex (delayed onset of 30 minutes; common in patients with spina bifida) can cause anaphylactic reactions.

■ Exercise-induced anaphylaxis (especially after ingestion of certain foods) has been reported.

■ Some allergens such as dust, pollen, and dander are inhaled.

■ Anaphylaxis may even be idiopathic. Without a known allergen, these patients must be managed with long-term oral steroid therapy. β-Blockers may increase the severity of anaphylaxis, blocking the response to endogenous catecholamines and exogenous epinephrine.

Pathophysiology

The manifestations of anaphylaxis are related to release of chemical mediators from mast cells. These mediators are released when antigens (allergens) bind to antigen-specific IgE attached to previously sensitized basophils and mast cells. In an anaphylactoid reaction, exposure to an antigen causes direct release of mediators, a process that is not mediated by IgE.

The most important mediators of anaphylaxis are histamines, leukotrienes, prostaglandins, thromboxanes, and bradykinins. These mediators contribute to vasodilation, increased capillary permeability, and airway constriction and produce the clinical signs of hypotension, angioedema, and bronchospasm. The sooner the reaction occurs after exposure, the more likely it is to be severe.

The location and concentration of the mast cells determine which organs are affected. The signs and symptoms are determined by the body system involved.

Signs and Symptoms

Signs and symptoms can be cutaneous, cardiovascular, respiratory, and gastrointestinal.

■ **Cutaneous.** These symptoms may include diffuse urticaria and conjunctivitis. The patient may appear either flushed or pale.

■ **Cardiovascular.** *Cardiovascular collapse* is the most common cause of death. Cardiac dysfunction is due principally to hypotension caused by both an *absolute* and a *relative* hypovolemia. Underlying cardiovascular disease can complicate the clinical presentation.

— *Absolute hypovolemia* is caused by intravascular volume loss from increased capillary permeability.

— *Relative hypovolemia* is caused by vasodilation.

■ **Respiratory.** Rhinitis is present. Upper airway (laryngeal) edema or lower airway edema or both may be present. Bronchospasm may develop in patients with preexisting asthma. Respiratory signs may develop acutely and become life-threatening.

■ **Gastrointestinal** symptoms include abdominal pain, vomiting, and diarrhea. These signs may be particularly prominent in children.

Differential Diagnosis

Patients with anaphylaxis can present with a wide variety of signs and symptoms. No single finding is pathognomonic. Many conditions can produce clinical signs that are similar to anaphylaxis but that require different treatments. To provide optimal therapy and avoid inappropriate treatment,[9] providers must differentiate between anaphylaxis and other diseases. The ACLS provider must recognize the following frequently encountered anaphylaxis "look-alikes."

■ **Urticaria** is characterized by distinctive small skin eruptions (*hives*) with well-defined borders and pale centers surrounded by patches of red skin (*wheal-and-flare reaction*). Typically these red areas are intensely itchy (*pruritus*).

■ **Angioedema** and urticaria are variable manifestations of the same pathologic process. This response is mediated by vasoactive substances, which cause the arterioles to dilate. Capillary fluid leak and edema develop in both conditions. Angioedema involves vessels in the subdermal skin layers. Urticaria is localized in skin layers superficial to the dermis. Angioedema results in areas of well-demarcated, localized, nonpitting edema. Although angioedema may be caused by anaphylaxis, the provider must consider other potential causes of angioedema and urticaria.

■ **Severe, life-threatening asthma.** Although bronchospasm is often a component of anaphylaxis, asthma and anaphylaxis are two distinct entities that require very different treatment. Failure to identify and treat either anaphylaxis or asthma could be fatal for the patient.[9]

■ **Vasovagal reactions.** Patients with classic "fainting" may appear to be either flushed or pale when they collapse or lose consciousness.

■ **Functional vocal cord dysfunction.** Change in voice or loss of voice can lead to a suspicion of the angioedema in the pharynx that occurs with allergic/anaphylactic reactions.

- **Scombroid poisoning.** This food-related illness often develops within 30 minutes of eating spoiled tuna, mackerel, or dolphin (mahi-mahi). Ingestion typically causes urticaria, nausea, vomiting, diarrhea, and headache. These symptoms are caused by histamine produced by bacteria on the fish. Histamine levels can be higher than 20 to 50 mg/100 g of toxic fish. Antihistamines (H_1 and H_2 blockers) are safe and are often effective in reducing or eliminating these symptoms.

- **Hereditary angioedema** (in which there is a family history of angioedema) does not cause urticaria but does cause gastrointestinal edema, which can lead to severe abdominal pain, or respiratory mucosal edema, which can lead to airway compromise. This form of angioedema is treated with fresh frozen plasma.

- **Angiotensin-converting enzyme (ACE) inhibitors** are associated with a reactive angioedema predominantly of the upper airway. This reaction can develop as late as days or years after ACE inhibitors are first used. The best medical treatment for this form of angioedema is unclear. ACLS providers must focus on aggressive early airway management.[10]

- **Panic disorder and panic attacks.** In some forms of panic attacks, functional stridor develops from forced adduction of the vocal cords. Panic attacks are not associated with urticaria, angioedema, or hypotension.

Treatment of Anaphylaxis

The treatment of anaphylaxis has not been standardized.[11] The etiology, clinical severity, clinical course, and organ involvement of anaphylactic reactions vary widely,[12] and randomized trials of treatment approaches are few. The following recommendations are commonly used and widely accepted but are based more on consensus than evidence.

- The mainstays of prearrest treatment are
  — Oxygen
  — Epinephrine
  — Aggressive fluid resuscitation
  — Antihistamines
  — H_2 blocking agents
  — Inhaled β_2-adrenergic agents
  — Corticosteroids

- **Oxygen.** Administer oxygen to all patients, and administer a high concentration of oxygen to patients with respiratory distress. Titrate oxygen administration based on pulse oximetry evaluation of oxyhemoglobin saturation. Be prepared to intubate the patient and provide mechanical ventilatory support if laryngeal edema produces severe upper airway obstruction or if bronchospasm causes severe respiratory distress (see "Special Considerations," below).

- **Epinephrine.** Administer epinephrine to all patients with clinical signs of shock, airway edema or constriction, or definite breathing difficulty.[13,14]
  — Give epinephrine IV if the anaphylactic reaction appears to be profound and life-threatening. The IV dose is 0.1 to 0.5 mg, given over 5 minutes. Use the more dilute solution of 1:10 000 (1 to 5 mL). An IV infusion (1 mg in 250 mL D_5W or 4 µg/mL) at a rate of 1 to 4 µg/min may eliminate the need for frequent repeat epinephrine doses.
  — Give epinephrine IM if vascular access is not available or anaphylaxis is less severe. The dose is 0.3 to 0.5 mg (1:1000; 0.3 to 0.5 mL). The dose may be repeated after 5 to 10 minutes if there is no clinical improvement.
  — Do not give epinephrine *subcutaneously* because absorption and achievement of maximum plasma concentration are delayed when systemic perfusion is poor.[15]

- **Aggressive fluid resuscitation.** Give isotonic *crystalloid* (normal saline) if hypotension is severe and does not respond rapidly to epinephrine. Give a *rapid infusion of 1 to 2 L* "wide-open." A total of 4 to 6 L may be needed. Monitor for the development of pulmonary edema and be prepared to support oxygenation and ventilation.

- **Antihistamines.** Administer antihistamines slowly by the IV or deep IM route (diphenhydramine 10 to 50 mg, no faster than 25 mg/min).

- **H_2 blockers.** Administer H_2 blockers such as cimetidine (300 mg PO, IM, or IV).[16]

- **Inhaled β-adrenergic agents.** Provide inhaled albuterol if bronchospasm is present. If the patient has both bronchospasm and hypotension, administer parenteral epinephrine before inhaled albuterol to minimize potential hypotensive effects of the albuterol. Inhaled ipratropium may be especially useful for treatment of bronchospasm in patients taking β-blockers.

- **Corticosteroids.** Infuse high-dose IV corticosteroids slowly or administer intramuscularly after severe attacks, especially in patients with asthma and those already receiving steroids. The beneficial effects may not be apparent for 4 to 6 hours.

- **Remove bee stinger and venom sac.**[17] Common first aid advice is to look for a bee stinger with an intact venom sac. Unlike wasps, bees leave their stingers in the skin with an attached venom sac. Remove the venom sac (stinger plus bee parts) by scraping with the dull side of a knife or a credit card, taking care not to compress it, which may release more toxins. Wash the area with soap and water and apply ice to relieve pain.

- **Glucagon.** Glucagon may be effective for patients who are unresponsive to epinephrine and may be particularly useful for patients receiving β-blockers. This agent is short-acting (1 to 2 mg

IV every 5 minutes or 1 to 5 mg/h). Nausea, vomiting, and hyperglycemia are common side effects.

- **Observation.** Observe the patient closely for up to 24 hours. Many patients do not respond promptly to therapy. Approximately 20% of patients that do respond to initial therapy demonstrate a second, or biphasic, anaphylactic response. In these patients an intervening asymptomatic period is followed by recurrence of symptoms within 8 to 24 hours.[18] In one retrospective study, patients who demonstrated a biphasic response required high doses of epinephrine to eliminate symptoms during the initial therapy.[18] It is important to note this potential for biphasic response if patients are discharged from the ED after an anaphylactic reaction.

Special Considerations in Anaphylaxis Management

Treatment of Severe Airway Obstruction

Monitor the patient's airway and breathing closely during therapy (see above). Perform early *elective* intubation if the patient develops hoarseness, lingual edema, posterior or oropharyngeal swelling, or severe bronchospasm. Be prepared to perform *semi-elective* (awake, sedated) tracheal intubation without paralytic agents when signs of distress develop and before respiratory arrest is imminent.

- *Provide assisted ventilation following intubation.* Patients with angioedema are at high risk for rapid deterioration. Most will present with some swelling of the face or lips. The patient with any hoarseness, lingual edema, or posterior or oropharyngeal swelling is at high risk for airway obstruction and respiratory compromise.

Early Tracheal Intubation: Some Precautions

If intubation is delayed, patients can deteriorate relatively quickly (within ½ to 3 hours) with development of progressive stridor, severe dysphonia or aphonia, laryngeal

edema, massive lingual swelling, facial and neck swelling, and hypoxemia. At this point both tracheal intubation and cricothyrotomy may be difficult or impossible. Attempts at tracheal intubation may only further increase laryngeal edema or compromise the airway with bleeding into the oropharynx and narrow glottic opening.

Hypoxia may lead to agitation and combativeness during administration of oxygen.

Initiation of paralysis before a tracheal intubation attempt may prove lethal in these patients. The glottic opening is narrow and difficult to visualize when lingual and oropharyngeal edema are present. Once paralyzing agents are administered, the patient will be unable to contribute to ventilation.

If tracheal intubation is unsuccessful, it may be impossible to provide effective bag-mask ventilation. Laryngeal edema prevents air entry. Facial edema prevents creation of an effective seal between the face and the bag-mask device. Pharmacologic paralysis at this point may deprive the patient of his/her only mechanism for ventilation, ie, spontaneous breathing attempts.

Treatment of Cardiac Arrest: Key Interventions and Modifications of BLS and ACLS

Cardiac arrest from anaphylaxis may be associated with profound vasodilation, total cardiovascular collapse, tissue hypoxia, and asystole. There is no research data to guide specific modifications in resuscitation procedures. Providers may find it difficult to achieve adequate volume replacement and ventilation. Consensus recommendations have been made following experience with nonfatal cases.

Death from anaphylaxis is usually due to cardiovascular collapse with massive vasodilation, cardiac pump failure, and progressive shock. The major clinical challenge is providing adequate volume replacement into a cardiovascular "tank" undergoing a life-threatening, but unknown, increase in capacity and capillary leak.

Airway, Oxygenation, and Ventilation

Cardiac arrest may result from angioedema and upper or lower airway obstruction. Bag-mask ventilation and tracheal intubation may be impossible. Cricothyrotomy may not be possible because landmarks are obliterated by severe swelling.

- Rapid sequence intubation, as described in the section on severe, life-threatening asthma (and in Volume 1, Chapter 8), should be initiated early rather than late. Note the precaution above about administration of paralyzing agents.

- In these desperate circumstances, consider the following airway techniques:

  — Fiberoptic tracheal intubation

  — Digital tracheal intubation, in which the fingers guide insertion of a small (<7.0 mm) tracheal tube

  — Needle cricothyrotomy followed by transtracheal oxygenation (ventilation will not be very effective unless a larger airway can be inserted)

  — Cricothyrotomy as described for patients with massive neck swelling[19]

Support of Circulation

- **Rapid volume expansion** is perhaps the most critical intervention. Anaphylaxis can produce profound vasodilation that greatly increases intravascular capacity, and capillary leak that produces intravascular volume loss.

  — Administer large volumes (a minimum of 2 to 4 L) of isotonic crystalloid as fast as possible.

  — Slow the rate of fluid administration as clinical response begins.

- **Give epinephrine early (1 mg); rapidly progress to high-dose levels IV (0.1 mg/kg)** for patients in full cardiac arrest.

  — Epinephrine is the drug of choice for treatment of both vasodilation/ hypotension and cardiac arrest.

  — One commonly used sequence is to give epinephrine in doses of 1 mg,

3 mg, and 5 mg IV, each 3 minutes apart. Following bolus administration, begin a constant infusion of epinephrine at 4 to 10 µg/min.

- **Antihistamines IV.** There is little data about the value of antihistamines in treatment of anaphylaxis with cardiac arrest. They are unlikely to be harmful.

- **Corticosteroid therapy.** Although steroids should have no effect if given during a cardiac arrest, their value may "kick in" hours later in the postresuscitation period.

- **Asystole and Pulseless Electrical Activity (PEA) Algorithms.** Because the arrest rhythm in anaphylaxis is often PEA or asystole, it is appropriate to initiate the remaining asystole and PEA interventions:

  — Atropine administration

  — Transcutaneous pacing

- **Prolonged CPR.** Cardiac arrest associated with anaphylaxis may respond to prolonged CPR attempts.

  — Often the patient is young with a healthy heart and cardiovascular system.

  — Simultaneous rapid correction of vasodilation and low blood volume is required for CPR to be effective.

  — CPR may maintain sufficient oxygen delivery to the brain and heart until the effects of the mediators triggered by the anaphylaxis subside.

Summary

- Management of anaphylaxis includes
  — Prevention
  — Early recognition
  — Anticipation of deterioration
  — Aggressive support of circulation with vasopressors and volume resuscitation
  — Aggressive support of airway, oxygenation, and ventilation
  — Early intubation and provision of mechanical ventilation

- These approaches may be successful even if cardiac arrest develops.

References

1. Cianferoni A, Novembre E, Mugnaini L, Lombardi E, Pucci N, Vierucci A. Clinical features of acute anaphylaxis in patients admitted to a university hospital: an 11-year retrospective review (1985-1996). *Ann Allergy Asthma Immunol.* 2001;87:27-32.

2. Stewart AG, Ewan PW. The incidence, aetiology and management of anaphylaxis presenting to an accident and emergency department. *QJM.* 1996;89:859-864.

3. Yocum MW, Butterfield JH, Klein JS, Volcheck GW, Schroeder DR, Silverstein MD. Epidemiology of anaphylaxis in Olmsted County: a population-based study. *J Allergy Clin Immunol.* 1999;104:452-456.

4. An epidemiologic study of severe anaphylactic and anaphylactoid reactions among hospital patients: methods and overall risks. The International Collaborative Study of Severe Anaphylaxis. *Epidemiology.* 1998;9:141-146.

5. Golden DB, Kagey-Sobotka A, Norman PS, Hamilton RG, Lichtenstein LM. Insect sting allergy with negative venom skin test responses. *J Allergy Clin Immunol.* 2001;107:897-901.

6. Reisman RE. Insect sting allergy: the dilemma of the negative skin test reactor. *J Allergy Clin Immunol.* 2001;107:781-782.

7. Hauk P, Friedl K, Kaufmehl K, Urbanek R, Forster J. Subsequent insect stings in children with hypersensitivity to Hymenoptera. *J Pediatr.* 1995;126:185-190.

8. Ewan PW. Clinical study of peanut and nut allergy in 62 consecutive patients: new features and associations. *BMJ.* 1996;312:1074-1078.

9. Brown AF. Anaphylaxis: quintessence, quarrels, and quandaries. *Emerg Med J.* 2001;18:328.

10. Ishoo E, Shah UK, Grillone GA, Stram JR, Fuleihan NS. Predicting airway risk in angioedema: staging system based on presentation. *Otolaryngol Head Neck Surg.* 1999;121:263-268.

11. Project Team of the Resuscitation Council. Emergency medical treatment of anaphylactic reactions. *J Accid Emerg Med.* 1999;16:243-247.

12. Gavalas M, Walford C, Sadana A, O'Donnell C. Medical treatment of anaphylaxis. *J Accid Emerg Med.* 2000;17:152; author reply 152-153.

13. Hughes G, Fitzharris P. Managing acute anaphylaxis. New guidelines emphasise importance of intramuscular adrenaline. *BMJ.* 1999;319:1-2.

14. Sadana A, O'Donnell C, Hunt MT, Gavalas M. Managing acute anaphylaxis. Intravenous adrenaline should be considered because of the urgency of the condition. *BMJ.* 2000;320:937-938.

15. Simons FE, Roberts JR, Gu X, Simons KJ. Epinephrine absorption in children with a history of anaphylaxis. *J Allergy Clin Immunol.* 1998;101:33-37.

16. Runge JW, Martinez JC, Caravati EM, Williamson SG, Hartsell SC. Histamine antagonists in the treatment of acute allergic reactions. *Ann Emerg Med.* 1992;21:237-242.

17. de Jong NW, Vermeulen AM, de Groot H. Allergy to bumblebee venom. III. Immunotherapy follow-up study (safety and efficacy) in patients with occupational bumblebee-venom anaphylaxis. *Allergy.* 1999;54:980-984.

18. Brazil E, MacNamara AF. "Not so immediate" hypersensitivity—the danger of biphasic anaphylactic reactions. *J Accid Emerg Med.* 1998;15:252-253.

19. Simon RR, Brenner BE. Airway procedures. In: *Emergency Procedures and Techniques.* Baltimore, Md: Williams & Wilkins; 1994:79.

Special Resuscitation Situations
Part 5: Cardiac Arrest Associated With Trauma

Introduction

In industrialized nations trauma is the leading cause of death from the age of 6 months through young adulthood.[1,2]

When anyone is severely injured, resuscitation must begin as soon as possible, preferably at the scene.[3] Early and effective support of airway, ventilation, oxygenation, and perfusion is vital because survival from out-of-hospital cardiac arrest secondary to blunt trauma is uniformly low in children and adults.[4-6] In some out-of-hospital and Emergency Department settings, resuscitative efforts are withheld when patients with blunt trauma are found in asystole or agonal electrical cardiac activity. Survival after cardiac arrest resulting from penetrating trauma is only slightly better. Following penetrating trauma, rapid transport to a trauma center is associated with better outcomes than prolonged resuscitative attempts in the field.[7]

BLS and ALS for the trauma patient are fundamentally the same as the care for a patient with a primary cardiac or respiratory arrest. In trauma resuscitation rescuers perform a "Primary Survey" to rapidly identify and immediately treat life-threatening conditions that will interfere with establishing an effective airway, oxygenation, ventilation, and circulation.[3] After completion of the Primary Survey, the rescuer should perform a more detailed Secondary Survey (also called the Focused History and Detailed Physical Examination). Terminology used to describe these assessments is presented in the Critical Concepts Box.

Cardiopulmonary deterioration associated with trauma has several possible causes. The management plan may vary for each. Potential causes of cardiopulmonary deterioration and arrest include the following:

- Severe central neurologic injury with secondary cardiovascular collapse

- Hypoxia secondary to respiratory insufficiency, resulting from neurologic injury, airway obstruction, large open pneumothorax, or severe tracheobronchial laceration or crush

- Direct and severe injury to vital structures such as the heart, aorta, or pulmonary arteries

- Underlying medical problems or other conditions that led to the injury, such as sudden cardiac arrest or stroke in the driver of a motor vehicle

- Severely diminished cardiac output from tension pneumothorax or pericardial tamponade

- Exsanguination leading to hypovolemia and severely diminished oxygen delivery

Critical Concepts: ATLS and NHTSA Terminology

Primary Survey = initial assessment

Secondary Survey = focused history and detailed physical examination

The National Highway Traffic Safety Administration (NHTSA) EMS National Standard Curricula uses some terms for the initial assessment and stabilization of the injured patient that differ slightly from those used in the Advanced Trauma Life Support Course (ATLS) offered by the American College of Surgeons. The ACLS provider should be familiar with the terms used by the two courses to describe the same rescuer actions and should be able to apply both sets of terms to the care of the injured patient.

Terminology:

Scene survey: Quick assessment to determine safety of scene.

General impression: A quick "from the door," "across the room," or "approaching the victim" assessment to determine if the patient looks "good" or "bad."

Primary survey (ATLS) or initial assessment (NHTSA): Rapid evaluation and stabilization of airway, breathing, circulation, disability (neurologic function), and exposure.

Secondary survey (ATLS) or focused history and detailed physical examination (NHTSA): A complete head-to-toe physical examination. The detailed physical examination of the NHTSA course includes a *focused history*. Use the AMPLE mnemonic to identify important aspects of the victim's history and presenting complaint:

- **A**llergies

- **M**edications

- **P**ast medical history

- **L**ast meal

- **E**vents leading up to the scenario

■ Injuries in a cold environment (eg, fractured leg) complicated by secondary severe hypothermia

In cases of cardiac arrest associated with uncontrolled internal hemorrhage or pericardial tamponade, the best outcomes are associated with rapid transport of the victim to an emergency facility with immediate operative capabilities.[7,8]

Despite rapid and effective out-of-hospital and trauma center response, survival is poor in patients with out-of-hospital cardiopulmonary arrest due to blunt trauma.[4-10] Patients who do survive out-of-hospital cardiopulmonary arrest associated with trauma generally are young, have penetrating injuries, receive early (out-of-hospital) tracheal intubation, and receive prompt transport by highly skilled paramedics to a definitive care facility.[9,11-13]

Trauma care should be provided within a planned system that promotes excellence in prehospital, in-hospital, and rehabilitative care. Such a system includes protocols for management of common complications of injury, early consultation with a surgeon when indicated, and an ongoing program of quality improvement. Detailed presentation of trauma management is beyond the scope of this textbook. Advanced courses are taught by several organizations, including the American College of Surgeons

(Advanced Trauma Life Support Course)[3] and the National Association of Emergency Medical Technicians (Pre-Hospital Trauma Life Support Course). Whenever possible, recommendations in this chapter were made consistent with the recommendations taught in those courses.

Initial Evaluation and Triage

Extricate and Evaluate

Specially trained rescuers should rapidly extricate the victim while immobilizing the cervical spine. Provide immediate BLS and ALS interventions to ensure adequate airway, oxygenation, ventilation, and circulation. Prepare the victim for rapid transport to a facility that provides definitive trauma care. Use lateral neck supports, strapping, and backboards throughout transport to minimize exacerbation of an occult neck or spinal cord injury.

Multicasualty Triage

When multiple victims have serious injuries, emergency personnel must establish priorities for care. When the number of victims with critical injuries exceeds the capability of the EMS providers at the scene, victims without a pulse are the lowest priority for care. Most EMS systems

have guidelines that permit out-of-hospital pronouncement of death or withholding of cardiac resuscitative efforts when there are multiple victims with critical injuries or when victims have injuries incompatible with life. EMS personnel should work within such guidelines when available.

Withholding or Terminating Resuscitation in Prehospital Traumatic Cardiopulmonary Arrest

In January 2003 the National Association of EMS Physicians and the American College of Surgeons Committee on Trauma published a position statement on withholding or terminating resuscitation in prehospital traumatic cardiopulmonary arrest.[14,15] These valuable guidelines are summarized in the Table. In addition, in 2001 the American College of Surgeons Committee on Advanced Trauma Life Support published their seventh edition of recommendations for Advanced Trauma Life Support.[3] Because these trauma guidelines were published after the international *ECC Guidelines 2000*, they have not yet been evaluated in the ECC Evidence Evaluation process. They are presented here as resource information for ACLS providers.

TABLE. Guidelines for Withholding or Terminating of Resuscitation in Prehospital Traumatic Cardiopulmonary Arrest

A. Specific Criteria and Recommendations by Type of Trauma		
Patient in Cardiac Arrest Associated With Trauma Upon Arrival of EMS Personnel		
Type of Trauma	**Specific Criteria**	**Recommendations**
Blunt	■ Thorough primary assessment finds patient to be apneic, pulseless, with no organized ECG activity	■ DO NOT START resuscitative efforts
Penetrating	■ Further assessment finds **POSITIVE** secondary signs of life (eg, pupillary reflexes, spontaneous movement, agonal respirations, organized ECG activity)	■ START resuscitative efforts ■ TRANSPORT to nearest ED or trauma center

Type of Trauma	Specific Criteria	Recommendations
Penetrating	■ Further assessment finds **NO** secondary signs of life (eg, pupillary reflexes, spontaneous movement, agonal respirations, organized ECG activity)	■ DO NOT START resuscitative efforts
Blunt or Penetrating	■ Injuries are obviously incompatible with life (eg, decapitation, hemicorporectomy)	■ DO NOT START resuscitative efforts
	■ Evidence of death (eg, dependent lividity, rigor mortis, decomposition)	
	■ Possible nontraumatic cardiac arrest: mechanism of injury does not correlate with clinical condition	■ START resuscitative efforts ■ TRANSPORT to nearest ED or trauma center
	■ No response, or no sustained response, to 15 minutes of resuscitation and CPR if EMS personnel witnessed arrest → *nonsalvageable*	■ STOP resuscitative efforts
	■ More than 15 minutes transport time to nearest ED or trauma center → *nonsalvageable*	

B. Guideline Elements and Recommendations

Guideline Element	Recommendations
System factors to consider	■ Average transport time within EMS system ■ Definitive care capabilities (trauma centers) within EMS system ■ Transport time based on accomplishment of IV access and airway management during transport
Special resuscitation situations	■ Give special consideration (following specific protocols) to victims of submersion, lightning strike, and significant hypothermia
Training	■ EMS providers must be thoroughly familiar with all guidelines and protocols for decisions to withhold or stop resuscitative efforts
Medical direction	■ EMS medical director should develop and implement all protocols ■ Online medical control should be available to help determine the appropriateness of withholding or stopping resuscitation
Notification policies and protocols	■ Procedures must include notification of appropriate law enforcement agencies, including medical examiners or coroners, about final disposition of the body
Survivor and provider support	■ The family of the deceased should have access to resources (eg, clergy, social workers, counseling personnel) as needed ■ EMS providers should have access to resources for debriefing and counseling as needed
Quality review	■ Polices and protocols for termination or withholding of resuscitation should be monitored through a quality review system

Modified from Hopson et al.[14,15]

Modifications in BLS for Cardiac Arrest Associated With Trauma

Establish Unresponsiveness

Head trauma, shock, or respiratory arrest may produce loss of consciousness. If spinal cord injury is present, the victim may be conscious but unable to move.

Throughout initial assessment and stabilization, the rescuer should monitor the victim's responsiveness. Deterioration could indicate either neurologic compromise or cardiorespiratory failure.

Airway

Cervical Spine Precautions

When head or neck injury or multisystem trauma is present, rescuers must immobilize the cervical spine throughout BLS maneuvers. Use a jaw thrust instead of a head tilt–chin lift to open the airway. If at all possible a second rescuer should be responsible for immobilizing the head and neck until spinal immobilization equipment is applied.

After opening the airway manually, clear the mouth of blood, vomitus, and other secretions. Remove this material with a (gloved) finger sweep, or use gauze or a towel to wipe the mouth. You may also use suction.

Breathing and Ventilation

Once you establish a patent airway, assess for breathing. If breathing is absent or grossly inadequate (eg, agonal or slow and extremely shallow), provide mouth-to–barrier device or bag-mask ventilation.

If there is a risk of cervical spine injury, immobilize the spine while providing rescue breathing. Maintain immobilization throughout the rescue attempt.

Deliver breaths slowly to avoid gastric inflation and possible regurgitation. If the chest does not expand during ventilation despite repeated attempts to open the airway with a jaw thrust, a tension pneumothorax or hemothorax may be present. These complications should be ruled out or treated by ACLS personnel.

Circulation

If the victim has no signs of circulation in response to the rescue breaths (no breathing, coughing, or movement) and no detectable carotid pulse, provide chest compressions.

Defibrillation

Sudden cardiac arrest associated with VF/pulseless VT may cause trauma. If the victim develops VF/pulseless VT, the victim will lose consciousness, and this can lead to falls and car crashes.

Cardiac arrest is an indication for use of an AED (or manual defibrillator in the hospital setting). Power on the AED, attach the electrode pads, and allow the AED to analyze for VF. The AED will evaluate the victim's cardiac rhythm and advise shock delivery if appropriate.

Disability

Throughout all interventions assess the victim's level of consciousness and general neurologic status. Monitor closely for signs of neurologic deterioration during BLS care. The Glasgow Coma Scale is useful and can be calculated in seconds (see Volume 1, Chapter 18: "Acute Stroke: Current Treatments and Paradigms").

Exposure

The victim may lose heat to the environment through conduction, convection, and evaporation. Such heat loss will be exacerbated when the victim's clothes are removed or if the victim is covered in blood or water. Take all practical actions to maintain the victim's temperature.

Modifications in ACLS for Cardiac Arrest Associated With Trauma

Airway

Indications for intubation in the injured patient include

- Respiratory arrest or apnea
- Respiratory failure, including severe hypoventilation, hypoxemia despite oxygen therapy, or respiratory acidosis
- Shock
- Severe head injury
- Inability to protect the upper airway (eg, loss of gag reflex, depressed level of consciousness, coma)
- Thoracic injuries (eg, flail chest, pulmonary contusion, penetrating trauma)
- Signs of airway obstruction
- Injuries associated with potential airway obstruction (eg, crushing facial or neck injuries)
- Anticipated need for mechanical ventilatory support

Perform tracheal intubation with cervical spine immobilization. Orotracheal intubation is the preferred method. You should avoid nasotracheal intubation, especially if you suspect cervical spine injury, because nasotracheal intubation is more likely than orotracheal intubation to require excessive manipulation of the cervical spine. Also avoid nasotracheal intubation if you suspect maxillofacial injury or basilar skull fracture. If the maxillofacial injury is associated with a dural tear, a nasogastric or tracheal tube placed through the nose may migrate intracranially.[16] Nasotracheal intubation also may result in introduction of bacteria through the dura.

ACLS providers should confirm proper tracheal tube placement by the primary and secondary confirmation techniques described in Volume 1, Chapter 8. Secondary confirmation techniques are exhaled CO_2 detectors or esophageal detector devices.

Maintain proper tube placement by use of commercial tracheal tube holders. Continuously confirm proper tube position by use of pulse oximetry and exhaled CO_2 monitoring during transport and after any transfer of the patient (eg, from ambulance to hospital gurney). In the prehospital setting, immobilization of the cervical spine with a collar or backboard or both can serve as an additional aid to prevent tube dislodgement, although the use and effect of these immobilizers on tube placement has not been reported.

The inability to intubate the trachea of the patient with massive facial injury and edema is an indication for a surgical airway. An emergent cricothyrotomy will provide an immediate, secure airway that supports oxygenation, although ventilation will be suboptimal. Commercial cricothyrotomy kits and transtracheal catheters are now widely available for use by prehospital and ED ACLS providers.

Complications

If CPR is needed after tracheal intubation, provision of simultaneous ventilations and compressions may cause a tension pneumothorax. The patient may require needle decompression and insertion of a 1-way valve.

There is a high risk for the development of a tension pneumothorax if lung injury has occurred, especially if the victim has fractured ribs or a fractured sternum. Synchronized ventilations and compressions in a ratio of 1 to 5 may be required if the thoracic cage is damaged.

Stomach Decompression

Insert a gastric tube to decompress the stomach. Insert an orogastric rather than a nasogastric tube in patients with severe head or maxillofacial injuries. If the dura is torn, a nasogastric tube can migrate into sinuses or even into the brain.[16] Always confirm proper oro- or nasogastric tube placement into the stomach by auscultation over the gastric region while injecting air through a syringe.

Ventilation

Provide high concentrations of oxygen even if the victim's oxygenation appears to be adequate. Once you ensure a patent airway, assess breath sounds and chest expansion.

Complications

Signs of a pneumothorax are unilateral decrease in breath sounds and inadequate chest expansion during positive-pressure ventilation. Assume that these signs are caused by a *tension pneumothorax* until that complication is either confirmed or ruled out.

Perform needle decompression of the pneumothorax immediately, and then insert a chest tube. Surgical exploration is indicated if thoracic decompression does not produce immediate hemodynamic improvement or if the patient has a penetrating thoracic wound.[12]

Rescuers should look for and seal any significant *open pneumothorax*. Tension pneumothorax may develop after sealing of an open pneumothorax, so decompression may be needed.[8]

A traumatic *hemothorax* also may interfere with ventilation and chest expansion. Treat significant hemothorax with blood replacement and chest tube insertion. If the hemorrhage is severe and continues, the patient may require surgical exploration.

If the victim has a significant *flail chest,* spontaneous ventilation likely will be inadequate to maintain oxygenation. Flail chest results from multiple fractures of adjacent ribs. These fractures cause instability of a portion of the chest wall. This instability may cause respiratory failure, particularly if the patient is breathing spontaneously. Treat flail chest with positive-pressure ventilation.

Circulation

Once airway, oxygenation, and ventilation are addressed, evaluate and manage circulation. In the setting of trauma and pulseless arrest, the outcome will be poor unless a reversible cause can be immediately identified and treated (eg, tension pneumothorax).

Control external bleeding with pressure. This control is particularly important in the prehospital setting when surgical intervention is not possible. If hypovolemic shock is present, establish vascular access with the largest bore catheter possible and administer boluses of isotonic crystalloids (see "Volume Resuscitation," below). Note that volume resuscitation is no substitute for manual or surgical control of hemorrhage.[3]

Volume Resuscitation

Volume resuscitation is an important but problematic part of trauma resuscitation. If hypovolemic shock is present in the prehospital setting, administer isotonic crystalloid by bolus. Aggressive volume replacement may be necessary to restore adequate systemic perfusion. Once the patient arrives in the hospital, replacement of blood loss is accomplished with a combination of packed red blood cells and isotonic crystalloids.

For patients with *penetrating* chest trauma who are located a short distance from the trauma center, aggressive fluid resuscitation in the field can prolong transport time, and it has been associated with lower survival than rapid transport with less aggressive fluid resuscitation.[7] Immediate surgical exploration is required if massive penetrating trauma or severe hemorrhage is present. Aggressive volume resuscitation in the field will delay arrival at the trauma center, delay surgical interventions to close bleeding vessels, increase blood pressure, and consequently accelerate the rate of blood loss.[7,17]

Rescuers must control bleeding as soon as possible to maintain adequate blood volume and oxygen-carrying capacity. If external pressure does not stop bleeding or internal bleeding continues, surgical exploration is required.

If the patient receives initial isotonic crystalloid resuscitation with up to 2 L of fluid in the field and remains hypotensive on arrival in the ED, blood replacement is often needed. Administer packed red blood cells. Fully crossmatched blood is the ideal blood replacement, but it typically requires too long to prepare. Most blood banks can provide type-specific blood within 10 minutes, and type O packed cells can be available immediately. In general, Rh-negative blood is reserved for girls and for women of childbearing age to reduce sensitization and later Rh incompatibility. Rh-positive blood is administered to male victims and women beyond childbearing age.[3]

Rhythms of Arrest

The most common terminal cardiac rhythms observed in trauma victims are PEA and bradyasystolic rhythms. Occasionally VF/VT occurs.

Treatment of PEA requires identification and treatment of reversible causes, such as severe hypovolemia, hypothermia, cardiac tamponade, or tension pneumothorax.[18] Development of bradyasystolic rhythms often indicates the presence of severe hypovolemia, severe hypoxemia, or cardiorespiratory failure. Treat VF/VT with defibrillation. Although epinephrine is typically administered during ACLS treatment of these arrhythmias, it may be ineffective in the presence of severe hypovolemia.

Emergency Thoracotomy

Open thoracotomy does not improve outcome from out-of-hospital *blunt trauma arrest.* But open thoracotomy can be lifesaving for patients with *penetrating chest trauma,* particularly penetrating wounds of the heart.[10,11] Emergency thoracotomy allows direct massage of the heart, relief of cardiac tamponade, control of thoracic and extrathoracic hemorrhage, and aortic cross-clamping.[10,11] For optimal effectiveness, you should perform open thoracotomy as soon as possible. Provide concurrent volume resuscitation during the thoracotomy.

Penetrating Cardiac Injury

Rescuers should suspect penetrating cardiac injury with any penetrating trauma to the left chest, particularly when the penetrating injury is associated with low cardiac output or signs of tamponade (eg, distended neck veins, hypotension, and decreased heart tones). Remember that bullet and stab wounds may cause thoracic and cardiac injury even when the entrance site is in the right chest, back, or abdomen.

The Focused Assessment Sonogram in Trauma (FAST) is a rapid and accurate method of imaging the heart and the pericardium that can be performed in the Emergency Department. When used by an experienced operator, the FAST may be 90% accurate for the diagnosis of pericardial fluid.[3] FAST, however, is not available in all hospitals.

Pericardiocentesis can be useful for both diagnosis and therapy of cardiac tamponade. In general, efforts to relieve pericardial tamponade due to penetrating injury should occur in the hospital. Pericardiocentesis can be used to stabilize the patient until exploration, pericardiotomy, and repair of the injury can be accomplished in the operating room.[3]

Cardiac Contusions

Cardiac contusions causing significant arrhythmias or impairing cardiac function are present in approximately 10% to 20% of adult victims of severe blunt chest trauma.[19] You should suspect myocardial contusion if the trauma victim has extreme tachycardia, arrhythmias, and ST-segment–T-wave changes.

The myocardial band fraction of creatine kinase (CK-MB) is frequently elevated in patients with blunt chest injuries, but the elevation has little diagnostic or prognostic significance. Patients with an elevated level are just as likely as others to do well, and patients with a normal level may still have significant cardiac dysfunction. An MB fraction >5% has been used historically to diagnose cardiac contusion, but

this isoenzyme is not a sensitive indicator of myocardial contusion.[20] Although cardiac troponins may signal the presence of cardiac injury, they do not provide more information than a 12-lead ECG.[3] Confirm the diagnosis of myocardial contusion by echocardiography or radionuclide angiography.

Indications for Surgical Exploration

Resuscitation may be impossible in the presence of severe, uncontrolled hemorrhage or in the presence of significant cardiac, thoracic, or abdominal injuries. Victims with such injuries require surgical intervention. The following conditions are generally thought to be indications for urgent surgical exploration.[3]

- Hemodynamic instability despite volume resuscitation

- Thoracic injury associated with

  — Excessive chest tube drainage (1.5 to 2 L or more total, or >300 mL/h for 3 or more hours)

  — Significant hemothorax on chest x-ray

  — Suspected cardiac or aortic injury. The helical, contrast-enhanced computed tomography of the chest is extremely accurate for diagnosis of aortic injury.[3]

- Gunshot wounds thought to traverse the peritoneal cavity or visceral/vascular retroperitoneum (note that the path of the bullet may be unpredictable)

- Penetrating torso trauma, particularly if associated with

  — Peritoneal perforation or hypotension

  — Bleeding from the stomach, rectum, or genitourinary tract

- Blunt abdominal trauma with the following:

  — Hypotension and clinical evidence of intraperitoneal bleeding

  — Positive diagnostic peritoneal lavage or ultrasound

- Significant solid-organ, diaphragm, or bowel injury or peritonitis

  — Contrast-enhanced CT indicates ruptured gastrointestinal tract, intraperitoneal bladder injury, renal pedicle injury, or severe visceral parenchymal injury after blunt or penetrating injury

  — Peritonitis (on presentation or as later complication)

  — Free air, retroperitoneal air, or rupture of the hemidiaphragm after blunt trauma

References

1. *World Health Statistical Annual, 1994.* Geneva, Switzerland: World Health Organization; 1994.

2. Anderson RN. Deaths: leading causes for 2000. *Natl Vital Stat Rep.* 2002;50:1-85.

3. Parks SN, ATLS Subcommittee, American College of Surgeons Committee on Trauma. *Advanced Trauma Life Support, Overview of Changes for 7th Edition.* Chicago, Ill: American College of Surgeons; 2001.

4. Rosemurgy AS, Norris PA, Olson SM, Hurst JM, Albrink MH. Prehospital traumatic cardiac arrest: the cost of futility. *J Trauma.* 1993;35:468-473; discussion 473-474.

5. Hazinski MF, Chahine AA, Holcomb GW III, Morris JA Jr. Outcome of cardiovascular collapse in pediatric blunt trauma. *Ann Emerg Med.* 1994;23:1229-1235.

6. Bouillon B, Walther T, Kramer M, Neugebauer E. Trauma and circulatory arrest: 224 preclinical resuscitations in Cologne in 1987-1990 [in German]. *Anaesthesist.* 1994;43:786-790.

7. Bickell WH, Wall MJ Jr, Pepe PE, Martin RR, Ginger VF, Allen MK, Mattox KL. Immediate versus delayed fluid resuscitation for hypotensive patients with penetrating torso injuries. *N Engl J Med.* 1994;331:1105-1109.

8. Pepe P. Emergency medical services systems and prehospital management of patients requiring critical care. In: Carlson RW, Geheb M, eds. *Principles and Practice of Medical Intensive Care.* Philadelphia, Pa: Saunders; 1993:9-24.

9. Copass MK, Oreskovich MR, Bladergroen MR, Carrico CJ. Prehospital cardiopulmonary resuscitation of the critically injured patient. *Am J Surg.* 1984;148:20-26.

10. Rozycki GS, Adams C, Champion HR, Kihn R. Resuscitative thoracotomy—trends in outcome [abstract]. *Ann Emerg Med.* 1990;19:462.

11. Durham LA III, Richardson RJ, Wall MJ Jr, Pepe PE, Mattox KL. Emergency center thoracotomy: impact of prehospital resuscitation. *J Trauma.* 1992;32:775-779.

12. Kloeck W, Kramer E. Prehospital advanced CPR in the trauma patient. *Trauma Emerg Med.* 1993;10:772-776.

13. Schmidt U, Frame SB, Nerlich ML, Rowe DW, Enderson BL, Maull KI, Tscherne H. On-scene helicopter transport of patients with multiple injuries—comparison of a German and an American system. *J Trauma.* 1992;33:548-553; discussion 553-555.

14. Hopson LR, Hirsh E, Delgado J, Domeier RM, McSwain NE Jr, Krohmer J. Guidelines for withholding or termination of resuscitation in prehospital traumatic cardiopulmonary arrest: a joint position paper from the National Association of EMS Physicians Standards and Clinical Practice Committee and the American College of Surgeons Committee on Trauma. *Prehosp Emerg Care.* 2003;7:141-146.

15. Hopson LR, Hirsh E, Delgado J, Domeier RM, McSwain NE, Krohmer J. Guidelines for withholding or termination of resuscitation in prehospital traumatic cardiopulmonary arrest: joint position statement of the national association of EMS physicians and the American College of Surgeons Committee on Trauma. *J Am Coll Surg.* 2003;196:106-112.

16. Baskaya MK. Inadvertent intracranial placement of a nasogastric tube in patients with head injuries. *Surg Neurol.* 1999;52:426-427.

17. Solomonov E, Hirsh M, Yahiya A, Krausz MM. The effect of vigorous fluid resuscitation in uncontrolled hemorrhagic shock after massive splenic injury. *Crit Care Med.* 2000;28:749-754.

18. Kloeck WG. A practical approach to the aetiology of pulseless electrical activity: a simple 10-step training mnemonic. *Resuscitation.* 1995;30:157-159.

19. McLean RF, Devitt JH, Dubbin J, McLellan BA. Incidence of abnormal RNA studies and dysrhythmias in patients with blunt chest trauma. *J Trauma.* 1991;31:968-970.

20. Paone RF, Peacock JB, Smith DL. Diagnosis of myocardial contusion. *South Med J.* 1993;86:867-870.

Special Resuscitation Situations Part 6: Cardiac Arrest Associated With Pregnancy

Background

Essential Facts

Pregnancy stimulates a variety of physiologic changes that make the pregnant woman more vulnerable to cardiovascular insult. These changes can complicate attempted resuscitation during cardiac arrest (see "Critical Concepts: Physiologic Changes of Pregnancy That May Affect Resuscitation"). The ACLS provider should be aware of the unique physiology of pregnancy and be able to adapt resuscitation techniques to support the mother and the child.

Frequency

Cardiovascular emergencies in pregnant women are uncommon. Death related to pregnancy itself is rare, occurring at an estimated rate of 3.3 pregnancy-related deaths for every 100 000 live births.[1-4] But when non–pregnancy-related deaths are included, the rate increases to 9.2 deaths of pregnant women per 100 000 live births.

In the United States the three leading causes of death in pregnant women are: homicide, suicide, and motor vehicle crashes.[5,6] In areas as disparate as North Carolina[6] and New York City,[5] homicide is the most common cause of death in pregnant women, exceeding any single pregnancy-related cause, preexisting medical condition, or obstetric complication.[7] The major subcategory for homicide is "domestic violence."

Pregnant women suffer the same problems of motor vehicle crashes, falls, assault, attempted suicide, and penetrating trauma (eg, stabbings and gunshot wounds) as the rest of modern society.[8] These injuries often require heroic interventions. Our response has been to craft harsh phrases to guide emergency care, such as "postmortem C-section," "perimortem delivery," "sacrifice mother or child," or "save mother

Critical Concepts: Physiologic Changes of Pregnancy That May Affect Resuscitation

Airway and Pulmonary Function

- The larynx is displaced anteriorly, with increased edema and blood flow.

- Oxygen consumption increases 20%.

- Elevation of the diaphragm causes decreased functional residual capacity and functional residual volume, which predispose to rapid desaturation during hypoxia.

- Tidal volume and minute ventilation are increased to support increased cardiac output and oxygen demand during pregnancy.

- The normal maternal arterial blood gases reflect a respiratory alkalosis with a mild compensatory metabolic acidosis. Mild maternal hypocarbia

($Paco_2$ 28 to 32 mm Hg) is needed to create a gradient in the placenta to facilitate removal of fetal CO_2. Because respiratory alkalosis is already present, the mother's ability to compensate for any new acid load is limited.

Circulation

- During most of the pregnancy there is a 40% increase in cardiac output and plasma volume; late in the third trimester, cardiac output decreases, particularly when the mother is supine.

- Physiologic anemia may reduce arterial oxygen content even if oxyhemoglobin saturation and Pao_2 are satisfactory.

- Systemic and pulmonary vascular resistance decrease.

- Beyond 20 weeks gestation the uterus compresses the inferior vena cava and aorta, compromising systemic venous return and systemic blood flow.

Gastrointestinal Function

- Hormonal changes contribute to an incompetent gastroesophageal sphincter even under normal conditions.

- An incompetent gastroesophageal sphincter predisposes the mother to regurgitation and the risk of aspiration with loss of consciousness.

—*Contributed by Carolyn M. Zelop, MD, St. Francis Hospital and Medical Center, Hartford, CT.*

or child," and "harvest the fetus."[9] We walk a thin line between aiding our memory and demeaning our patients. These guidelines will avoid such phrases as much as possible.

Much of the literature on cardiac arrest associated with pregnancy comes from the specialties of emergency medicine and trauma[7,10] rather than obstetrics and anesthesiology.[11] The ACLS Course for Experienced Providers includes a teaching scenario dealing with attempted resuscitation of a pregnant woman with traumatic cardiac arrest.

The Second Victim

A cardiovascular emergency in a pregnant woman creates a special situation for the ACLS provider. This emergency involves 2 potential patients, the mother and the fetus. You must always consider the fetus when an adverse cardiovascular event occurs in a pregnant woman:

- At a gestational age of approximately ≥20 weeks, the size of the uterus begins to adversely affect the attempted resuscitation.

- At a gestational age of approximately 24 to 25 weeks, the fetus may survive outside the womb.

Decisions About Cesarean Delivery

The decision of whether to perform an emergency cesarean delivery must be made quickly when the mother is in cardiac arrest. Emergency cesarean delivery—also known as hysterotomy—may improve the outcome for both mother and child.[12]

Causes of Maternal Cardiopulmonary Arrest

The many causes of cardiac arrest in pregnant women can be grouped into several defining categories (see Table 1 for a detailed list):

- Injury/trauma
- Obstetric complications at the time of delivery
- Iatrogenic complications
- Medical conditions related to pregnancy
- Preexisting medical conditions

"The terminology we employ influences our perceptions. . . . The term 'cesarean section' should be abandoned. A medical procedure is rarely named after a historic figure, and almost never after an ancient Roman law. *Cesarean section* has recently been amended to *cesarean birth* [emphasis added]; however, the term is still inadequate. The word "hysterotomy" more appropriately describes the procedure we regularly perform. The adjectives used to describe cesarean birth should also be reevaluated. . . . Such revision of our terminology will keep obstetrics at the forefront of medical science and bring us most efficiently into the 21st century."

—From Katz et al, "Cesarean Delivery: A Reconsideration of Terminology."[12]

Changes in Maternal and Fetal Physiology: Relation to Cardiac Arrest

Uterine-Placental Blood Flow

During pregnancy the mother's cardiac output and plasma volume increase by 40%, and one third of maternal cardiac output flows through the uteroplacental unit. During pregnancy the uterus and placenta form a passive, low-resistance system. Maternal perfusion pressure is the sole determinant of uteroplacental and fetal blood flow. Consequently any cardiovascular compromise in the mother can severely impair blood flow to the uterus, placenta, and fetus. Restoration and support of maternal systemic perfusion is essential for the mother and the fetus.

Effect of the Enlarging Uterus

By the 20th week of pregnancy the gravid uterus is large enough to significantly compress the inferior vena cava and the aorta.[13] Compression of the inferior vena cava reduces venous return to the heart,

Relevant Research

In a study published in 1969, Uleland and colleagues[13] performed serial cardiovascular studies in 11 pregnant patients. They studied normal hemodynamics and the effects of changes in patient position and exercise during the course of normal pregnancy. This is still considered the definitive study of hemodynamics of pregnancy. Uleland and colleagues noted the effects of the gravid uterus on normal maternal cardiac output and the importance of the lateral decubitus position:

In this study it became apparent that cardiac output was elevated early in pregnancy and was maintained at a high level for a considerable length of time. Late in gestation cardiac output declines toward nonpregnant levels, regardless of maternal position. . . . The increasing influence of the enlarging uterus as pregnancy advances is apparent from our data; a change in position from the supine to lying on the side produced a . . . rise[15] of 8 percent . . . at 20 to 24 weeks' gestation, 13.6 percent at 28 to 32 weeks' gestation, and 28.5 percent ($P<0.01$) at term.

and compression of the aorta compromises forward flow. These factors can compromise cardiac output even in a normal pregnancy, particularly when the mother is supine.[13]

If cardiac arrest develops, the gravid uterus can compromise the effectiveness of resuscitation. Because there is obstruction of venous return, you should not administer resuscitation medications through a subdiaphragmatic vein. During cardiac arrest these medications may not reach the mother's heart unless or until the fetus is delivered.

| **TABLE 1.** | **Potential Causes of Maternal Cardiopulmonary Arrest[7,11]** |

Injury/trauma:
- Homicide
- Suicide
- Motor vehicle crash
- Illicit drug use, unintentional overdose

Obstetric complications at the time of delivery:
- Amniotic fluid embolism
- Hemorrhagic events:
  — Placenta previa, accreta, increta, or percreta
  — Placental abruption
  — Uterine atony
  — Disseminated intravascular coagulopathy
- Pregnancy-induced malignant hypertension
- Idiopathic peripartum cardiomyopathy

Iatrogenic complications:
- Intubation errors
- Pulmonary aspiration
- Anesthetic overdose (intrathecal, intravascular)
- Medication-related errors (overdose, allergies)
- Hypermagnesemia

Medical conditions related to pregnancy (increased risk during pregnancy):
- Pulmonary embolism from thrombus, air, or fat (most common nontraumatic cause)
- Infection or sepsis

Preexisting medical conditions:
- Asthma
- Cerebral hemorrhage
- Cerebral aneurysm
- Cerebral thrombosis
- Malignant hyperthermia
- Cardiac pathology:
  — Acute coronary syndromes
  — Arrhythmias
  — Congenital or vascular heart disease

Maternal Physiology

A number of factors can compromise maternal oxygen delivery and ability to compensate for hypoxia and acidosis:

- If the mother is anemic, arterial oxygen content will be reduced even when oxyhemoglobin saturation and PaO_2 are adequate.

- By the third trimester the gravid uterus pushes the diaphragm up enough to significantly reduce the functional residual capacity and functional residual volume. The decrease in these lung volumes coupled with the high oxygen consumption that exists during pregnancy can predispose the mother to rapid arterial oxygen desaturation if hypoxia develops. If the mother is supine during cardiac arrest, this reduction in functional residual capacity limits the effectiveness of efforts to oxygenate and ventilate the victim.

- Because the pregnant woman maintains a respiratory alkalosis with mild compensatory acidosis, the mother will have limited ability to buffer an acid load.

- The high level of progesterone during pregnancy reduces the tone of the lower esophageal sphincter. Incompetence of this sphincter increases the risk that positive-pressure ventilation during CPR will cause regurgitation and aspiration of gastric contents. For this reason the ACLS provider should establish a protected airway early in resuscitation.

- Maternal laryngeal edema may make intubation more difficult and may require use of a smaller tracheal tube.

- Increased laryngeal blood flow increases the risk of bleeding when any tube (orogastric, nasogastric, nasopharyngeal, tracheal) tube is inserted into the oro- or nasopharynx.

Fetal Physiology

Fetal physiology may offer the fetus some protection during the first minutes of maternal hypoxia or cardiac arrest:

- Fetal hemoglobin differs from "adult" hemoglobin in that it binds more readily with oxygen. For this reason it is better saturated at lower arterial oxygen tension. As a result fetal arterial oxygen content is higher at a given PaO_2.

- Fetal cardiac output is higher per kilogram of body weight than newborn cardiac output.

There has been a single case report of intact newborn survival after 20 minutes of maternal cardiac arrest (but not more than 25 minutes).[14] In this case the mother received uninterrupted CPR during the emergency cesarean delivery and for several minutes afterward.

The effects of maternal CPR on fetal blood flow has not been studied in humans.[10] Decades-old laboratory research showed that primate fetuses can survive up to 7 minutes of in utero asphyxiation without evidence of neurologic damage after birth.[16] But this laboratory experience contradicts anecdotal reports of human perimortem cesarean delivery. For the human fetus the window of reversible damage appears to be no wider than 4 to 5 minutes.[10]

Resuscitation of the Pregnant Woman in Cardiac Arrest

Basic Life Support

Effect of the Uterus on Blood Flow

In an emergency the simplest and most effective action may be overlooked. Many cardiovascular problems associated with pregnancy are due to nothing more than anatomy interacting with gravity. The pregnant woman's uterus may press down against the inferior vena cava and aorta, impeding venous return and cardiac output.

Uterine obstruction of venous return can produce prearrest hypotension or shock.[17,18] With cardiac arrest the compromise in venous return and aortic flow can limit the effectiveness of chest compressions.

Shifting the Gravid Uterus

Manual Displacement

Relieve compression of the inferior vena cava and the aorta by shifting the gravid uterus to the left:

- Stand on the left side of the patient, level with the top of the uterus.

- Reach across the midline with both hands, and pull the gravid uterus toward your abdomen.

- Pull until the patient's right hip/buttock begins to rise from the surface where the woman is lying.

Mechanical Techniques

The "Cardiff wedge" is a firm, wedge-shaped cushion that is available commercially.[19] Such firm, wedge-shaped supports not only shift the uterus to the left but also provide a wide, firm, angled surface to support the tilted torso during chest compressions. In emergency circumstances such single-purpose equipment is often unavailable.

Alternative means of support are the angled backs of 2 or 3 chairs or the angled thighs of several rescuers.[19] Overturn a 4-legged chair so that the top of the chair back touches the floor. Align 1 or 2 more overturned chairs on either side of the first so that all are tilted in the same manner.

Place the woman on her left side, align her torso parallel with the chair backs, and begin chest compressions (see Figure).

Chest Compressions

Perform chest compressions higher on the sternum. This shift in hand placement will adjust for the elevation of the diaphragm and abdominal contents by the gravid uterus. We lack clear guidelines on how far the compression point should be shifted. Use the pulse check during chest compressions to adjust the sternal compression point.

Complications of CPR in the Pregnant Woman

The physical changes associated with pregnancy and the challenges of performing modified chest compressions increase the risk of several CPR complications, including liver lacerations, uterine rupture, hemothorax, and hemopericardium.

Defibrillation

If the pregnant woman has ventricular fibrillation, administer defibrillation shocks at the doses recommended in the ACLS guidelines. There is no evidence that shocks from a direct-current defibrillator have adverse effects on the heart of the fetus. If fetal or uterine monitors are in place, remove them before you deliver shocks.

Advanced Cardiac Life Support

There are no substantive changes to standard ACLS algorithms for defibrillation, medications, and intubation in pregnant women (see Table 2).

Airway

- Secure the airway early in resuscitation. Hormonal changes promote insufficiency of the gastroesophageal sphincter and increase the risk of regurgitation.

- Intubation of a pregnant woman during attempted resuscitation can be difficult.

  — A provider experienced in intubation should perform the procedure.

FIGURE. Left lateral position for pregnant woman.

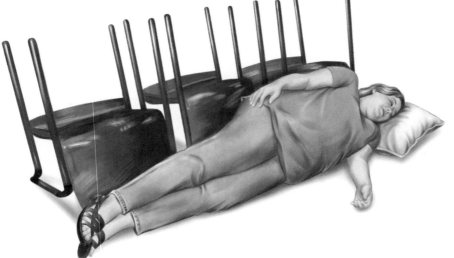

TABLE 2. Primary and Secondary ABCD Surveys: Modifications for Pregnant Women

ACLS Approach	Modifications to BLS and ACLS Guidelines
Primary ABCD Survey	**Airway** ■ No modifications. **Breathing** ■ No modifications. **Circulation** ■ Place the woman on her left side with her back angled 30° to 45° from the floor or bed surface. Then start chest compressions. 　　**or** ■ Place a wedge under the woman's right side (so that she tilts toward her left side). 　　**or** ■ Have one rescuer kneel next to the woman's left side and pull the gravid uterus laterally. This maneuver will relieve pressure on the inferior vena cava. **Defibrillation** ■ No modifications in dose or pad position. ■ Defibrillation shocks transfer no significant current to the fetus. ■ Remove any fetal or uterine monitors before shock delivery.
Secondary ABCD Survey	**Airway** ■ Secure the airway early in resuscitation to reduce the risk of regurgitation and aspiration. ■ Airway edema and swelling may reduce the diameter of the trachea. Be prepared to use a tracheal tube that is slightly smaller than the one you would use for a nonpregnant woman of similar size. ■ Monitor for excessive bleeding following insertion of any tube into the oro- or nasopharynx. ■ No modifications to intubation techniques. A provider experienced in intubation should insert the tracheal tube. 　— Effective preoxygenation is critical because hypoxia can develop quickly. 　— Rapid sequence intubation with continuous cricoid pressure is the preferred technique. 　— Etomidate or thiopental are preferred agents for anesthesia or deep sedation. **Breathing** ■ No modifications to secondary confirmation of successful intubation. Note that the esophageal detector device may suggest esophageal placement despite correct tracheal tube placement (see discussion in this chapter and Volume 1, Chapter 8, Table 6). ■ The gravid uterus elevates the diaphragm: 　— Functional residual capacity and functional residual volume are decreased. Minute ventilation and tidal volume are increased. 　— Tailor ventilatory support to produce effective oxygenation and ventilation. **Circulation** ■ Follow standard ACLS recommendations for administration of all resuscitation medications. ■ Do not use the femoral vein or other lower extremity sites for venous access. Drugs administered through these sites may not reach the maternal heart unless or until the fetus is delivered. **Differential Diagnosis and Decisions** ■ Decide whether to perform emergency hysterotomy (see Table 3). ■ Identify and treat reversible causes of the arrest. Consider causes related to pregnancy and causes considered for all ACLS patients (see the 6 H's and 6 T's, Chapter 1 of this volume).

— Edema and swelling may narrow the woman's airway. It may be necessary to use a tracheal tube that is slightly smaller (0.5 to 1 mm smaller ID) than the one used for a nonpregnant woman of similar size. The provider must be aware that a smaller tube will increase resistance to air flow and work of breathing during spontaneous ventilation.

— Effective preoxygenation before each intubation attempt is especially important because the decrease in functional residual capacity and functional residual volume predispose to rapid development of hypoxia.

— Rapid sequence intubation with continuous cricoid pressure is the preferred technique. Etomidate or thiopental is preferred for anesthesia or deep sedation.

■ Blood flow to the larynx increases during pregnancy. Watch for excessive bleeding in the airway following insertion of any tube into the oro- or nasopharynx.

Breathing

■ Verify correct tracheal tube placement using primary and secondary confirmation techniques. Note that in late pregnancy the esophageal detector device may suggest esophageal placement (the aspirating bulb does not reinflate after compression) when the tube is actually in the trachea. This false-positive result could lead the provider to remove a properly placed tracheal tube.

■ Pregnancy decreases functional residual capacity and functional residual volume, but the tidal volume and minute ventilation are increased. As a result, you must tailor ventilatory support based on evaluation of oxygenation and ventilation.

Circulation

■ Follow the ACLS guidelines for choice of resuscitation medications.

■ Pressor agents such as epinephrine, vasopressin, and dopamine will significantly decrease blood flow to the uterus. But there are no alternatives to using all indicated medications in recommended doses. You must resuscitate the mother or the chance of resuscitating the fetus vanishes. Recall the time-honored clinical aphorism that "maternal resuscitation is the best method for fetal resuscitation."

■ The ACLS guidelines do not recommend routine use of sodium bicarbonate. The use of sodium bicarbonate creates particular problems in attempted resuscitation during pregnancy. It is unlikely to buffer the fetal pH but may temporarily buffer maternal pH, so it may mask the severity of the fetal acidosis.

Differential Diagnosis

Consider the reversible causes of cardiac arrest during pregnancy and the reversible causes considered for any adult cardiac arrest; the "6 H's and 6 T's": the 6 H's are hypovolemia, hypoxia, hydrogen ion, hyper-/hypoelectrolytes, hyper-/hypoglycemia, hyper-/hypothermia; the 6 T's are tablets, tamponade, tension (pneumothorax), thrombosis (coronary), thrombosis (pulmonary), trauma.

■ Administer *calcium gluconate* (1 ampule or 1 g) or *glucagon* to counteract the effects of magnesium sulfate in eclamptic women who may have inadvertently received an excessive amount of magnesium.

■ *Fibrinolytics* are relatively contraindicated in pregnancy. Women who suffer an acute coronary syndrome in association with pregnancy may experience a VF arrest from which they are resuscitated. In such patients percutaneous coronary interventions are the reperfusion strategy of choice.[10] But there are reports of successful use of fibrinolytics for massive, life-threatening pulmonary embolism in pregnant women.[20]

> ### The 6 H's and the 6 T's
> Hypovolemia
> Hypoxia
> Hydrogen ion
> Hypo-/hyperelectrolytes
> Hypo-/hyperglycemia
> Hypo-/hyperthermia
>
> Tablets (drug overdoses)
> Trauma
> Tamponade, cardiac
> Tension pneumothorax
> Thrombosis, coronary
> Thrombosis, pulmonary

■ Clinicians have reported successful application of cardiopulmonary bypass for women suffering life-threatening amniotic fluid embolism during labor and delivery.[21]

Emergency Hysterotomy (Cesarean Delivery) for the Pregnant Woman in Cardiac Arrest

Maternal Cardiac Arrest Persists After Several Minutes of BLS and ACLS

The 2 Victims. Clinicians treating a pregnant woman in cardiac arrest must never forget the second victim, the unborn child. With the mother in cardiac arrest, the blood supply to the fetus becomes hypoxic and acidotic. This will prove fatal to the fetus without rapid restoration of the mother's spontaneous circulation. *The key to resuscitation of the infant is resuscitation of the mother.* After approximately 20 to 23 gestational weeks, however, the *key to resuscitation of the mother is removal of the fetus from the gravid uterus.* After 20 to 23 weeks the gravid uterus obstructs the inferior vena cava, preventing venous return to the heart, and compresses the aorta, threatening arterial blood flow to critical organs.

A Solomon-like Solution? The emergency ("crash") hysterotomy or cesarean delivery has gained general acceptance as a way of resuscitating a pregnant woman who remains in cardiac arrest after the initial few minutes of BLS and ACLS. Although the crash hysterotomy also offers the best chance of resuscitating the gestationally advanced fetus, cesarean delivery mandates sacrifice of a fetus below the gestational age of 20 to 23 weeks. The ECC guidelines first recommended the crash hysterotomy in 1992.[22] The evidence for this recommendation consisted of a small number of case reports.[15,23,24] With candid acknowledgement of the lack of definitive evidence from large-scale studies, the crash hysterotomy, as detailed below, has become widely cited and adopted.[7,8,10,11,25] The updated guidelines 2000[26] retain this recommendation. Candor, however, requires acknowledging that the published evidence leaves the crash hysterotomy as a generally accepted *intervention of desperation* for both the mother and the fetus. Designating the crash hysterotomy the "standard of care" for all emergency settings must await further published evidence.

Recommendations Based on Gestational Age

Hysterotomy allows access to the infant so that newborn resuscitation can begin. It also leads to immediate correction of much of the abnormal physiology of the full-term mother. The critical point to remember is that *both mother and infant will die if you cannot restore blood flow to the mother's heart.*[27]

Once the fetus is delivered, the uterus is decompressed and the abdominal incision may enable direct massage of the mother's heart through the diaphragm. Internal cardiac compression through a thoracotomy may also be attempted. Evidence to support these interventions is lacking.

The gravid uterus reaches a size that will begin to compromise aortocaval blood flow at approximately 20 weeks' gestation for the single fetus.[13] Fetal viability is estimated to begin at approximately 24 to 25 weeks. Consequently there is general acceptance of the following recommendations:

■ **Attempt to determine gestational age from history and examination:** As a rule the uterus is palpable at the maternal umbilicus at approximately 20 weeks' gestation. For every centimeter above the umbilicus that the uterus is palpable, add 1 week to the estimated gestational age. Note that this estimate applies only to the single fetus. The uterus will be larger earlier in gestation if there is more than one fetus in the uterus.

■ **Gestational age <20 weeks:** Resuscitation protocols should focus on the mother. If there is a single fetus, there is no need to consider urgent hysterotomy. The size of the uterus is unlikely to significantly compromise maternal venous return and cardiac output. But if there is more than one fetus, the uterus may compromise maternal blood flow, and emergency hysterotomy may be advisable.

■ **Gestational age approximately 20 to 23 weeks:** Perform emergency hysterotomy and deliver the fetus to save the life of the mother. If the mother remains in cardiac arrest, unresponsive to BLS and ACLS for more than 5 minutes, delivery of the fetus will relieve the obstruction on the inferior vena cava and the aorta and may enable successful resuscitation of the mother. Survival of the newborn infant is unlikely.

■ **Gestational age approximately >24 to 25 weeks:** After consideration of the factors listed in Table 3, perform emergency hysterotomy to save the life of both the mother and the fetus.

■ **Consider infant factors that influence infant survival:** The factors that influence the newborn's chance of survival are gestational age, birth weight, and lung maturity. Survival is unlikely for the infant born at a gestational age less than 24 to 25 weeks and a birth weight less than 500 g.[17,18,27-30]

■ **Several factors related to the survival of a cardiac arrest infant:** The following arrest conditions have been linked with increased infant survival:

— Short interval between the mother's arrest and delivery of the infant:

● <5 minutes: Excellent probability of survival

● 5 to <10 minutes: Good survival

● 10 to <15 minutes: Fair survival

● 15 to <20 minutes: Poor survival

● 20 minutes: Only 1 case report[16]

— Mother's cardiac arrest is not associated with sustained prearrest hypoxia

— No or minimal signs of fetal distress at the time of the mother's cardiac arrest[31]

— Mother's resuscitation is conducted effectively and aggressively

— Hysterotomy occurs in a medical center with a neonatal intensive care unit

Factors to Consider

Table 3 lists the many factors to consider in a very short time during a maternal cardiac arrest and attempted resuscitation.

Resuscitation of a pregnant patient can become a chaotic event. Particularly in major centers, there may be other specialist involved, including pediatricians, neonatologists, anesthesiologists, obstetricians, and possibly others. These specialists have unique skills and experience that will help in the resuscitation. However, many of the specialists are poorly versed in emergency medicine and advanced cardiac life support protocols. It is particularly important that the team leader of the resuscitation take strict control of the events and the order in which they occur. The other specialists involved should not be allowed to deviate from the proper process. . . . The emergency physician must be the director of the resuscitation and take firm control.

—From Datner and Promes, "Resuscitation Issues in Pregnancy."[7]

TABLE 3. The Emergency Hysterotomy (Cesarean Delivery) Decision: Factors to Consider Upon Maternal Arrest

Factors to Consider	Comments
Arrest Factors ■ If the mother fails to respond to initial resuscitative efforts and the gestational age is >20 weeks, ask that personnel and equipment be assembled for emergency hysterotomy. This will allow simultaneous continuation of resuscitative efforts and preparation for the cesarean delivery. ■ Is the mother receiving appropriate BLS and ACLS care, including — CPR with compressions performed with the mother angled to the left? — Early intubation with verification of proper placement of the tracheal tube? — Administration of indicated IV medications to a venous site above the diaphragm? ■ Has the mother responded to arrest interventions? ■ Are there any potentially reversible causes of arrest?	**Arrest Factors** ■ Survival probabilities for the mother and fetus decrease as the interval from maternal arrest increases. ■ Aim for an interval of 5 minutes or less from maternal arrest to delivery of the fetus. This goal requires efficient assembly of personnel and equipment. ■ Do *not* wait until 5 minutes of unsuccessful resuscitation have passed before you begin to consider the need to deliver the fetus emergently. You should consider the need for hysterotomy within minutes to enable assembly of personnel and equipment. ■ Ensure that the mother has received superior resuscitative efforts. She cannot be declared "refractory" to CPR and ACLS unless all interventions have been implemented and implemented well.
Mother-Infant Factors ■ Is the fetus old enough to survive? ■ Has too much time passed for the mother to survive? ■ Is the mother's cardiac arrest due to a chronic hypoxic state? ■ What is the status of the fetus at the time of the mother's cardiac arrest?	**Mother-Infant Factors** ■ This question recognizes the critical importance of gestational age. Survival is unlikely for the infant born at a gestational age less than approximately 24 to 25 weeks and a birth weight less than 500 g. ■ Do not lose site of the goal of this dramatic event: a live, neurologically intact infant and mother. ■ Carefully consider the future before pushing the margins of survivability. ■ Even if the fetus is unlikely to survive (gestational age of 20 to 23 weeks), the mother may benefit from emergency hysterotomy.
Setting and Personnel ■ Are appropriate equipment and supplies available? ■ Is hysterotomy within the rescuer's skill "comfort zone"? ■ Are skilled neonatal or pediatric support personnel available to care for the infant, especially if it is not at full term? ■ Are obstetric personnel immediately available to support the mother after delivery? ■ In both in-hospital and out-of-hospital settings, is there adequate staff and equipment support? In out-of-hospital settings, is bystander support available?	
Differential Diagnosis ■ Consider whether persistent arrest is due to an immediately reversible problem (eg, excess anesthesia, reaction to analgesia, or severe bronchospasm). If it is, correct the problem and there may be no need for hysterotomy. ■ Consider whether persistent arrest is due to a fatal, untreatable problem (eg, massive amniotic fluid embolism). If it is, an immediate hysterotomy may save the fetus.	

Every Emergency Department should rehearse its plan of action for this type of event, including location of supplies, sources of extra equipment, and best methods for obtaining subspecialty assistance. All planning should be done in collaboration with obstetrical and neonatal or pediatric specialists.

Avoid chaos. Cardiac arrest in the pregnant woman, especially if it occurs outside the operating room or labor and delivery suites, can become a chaotic event. The following quotation describes an all too common reality:

References

1. Berg CJ, Atrash HK, Koonin LM, Tucker M. Pregnancy-related mortality in the United States, 1987-1990. *Obstet Gynecol.* 1996;88: 161-167.

2. Beasley JW, Damos JR, Roberts RG, Nesbitt TS. The advanced life support in obstetrics course. A national program to enhance obstetric emergency skills and to support maternity care practice. *Arch Fam Med.* 1994;3:1037-1041.

3. Beasley JW, Byrd JE, Damos JR, Roberts RG, Koller WS. Advanced life support in obstetrics course. *Am Fam Physician.* 1993;47:579-580.

4. Wolcomir M. *Advanced Life Support for Obstetrics.* Kansas City, Mo: American Academy of Family Physicians; 1996.

5. Dannenberg AL, Carter DM, Lawson HW, Ashton DM, Dorfman SF, Graham EH. Homicide and other injuries as causes of maternal death in New York City, 1987 through 1991. *Am J Obstet Gynecol.* 1995;172:1557-1564.

6. Harper M, Parsons L. Maternal deaths due to homicide and other injuries in North Carolina: 1992-1994. *Obstet Gynecol.* 1997;90:920-923.

7. Datner EM, Promes SB. Resuscitation issues in pregnancy. In: Rosen P, Barkin R, eds. *Emergency Medicine: Concepts and Clinical Practice.* 4th ed. St Louis, Mo: Mosby; 1998: 71-76.

8. Kupas DF, Harter SC, Vosk A. Out-of-hospital perimortem cesarean section. *Prehosp Emerg Care.* 1998;2:206-208.

9. Kam CW. Perimortem caesarean sections (PMCS). *J Accid Emerg Med.* 1994;11:57-58.

10. Doan-Wiggins L. Resuscitation of the pregnant patient suffering sudden death. In: Paradis NA, Halperin HR, Nowak RM, eds. *Cardiac Arrest: The Science and Practice of Resuscitation Medicine.* Baltimore, Md: Williams & Wilkins; 1997:812-819.

11. Johnson MD, Luppi CJ, Over DC. Cardiopulmonary resuscitation. In: Douglas MJ, ed. *Obstetric Anesthesia and Uncommon Disorders.* Philadelphia, Pa: WB Saunders; 1998:51-74.

12. Katz VL, Wells SR, Kuller JA, Hansen WF, McMahon MJ, Bowes WA Jr. Cesarean delivery: a reconsideration of terminology. *Obstet Gynecol.* 1995;86:152-153.

13. Uleland K. Maternal cardiovascular dynamics: the influence of gestational age. *Am J Obstet Gynecol.* 1969;104:856-864.

14. Van der Touw T, Tully A, Amis TC, Brancatisano A, Rynn M, Mudaliar Y, Engel LA. Cardiorespiratory consequences of expiratory chest wall compression during mechanical ventilation and severe hyperinflation. *Crit Care Med.* 1993;21:1908-1914.

15. Oates S, Williams GL, Rees GA. Cardiopulmonary resuscitation in late pregnancy. *BMJ.* 1988;297:404-405.

16. Windle WF. Brain damage at birth: functional and structural modifications with time. *JAMA.* 1968;206:1967-1972.

17. Page-Rodriguez A, Gonzalez-Sanchez JA. Perimortem cesarean section of twin pregnancy: case report and review of the literature. *Acad Emerg Med.* 1999;6:1072-1074.

18. Cardosi RJ, Porter KB. Cesarean delivery of twins during maternal cardiopulmonary arrest. *Obstet Gynecol.* 1998;92:695-697.

19. Goodwin AP, Pearce AJ. The human wedge: a manoeuvre to relieve aortocaval compression during resuscitation in late pregnancy. *Anaesthesia.* 1992;47:433-434.

20. Turrentine MA, Braems G, Ramirez MM. Use of thrombolytics for the treatment of thromboembolic disease during pregnancy. *Obstet Gynecol Surv.* 1995;50:534-541.

21. Esposito RA, Grossi EA, Coppa G, Giangola G, Ferri DP, Angelides EM, Andriakos P. Successful treatment of postpartum shock caused by amniotic fluid embolism with cardiopulmonary bypass and pulmonary artery thromboembolectomy. *Am J Obstet Gynecol.* 1990;163:572-574.

22. Emergency Cardiac Care Committee and Subcommittees, American Heart Association. Guidelines for cardiopulmonary resuscitation and emergency cardiac care, part IV: special resuscitation situations: pregnancy. *JAMA.* 1992;268:2249-2250.

23. Strong TH Jr, Lowe RA. Perimortem cesarean section. *Am J Emerg Med.* 1989;7:489-494.

24. Katz VL, Dotters DJ, Droegemueller W. Perimortem cesarean delivery. *Obstet Gynecol.* 1986;68:571-576.

25. Whitten M, Irvine LM. Postmortem and perimortem caesarean section: what are the indications? *J R Soc Med.* 2000;93:6-9.

26. American Heart Association in collaboration with International Liaison Committee on Resuscitation. Guidelines 2000 for Cardiopulmonary Resuscitation and Emergency Cardiovascular Care: International Consensus on Science, Part 8: Advanced Challenges in Resuscitation: Section 3: Special Challenges in ECC. *Circulation.* 2000;102(suppl I):I229-I252.

27. Lanoix R, Akkapeddi V, Goldfeder B. Perimortem cesarean section: case reports and recommendations. *Acad Emerg Med.* 1995; 2:1063-1067.

28. Parker J, Balis N, Chester S, Adey D. Cardiopulmonary arrest in pregnancy: successful resuscitation of mother and infant following immediate caesarean section in labour ward. *Aust N Z J Obstet Gynaecol.* 1996;36:207-210.

29. Tang G, Nada W, Gyaneshwar R, Crooke D. Perimortem caesarean section: two case reports and a management protocol. *Aust N Z J Obstet Gynaecol.* 2000;40:405-408.

30. Finegold H, Darwich A, Romeo R, Vallejo M, Ramanathan S. Successful resuscitation after maternal cardiac arrest by immediate cesarean section in the labor room [letter]. *Anesthesiology.* 2002;96:1278.

31. Morris JA Jr, Rosenbower TJ, Jurkovich GJ, Hoyt DB, Harviel JD, Knudson MM, Miller RS, Burch JM, Meredith JW, Ross SE, Jenkins JM, Bass JG. Infant survival after cesarean section for trauma. *Ann Surg.* 1996;223:481-488; discussion 488-491.

Special Resuscitation Situations Part 7: Electric Shock and Lightning Strikes

Background

With both electric shock and lightning strike injuries, electric current enters the body, causing damage from current and from conversion of the electrical energy into thermal energy. The severity of injury can range from unpleasant tingling sensation to cardiac arrest, and both internal and external thermal burns may be present. The ACLS provider who treats cardiac arrest caused by electrical shock or lightning strike must provide CPR and trauma and burn care. In general, more prolonged resuscitative efforts and more aggressive fluid resuscitation are indicated for these patients than for other patients in cardiac arrest.

Electric injuries have played a significant role in the development of ACLS care. In the 1930s to 1950s the utility companies stimulated the development of prehospital defibrillators to treat utility workers who sustained fatal electric shock injuries. In fact, the early term for defibrillation was *countershock,* in acknowledgement of its use in treatment of cardiac arrest induced by high-voltage shocks in humans and in laboratory animals.

Perspective on Risk

Electric shock injuries cause approximately 500 deaths annually in the United States,[1] and lightning strikes cause approximately 150 to 300 deaths in the United States per year.[2] Although these are not common causes of traumatic death (Table),[3] they are responsible for an estimated 52 000 trauma admissions per year and 4% to 7% of burn center admissions.[2] Many victims who survive electric shock and lightning strike have permanent sequelae.[2]

Electric Shock

Essential Facts

Electric shock injuries can be caused by high-voltage sources encountered by utility workers and by low-voltage current sources typically seen in the home.

- **Setting:** One third of all electric shock injuries and most high-voltage electric shocks occur at the worksite,[4] caused by contact with power lines. Other occupational electric shock injuries occur during use of electric tools or machines.[2] Electric injuries in the home account for nearly half of the annual deaths from electric shock.[2] They result from failure to properly ground tools or appliances or from using electric appliances near water.[2]

Pediatric electric shock injuries typically occur around the home, when the child bites an electrical wire, places an

TABLE. Estimated Lifetime Risk of Death (by Age 70) From Various Causes

Cause of Death	Lifetime Risk* (numerator/denominator) Interpretation: a total of (numerator) people will die from (cause of death) before reaching age 70 in a population of (denominator)
Measles	1.5/1 000 000
Smallpox vaccination	5/1 000 000
Lightning strike	3/100 000
Electrocution	3/10 000
Drowning	2.5/1000
Falls	6/1000
Motor vehicle crash	1.5/100

*These estimates are based on actuarial data and represent "best estimates" of risk rather than "upper bounds" of risk. Lifetime risks are derived by multiplying annual deaths by 70 years, then dividing the product by the total US population.[3]

object in an electrical socket, contacts an exposed low-voltage wire or appliance, or touches a high-voltage wire outdoors.[5] Adolescents are injured when climbing utility poles, playing near electric railway lines, or entering transformer substations.[2]

■ **Determinants of severity:** Several factors determine the nature and severity of electric trauma: the magnitude of energy delivered, resistance to current flow, type of current, duration of contact with the current source, and current pathway. The damage caused by the electric injury is proportional to the magnitude and intensity of the current delivered. The current flow is related to the voltage from the original source and is inversely related to the resistance in the current path.[2]

In electric injuries the power source can usually be identified, so the magnitude of the current exposure is known. High-voltage current (>1000 volts) generally causes the most serious injuries, but fatal electrocutions may occur with low voltage (<1000 volts). In fact, many fatal electrocutions occur with household current (110 V in the United States and Canada; 220 V in Europe, Australia, Asia, and many other areas).[6]

The body tissues vary in the amount of resistance they offer to current flow. Bone and skin are most resistant to the passage of electric current. Muscle, blood vessels, and nerves conduct with the least resistance.[7] Skin resistance is the most important factor impeding current flow because it is the surface through which the current must pass to enter the body. Skin resistance can be reduced substantially by moisture. Moisture can convert what ordinarily would be a minor injury into a life-threatening one.

Transthoracic current flow (eg, a hand-to-hand pathway) is more likely to be fatal than a vertical (hand-to-foot) or straddle (foot-to-foot) current pathway[8]

because transthoracic flow often causes ventricular fibrillation. Current flow through a vertical pathway can actually cause more myocardial injury than would result from a horizontal path. Investigators attribute this myocardial injury to the direct effects of current and coronary artery spasm and to the fact that current is in transit for a longer period of time in a vertical path and creates a wider path through the body with greater risk of organ injury than would result from a horizontal path.[9-11]

Long exposure to current flow causes more severe damage than a short exposure. Contact with alternating current at 60 cycles per second (the frequency used in most household and commercial sources of electricity) may cause tetanic contractions of skeletal muscle and prevent self-release from the source of electricity, prolonging exposure. The longer the duration of exposure to alternating current, the greater the likelihood that current will flow through the heart during the vulnerable period. This exposure can precipitate VF, analogous to the R-on-T phenomenon.[12]

■ **Pathophysiology:** Electric shock injuries result from the direct effects of current on cell membranes and vascular smooth muscle. Injuries also occur with the conversion of electric energy into thermal energy as current passes through body tissues.

Life-threatening arrhythmias including ventricular tachycardia or ventricular ectopy may result from either low- or high-intensity electric current, and cardiopulmonary arrest may result. Low-voltage alternating current typically causes ventricular fibrillation, while high-intensity current can cause asystole. In addition to arrhythmias, the current may create a brief but substantial inotropic stimulus, widespread muscle contraction and probable muscle cell rupture, myocardial cell damage, coronary artery spasm, and decreased coronary artery perfusion.[2,8,9,12] These

factors can contribute to cardiopulmonary arrest, post-shock arrhythmias, and persistent myocardial dysfunction.

Respiratory arrest can be caused by the passage of electric current through the brain, by contraction of the diaphragm and chest wall muscles, from prolonged paralysis of the respiratory muscles, and by cessation of brain perfusion secondary to cardiac arrest. The respiratory arrest may persist even after circulation is restored.[2]

Metabolic and systemic complications of electric injury include organ, muscle, and joint injuries and burns. Fractures of long bones and joint dislocations following electric shock have been reported resulting from severe muscle contractions or falls. Many patients demonstrate hypovolemia and metabolic acidosis from fluid loss through skin damage and tissue destruction.[2] Rhabdomyolysis may result from muscle injury and may lead to renal failure. Vascular complications may compromise perfusion to extremities, and neurologic injuries can range from coma or altered level of consciousness to peripheral nerve damage.[2]

Lightning Strike
Essential Facts

Lightning strike is a leading environmental cause of cardiac arrest. It exposes the victim to a potentially very large current for a very short time. Victims may be injured by a direct strike or through a side flash or splash, or from shock waves created in the surrounding air. In many cases of apparent direct strike, victims who receive immediate resuscitation can survive because much of the lightning current "flashes over" the outside of the victim with only a small amount of the current entering the victim.[2] Figures 1 and 2 display 2 examples of the unique "ferning pattern" that can be produced on the skin when this "flash-over" phenomenon occurs with a direct lightning strike.

■ **Frequency:** Lightning strikes kill hundreds of people internationally every year and injure many times that number. Approximately 30% of victims of lightning strike die, and up to 70% of survivors sustain significant and permanent sequelae.[2,13-15]

■ **Clinical presentations:** The presentation of lightning strike injuries varies widely, even among people struck at the same time.[16] (See below for a discussion of the concept of *reverse triage*.) Some victims have mild symptoms and may not require hospitalization; others die from the injury.[7,17]

Immediately after electrocution or lightning strike, the victim's respiratory function, circulation, or both may fail. The patient may be apneic, mottled, unconscious, and in cardiac arrest from VF or asystole.

FIGURE 1. A 54-year-old man struck by lightning with initial stupor but rapid return of consciousness and eventual full recovery. His back displays an erythematous, fern-leaf pattern that was painless. This pattern has been referred to as "Lichtenberg figures." No blistering occurred and the marks disappeared completely within 48 hours. Reprinted with permission from *The New England Journal of Medicine.* 2000;343:1536. Copyright 2000 Massachusetts Medical Society. All rights reserved.

■ **Pathophysiology:** The most common cause of death in fatal lightning strike is cardiac arrest.[18,19] The arrest may be associated with primary VF or asystole.[7,17,20,21]

Lightning acts as an instantaneous, massive, direct-current shock that depolarizes the entire myocardium at once.[7,22] In the 70% of lightning strike victims who survive, cardiac automaticity resumes spontaneously. Organized cardiac activity and a perfusing rhythm soon follow.

Victims of lightning strike frequently suffer acute respiratory arrest. If apnea continues for more than 1 to 4 minutes, secondary hypoxic cardiac arrest will occur. This cessation of breathing may be caused by a variety of mechanisms:

— Electric current passing through the brain and stopping further respiratory center activity in the medulla

— Tetanic contraction of the diaphragm and chest wall musculature during exposure to the current

— Prolonged paralysis of respiratory muscles, which may continue for minutes after the electric shock has ended

Respiratory arrest due to thoracic muscle spasm or suppression of the respiratory center may persist after return of spontaneous circulation. Unless ventilatory assistance is provided, a secondary hypoxic cardiac arrest may occur.[23]

Lightning strikes have widespread effects on the cardiovascular system. The strikes produce extensive catecholamine release, stimulating the autonomic nervous system. If cardiac arrest does not occur, the victim may develop hypertension, tachycardia, and nonspecific ECG changes (including prolongation of the QT interval and transient T-wave inversion). Myocardial necrosis

FIGURE 2. A 24-year-old woman, in her 26th week of pregnancy, struck by lightning while standing under a tree during a thunderstorm. The lightning entered her body through a necklace on the right side of her neck. As the lightning traveled to the ground it encountered the baby's head and was deflected to the left. An erythematous fern-leaf "print" of the lightning marks her skin. Although the woman survived, the baby died. Reprinted with permission from *The New England Journal of Medicine.* 1994;330:1492. Copyright 1994 Massachusetts Medical Society. All rights reserved.

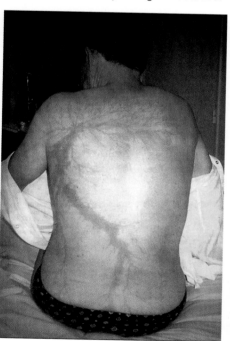

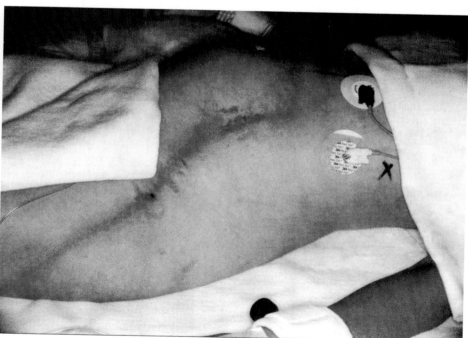

with release of creatine kinase-MB fraction may occur. Right and left ventricular ejection fractions may also be depressed, but this effect appears to be reversible.[20]

Lightning can produce a wide spectrum of neurologic injuries. Injuries may be primary, resulting from effects on the brain, or secondary, developing as complications of cardiac arrest and hypoxia.[14] The current can produce brain hemorrhage, edema, and small-vessel and neuronal injury. Hypoxic encephalopathy can result from cardiac arrest. A lightning strike can also damage myelin of peripheral nerves.[14]

■ **The concept of reverse triage:** In multiple-casualty emergencies, especially from traumatic events, victims in cardiac arrest are given the lowest priority (see Part 6 of this chapter: "Cardiac Arrest Associated With Trauma"). The harsh but evidence-based principle is that these victims have a very low probability of survival even with aggressive resuscitative efforts. Emergency personnel, especially if they are limited in numbers, will save more lives if they support victims who are not in cardiac arrest.

But in a multi-casualty lightning strike event, the victim who develops immediate cardiac arrest has a high probability of survival and recovery *if* BLS is provided without delay. When multiple victims suffer simultaneous lightning strike, rescuers should give highest priority to victims who are in respiratory or cardiac arrest. Victims of lightning strike who do not suffer immediate cardiopulmonary arrest are unlikely to do so. They have an excellent chance of recovery with little additional treatment. Survival is high when victims with cardiac or respiratory arrest receive immediate resuscitation. This is true even when the presenting rhythm is asystole or when prolonged efforts are required.

Modifications of BLS for Cardiopulmonary Arrest Caused by Electric Shock or Lightning Strike

■ **Expect success:** For victims in cardiopulmonary arrest, start BLS as soon as it is safe to approach the victim. Provide cervical spine immobilization throughout BLS maneuvers. The goal is to oxygenate the heart and brain adequately until cardiac activity resumes. Victims in respiratory arrest may require only ventilation and oxygenation to avoid secondary hypoxic cardiac arrest.

If immediate resuscitation is provided, survival from cardiac arrest caused by lightning strike is higher than that reported following cardiac arrest from other non-VF causes. Aggressive and persistent resuscitation efforts are justified even when the interval between collapse and the start of resuscitation is prolonged or when cardiac arrest persists despite initial efforts.[23]

■ **Rescuer safety:** All rescuers must be certain that rescue efforts will not put them in danger of electric shock. Ensure that authorized personnel turn off electrical power or safely clear the source of electricity from the victim. Rescuers should note that any material can conduct high-voltage current, and current can flow through the ground surrounding the victim. For these reasons the rescuer should not approach the victim until a high-voltage power source is turned off.

Carefully remove any hot or smoldering clothing, shoes, and belts. This precaution will help prevent further burns.

■ **Extrication:** When electric shock occurs in a location not readily accessible, such as on a utility pole, rescuers must lower the victim to the ground as quickly as possible. *Note: Special precautions must be followed if the rescue efforts require personnel to go near live current. Only rescuers specifically trained to execute such tasks should attempt them.*

■ **Cervical spine immobilization:** Maintain spinal protection and immobilization during extrication and treatment if there is any possibility of head or neck trauma.[24,25] Electrical injuries often cause musculoskeletal trauma, spinal injuries, muscle strains, and fractures. These injuries are often due to the tetanic contraction of skeletal muscles.[25]

■ **Primary ABCD Survey:** Immediately after the electric or lightning strike injury, spontaneous respiration, circulation, or both may fail. The patient may be apneic, mottled, and unconscious. The victim may be in circulatory collapse with VF/pulseless VT, PEA, or asystole.[24]

Assess and manage the airway, breathing, and circulation, and provide defibrillation as needed according to the ACLS guidelines. Continue vigorous resuscitative measures for longer than usual, even for victims who appear dead on initial evaluation. The prognosis for recovery from electric shock or lightning strike cannot be predicted accurately. The important factors of current flow and duration of the charge are usually unknown. But many victims are young with no pre-existing cardiopulmonary disease. They have a reasonable chance of survival if immediate support of cardiopulmonary function is provided.

Modifications of ACLS for Arrest Caused by Electric Shock or Lightning Strike

Initiate the ACLS interventions of the Secondary ABCD Survey with several important precautions:

■ **Airway:** It may be difficult to establish an airway if the victim has burns or immediate edema of the face, mouth, or airway. It is important to intubate early if there is a risk of development of extensive soft tissue swelling following the injury. ACLS providers should be prepared to provide respiratory support if respiratory arrest persists even after return of spontaneous circulation.

- **Circulation:** Initial support of cardiovascular function requires treatment of arrest rhythms and then treatment of any life-threatening arrhythmias. Once spontaneous perfusion is restored, the victim may require fluid therapy and inotropic or vasopressor support.

Victims with electric injuries have greater fluid requirements than those with thermal burns and will require rapid intravascular fluid administration to replace ongoing fluid losses and prevent hemodynamic compromise. Administer fluids at a rate and volume to maintain a brisk diuresis. Fluid replacement will facilitate renal excretion of myoglobin, potassium, and other byproducts of tissue destruction.[22]

- **Differential diagnosis:** Increased capillary permeability will occur in association with tissue injury. Expect the development of local tissue edema at the site of injury.

Compartment syndromes can rapidly develop in any extremity, especially if circumferential burns are present. This severe tissue edema can produce local areas of vascular compromise and tissue necrosis.

Electrothermal burns and underlying tissue injury may require surgical attention for debridement or fasciotomies. Seek early consultation with a physician skilled in treatment of electrical injuries.

References

1. National Safety Council. *1999 Injury Facts.* Itasca, Il; 1999:17.

2. Fontanarosa PB. Electrical shock and lightning strike. *Ann Emerg Med.* 1993;22:378-387.

3. Klaassen C, Eaton E. Principles of toxicology. In: Klaassen C, ed. *Casarett and Doull's Toxicology: The Basic Science of Poisons.* 4th ed. New York: McGraw-Hill; 1993:12-49.

4. Cooper MA. Electrical and lightning injuries. *Emerg Med Clin North Am.* 1984;2:489-501.

5. Kobernick M. Electrical injuries: pathophysiology and emergency management. *Ann Emerg Med.* 1982;11:633-638.

6. Budnick LD. Bathtub-related electrocutions in the United States, 1979 to 1982. *JAMA.* 1984;252:918-920.

7. Browne BJ, Gaasch WR. Electrical injuries and lightning. *Emerg Med Clin North Am.* 1992;10:211-229.

8. Thompson JC, Ashwal S. Electrical injuries in children. *Am J Dis Child.* 1983;137:231-235.

9. Chandra NC, Siu CO, Munster AM. Clinical predictors of myocardial damage after high voltage electrical injury. *Crit Care Med.* 1990;18:293-297.

10. Ku CS, Lin SL, Hsu TL, Wang SP, Chang MS. Myocardial damage associated with electrical injury. *Am Heart J.* 1989;118:621-624.

11. Xenopoulos N, Movahed A, Hudson P, Reeves WC. Myocardial injury in electrocution. *Am Heart J.* 1991;122:1481-1484.

12. Geddes LA, Bourland JD, Ford G. The mechanism underlying sudden death from electric shock. *Med Instrum.* 1986;20:303-315.

13. Cooper MA. Lightning injuries: prognostic signs for death. *Ann Emerg Med.* 1980;9: 134-138.

14. Kleinschmidt-DeMasters BK. Neuropathology of lightning strike injuries. *Semin Neurol.* 1995;15:323-328.

15. Stewart CE. When lightning strikes. *Emerg Med Serv.* 2000;29:57-67, quiz 103.

16. Fahmy FS, Brinsden MD, Smith J, Frame JD. Lightning: the multisystem group injuries. *J Trauma.* 1999;46:937-940.

17. Patten BM. Lightning and electrical injuries. *Neurol Clin.* 1992;10:1047-1058.

18. Jensen PJ, Thomsen PE, Bagger JP, Norgaard A, Baandrup U. Electrical injury causing ventricular arrhythmias. *Br Heart J.* 1987;57: 279-283.

19. Homma S, Gillam LD, Weyman AE. Echocardiographic observations in survivors of acute electrical injury. *Chest.* 1990;97:103-105.

20. Lichtenberg R, Dries D, Ward K, Marshall W, Scanlon P. Cardiovascular effects of lightning strikes. *J Am Coll Cardiol.* 1993;21:531-536.

21. Kleiner JP, Wilkin JH. Cardiac effects of lightning stroke. *JAMA.* 1978;240:2757-2759.

22. Cooper MA. Emergent care of lightning and electrical injuries. *Semin Neurol.* 1995;15: 268-278.

23. Milzman DP, Moskowitz L, Hardel M. Lightning strikes at a mass gathering. *South Med J.* 1999;92:708-710.

24. Duclos PJ, Sanderson LM. An epidemiological description of lightning-related deaths in the United States. *Int J Epidemiol.* 1990;19: 673-679.

25. Epperly TD, Stewart JR. The physical effects of lightning injury. *J Fam Pract.* 1989;29: 267-272.

Life-Threatening Electrolyte and Acid-Base Abnormalities

Introduction

This chapter presents the common causes of electrolyte and acid-base abnormalities and their diagnosis and treatment. A critical clinical goal for ACLS providers is to prevent deterioration of a stable patient to the unstable "arrest" condition. This chapter provides recommendations for recognition and treatment of life-threatening electrolyte and acid-base abnormalities *before* they cause cardiac arrest.

Electrolyte and acid-base abnormalities are commonly associated with cardiovascular emergencies. Identified abnormalities probably represent only the "tip of the iceberg"—the numerator of a much larger, unrecognized denominator. The true frequency of a causative role of electrolyte and acid-base abnormalities in periarrest emergencies remains unknown.

When faced with an unexplained cardiovascular emergency, healthcare professionals should suspect that the origin lies in electrolyte and acid-base problems. When patients with underlying conditions develop unexpected cardiovascular deterioration, the astute clinician should remember to search for the explanation in the original condition. Conditions that can frequently cause electrolyte and acid-base abnormalities are listed in Table 1.

If you identify predisposing conditions you may be able to provide *anticipatory therapy* to prevent development of life-threatening electrolyte and acid-base

disorders. You may need to start empiric treatment on the basis of history, physical examination, and objective signs before laboratory results become available.

This chapter refers to electrolyte values that are above or below the normal range. For ease of reference, Table 2 presents the normal range for a number of relevant clinical parameters. Table 2 also contains the various diagnostic and therapeutic equations presented throughout the chapter.

TABLE 1. Conditions Frequently Associated With Life-Threatening Electrolyte or Acid-Base Abnormalities

Possible Presenting Signs and Symptoms	
■ Vomiting	■ Confusion, lethargy, irritability
■ Diarrhea, constipation	■ Weakness, fatigue

Acute Conditions	
■ Anorexia	■ Poor oral intake
■ Use of multiple medications	■ Recent seizures
■ Alcohol abuse, acute	■ Recent surgery
■ Pancreatitis	■ Peritonitis

Chronic Medical Problems	
■ Renal failure	■ Nephrotic syndrome
■ Renal dialysis	■ Older age (>65 y)
■ Drug abuse	■ Insulin-dependent diabetes
■ Metastatic cancer	■ Hypertension
■ Immobilization	■ Cirrhosis
■ Alcohol abuse, chronic	■ Congestive heart failure
■ Hyperalimentation	■ Weight loss, chronic
■ Malnutrition, chronic	

Potassium

Physiology

■ Potassium is a positive ion that is present in much higher concentration inside cells than in the extracellular space that includes the serum. The difference in potassium concentration between the inside and outside of cells is called the *potassium gradient*. Maintaining the potassium gradient across cell membranes is critical for muscular and neurologic function.

TABLE 2. A, Normal Values of Electrolytes. B, Diagnostic and Therapeutic Equations

Table 2A. Normal Values

Parameter (Symbol)	Reference Range (Normal)	Parameter (Symbol)	Reference Range (Normal)
Sodium (Na^+)	135 to 145 mEq/L	**Arterial Blood Gases (Room Air)**	
Potassium (K^+)	3.5 to 5 mEq/L	pH	7.35 to 7.45
Chloride (Cl^-)	98 to 108 mEq/L	Pco_2	35 to 45 mm Hg
Carbon dioxide (HCO_3^-)	22 to 32 mEq/L	Base excess	> + 2 = Metabolic alkalosis
Anion gap	10 to 15 mEq/L	Base deficit	< − 2 = Metabolic acidosis
Glucose	62 to 125 mg/dL	Calculated vs measured pH	See below
Urea nitrogen (BUN)	8 to 21 mg/dL		
Creatinine	0.3 to 1.2 mg/dL		
Calcium, total (Ca^{2+})	8.5 to 10.5 mg/dL		
Calcium, ionized	4.2 to 4.8 mg/dL		
Magnesium (Mg^{2+})	1.3 to 2.2 mEq/L		
Urine specific gravity	1.005 to 1.030 mg/mL		
Albumin	3.5 to 5.2 g/dL		
Protein, total	6 to 8.2 g/dL		
Osmolality, serum	275 to 295 mOsm/L		

Table 2B. Useful Calculations and Formulae*

Calculation	Formula	Comments
Anion gap (serum concentration in mEq/L)	$[Na^+] - ([Cl^-] + [HCO_3^-])$	Normal range: 10 to 15 mEq/L. A gap >15 suggests metabolic acidosis.
Osmolal gap	$Osmolality_{measured} - Osmolality_{calculated}$ Normal = <10	Osmolal gap normally <10. If osmolal gap is >10, suspect unknown osmotically active substances.
Calculated osmolality (in mOsm/L)	$(2 \times [Na^+]) + ([Glucose] \div 18) + ([BUN] \div 2.8)$	Simplified to give *effective* osmolality. Normal = 272 to 300 mOsm/L
Total free water deficit (in L)	$$\frac{([Na^+]_{measured} - 140) \times TBW}{140}$$ $TBW_{in\,L} = (0.6_{men}$ or $0.5_{women}) \times Weight_{in\,kg}$	Use to calculate quantity of water needed to correct water deficit in hypernatremia.
Sodium deficit (in total mEq)	$([Na^+]_{desired} - [Na^+]_{measured}) \times TBW_{in\,L}$ $TBW_{in\,L} = (0.6_{men}$ or $0.5_{women}) \times Weight_{in\,kg}$	Use to calculate sodium deficit to replace with 3% saline in severe hyponatremia (3% saline contains 513 mEq sodium per liter).
Determination of *predicted* pH	$(40 - Pco_2) \times 0.008 =$ $\pm\Delta$ in pH from 7.4	For every 1 mm Hg change in Pco_2 from 40, pH will change by 0.008. Measured pH less than calculated pH: metabolic acidosis is present. Measured pH greater than predicted pH: metabolic alkalosis is present.

*See text for details. Concentration units are the same as listed above.

- Minor changes in the serum potassium concentration can have major effects on the excitability of the heart and conduction within it. Of all significant electrolyte abnormalities, rapid changes in serum potassium are the most likely to be life-threatening.

Hyperkalemia

Normal potassium range: 3.5 to 5 mEq/L

Causes

- Early recognition of conditions that cause hyperkalemia may prevent or minimize hyperkalemic cardiac arrhythmias.[1-3] Table 3 lists the most common causes of hyperkalemia.

  — In general, hyperkalemia is caused by either increased K[+] release from cells or impaired excretion by the kidneys.

  — The most common cause of severe, life-threatening hyperkalemia is kidney failure—classically in a dialysis patient who misses scheduled dialysis appointments and presents with severe weakness.[4] These patients can experience good outcomes if resuscitation includes concomitant hemodialysis.[5]

- A change in pH results in redistribution of the potassium[6] as follows:

  — A fall in pH (acidosis) shifts potassium out of cells, raising serum potassium.

  — A rise in pH (alkalosis) shifts potassium back into cells, lowering serum potassium.

  — A good way to remember the relationship between pH and serum potassium is that the *serum potassium changes in a direction opposite the serum pH.*

- Medications are the most frequent *exogenous* cause of hyperkalemia.

  — Potassium supplements prescribed to prevent *hypo*kalemia are the most frequent cause of hyperkalemia in hospitalized patients.

  — Potassium-sparing diuretics, such as spironolactone, triamterene, and amiloride, are another well-recognized cause of hyperkalemia.

  — Use of angiotensin-converting enzyme (ACE) inhibitors (eg, captopril) can also lead to elevation of serum potassium, particularly when combined with oral potassium supplements.

  — Nonsteroidal anti-inflammatory agents (eg, ibuprofen) can cause hyperkalemia through direct effects on the kidney.

Diagnosis

- The most common symptoms of hyperkalemia are *weakness, hypotension, paresthesias,* and *ascending paralysis.*

- The physical examination, the 12-lead ECG, and serum potassium concentration provide important (though indirect) information about the significance of the hyperkalemia. These evaluations must be performed promptly for critically ill patients.

- As the hyperkalemia worsens, the ECG becomes abnormal. Table 4 lists these changes in roughly the sequence in which they occur.

- The appearance of widened QRS complexes heralds significant cardiac dysfunction. If untreated at this point, progressive hyperkalemia leads to sine-wave–like complexes, unstable and symptomatic arrhythmias, and finally asystole and death.

Treatment

- The first critical action in treating hyperkalemia is to reduce potassium intake as much as possible.

  — Stop any potassium supplementation.

  — Identify and discontinue any prescribed or over-the-counter drugs that can cause hyperkalemia. If necessary call the patient's pharmacist to determine which medications may be involved.

- Further treatment of hyperkalemia varies by the level of serum potassium and the severity of the patient's clinical status.[4]

TABLE 3. Common Causes of Hyperkalemia

Endogenous Causes
■ Chronic renal failure
■ Metabolic acidosis (eg, diabetic ketoacidosis)
■ Pseudohypoaldosteronism type II (also known as Gordon's syndrome; familial hyperkalemia and hypertension)
■ Chemotherapy causing tumor lysis
■ Muscle breakdown (rhabdomyolysis)
■ Renal tubular acidosis
■ Hemolysis
■ Hypoaldosteronism (Addison's disease, hyporeninemia)
■ Hyperkalemic periodic paralysis

Exogenous Causes
■ Medications: K[+]-sparing diuretics, ACE inhibitors, nonsteroidal anti-inflammatory drugs, potassium supplements, penicillin derivatives, succinylcholine (in paralyzed patients), β-blockers
■ Blood administration (particularly with older "bank" blood)
■ Diet (rarely the sole cause), salt substitutes
■ Pseudohyperkalemia (due to blood sampling or hemolysis, high white blood cell count, high platelets, tumor lysis syndrome)

TABLE 4. Increasing Serum Potassium Levels and Most Frequently Associated ECG Findings

Serum Potassium Range (mEq/L)	Frequent ECG Findings
5.5 to <6	■ Peaking (tenting) of T waves (most prominent early ECG change)
6 to <6.5	■ Increasing PR and QT intervals
6.5 to <7	■ Flattened P waves and ST segments
7 to <7.5	■ Widened QRS complexes
7.5 to <8	■ Deepening S waves, merging of S and T waves
8 to <10	■ Sine-wave shaped complexes begin; idioventricular complexes and rhythms; VT-like appearance
≥10	■ PEA (often with a "sine wave" appearance), VF/VT, asystole

— **Mild hyperkalemia (5 to 6 mEq/L):** Remove potassium from the body by one or more of the following therapies:

- Diuretics: Furosemide 1 mg/kg slow IV

- Resins: Kayexalate 15 to 30 g in 50 to 100 mL of 20% sorbitol, either orally or by retention enema

- Dialysis: Peritoneal or hemodialysis (usually reserved for more severe cases, but mentioned in this group for completeness)

— **Moderate elevation (6 to 7 mEq/L):** Initiate a temporary intracellular shift of potassium using the following agents:

- Sodium bicarbonate: 50 mEq IV or up to 1 mEq/kg over 5 minutes

- Glucose/insulin: Mix 10 U regular insulin and 25 g (50 mL of D_{50}) glucose, and give IV over 15 to 30 minutes

- Nebulized albuterol: 5 to 20 mg over 15 minutes

The Periarrest Hyperkalemic Patient

■ Hyperkalemic patients in periarrest usually have renal failure. Often they are patients on renal dialysis who have missed one or more treatments. (Hyperkalemic patients who develop cardiac arrest have been successfully resuscitated using either hemodialysis[5] or peritoneal dialysis.[1])

■ Patients with severe potassium elevation (>7 mEq/L), especially those with widened QRS complexes, require urgent care.

■ **Severe elevation (>7 mEq/L with potassium-induced ECG changes):**

— First and most urgent, give 5 to 10 mL of 10% calcium chloride IV over 2 to 5 minutes. Calcium chloride will antagonize the toxic effects of potassium at the myocardial cell membrane, lowering the risk of VF.

— Second, initiate a rapid shift of K^+ into cells with sodium bicarbonate, glucose plus insulin, and nebulized albuterol (as for moderate hyperkalemia; see Table 5).

— Third, begin removal of K^+ from the body with diuretics, resins, or dialysis as described for mild hyperkalemia. Dialysis is the treatment of choice for patients with renal failure.

■ The clinical case on the next page illustrates the critical actions necessary for severe hyperkalemia. Table 5 summarizes the emergency treatments and treatment sequence recommended for hyperkalemia.

Hypokalemia

Normal potassium range: 3.5 to 5 mEq/L

Causes

■ Hypokalemia results from one or more of the following:

— Decreased dietary intake

— Redistribution: potassium shift from extracellular to intracellular space

— Increased potassium loss from the body

■ Table 6 lists the most common causes of low serum potassium.

Diagnosis

■ The major effects of hypokalemia are on neurologic and muscular (including myocardial) function. The myocardium is extremely sensitive to the effects of hypokalemia, particularly if the patient has preexisting coronary artery disease.

— In one survey severe hypokalemia (potassium <3.0 mEq/L) was present in 2.6% of hospitalized patients and was associated with a 21% mortality rate.[11]

— Hypokalemia in patients hospitalized with acute myocardial infarction is an independent risk factor for VF.[12]

TABLE 5. Emergency Treatments and Treatment Sequence for Hyperkalemia

Therapy	Dose	Effect Mechanism	Onset of Effect	Duration of Effect
Calcium chloride	■ 5 to 10 mL IV 10% solution (500 to 1000 mg)	■ Antagonism of toxic effects of hyperkalemia at cell membrane	■ 1 to 3 min	■ 30 to 60 min
Sodium bicarbonate	■ Begin with 1 ampule; give up to 1 mEq/kg Repeat in 15 min ■ Then give 2 ampules (100 mEq) in 1 L D_5W IV prn over next 1 to 2 hours	■ Redistribution: intracellular shift	■ 5 to 10 min	■ 1 to 2 h
Insulin plus glucose (use 1 U insulin per 5 g glucose)	■ 10 U regular insulin IV plus 1 ampule (50 mL) D_{50} (25 g) ■ Then give 10 to 20 U regular insulin and 500 mL $D_{10}W$ IV over 1 hr PRN	■ Redistribution: intracellular shift	■ 30 min	■ 4 to 6 h
Nebulized albuterol	■ 10 to 20 mg over 15 min ■ May repeat	■ Redistribution: intracellular shift	■ 15 min	■ 15 to 90 min
Diuresis with furosemide	■ 40 to 80 mg IV bolus	■ Removal from body	■ At start of diuresis	■ Until end of diuresis
Cation-exchange resin (Kayexalate)	■ 15 to 50 g PO or PR plus sorbitol	■ Removal from body	■ 1 to 2 h	■ 4 to 6 h
Peritoneal or hemodialysis	■ Per institutional protocol	■ Removal from body	■ At start of dialysis	■ Until end of dialysis

Clinical Case: Hyperkalemia in Patient With End-Stage Renal Failure

A 24-year-old man with type I diabetes mellitus and dialysis-dependent kidney failure presents to the ED. The patient reports severe weakness, shortness of breath, nausea, vomiting, and dizziness. He missed his last two scheduled dialysis sessions while out of town on vacation. On examination the patient looks ill and uncomfortable. Vital signs are as follows: temperature 35.3°C, pulse 108/min, BP 175/110 mm Hg, RR 32/min and labored, and oxyhemoglobin saturation per pulse oximetry is 93% on room air. Auscultation reveals bibasilar rales and an S_3 gallop.

Findings of the initial exam are consistent with volume overload. *Initiate O_2–IV–monitor.* A 12-lead ECG shows

wide-complex sinus tachycardia. STAT laboratory studies (including serum K^+) are pending.

In view of the wide QRS complexes, the situation is critical. *Immediate therapy for hyperkalemia is warranted,* so do not delay treatment while waiting for the lab results.

Administer IV calcium chloride 10% solution (500 to 1000 mg) over 2 to 5 minutes to antagonize the effects of potassium at the cell membrane.

Next give medications that shift K^+ into the cells. In end-stage renal disease, sodium bicarbonate has little effect.[6] Moreover, the Na^+ load associated with use of bicarbonate can worsen existing volume overload.

■ In this case 10 U of regular insulin IV plus 50 mL of D_{50} glucose should shift K^+ intracellularly.

■ Nebulized albuterol (10 to 20 mg over 15 minutes) also shifts K^+ intracellularly through the mechanism of adrenergic stimulation, an effect known for nearly 3 decades.[7] Albuterol inhalation is particularly effective in patients with renal failure.[8-10] It also helps prevent the hypoglycemia associated with use of glucose/insulin.

Finally, initiate agents and methods to remove K^+ from the body, such as diuresis with furosemide (though it may not work in end-stage renal disease), Kayexalate, and urgent dialysis.

■ Signs and symptoms of hypokalemia correlate with both the level of serum potassium and the speed of the fall in serum potassium[13]:

— Mild (3 to 3.5 mEq/L): often no symptoms

— Moderate (2.5 to <3.0 mEq/L): generalized weakness, fatigue, lassitude, constipation, leg cramps

— Severe (2.0 to <2.5 mEq/L): muscle breakdown (rhabdomyolysis), paralytic ileus, bowel obstruction

— Life-threatening (<2.0 mEq/L): development of ascending paralysis, impairment of respiratory function, unstable cardiac arrhythmias

■ Patients with cardiac ischemia, heart failure, or ventricular hypertrophy have an increased risk of cardiac arrhythmias even with mild to moderate hypokalemia.[14]

■ Hypokalemia is suggested by changes in the ECG (see Table 7).

Treatment

■ Treatment of hypokalemia includes limiting further potassium loss and replacing the body's potassium stores. Potassium administration may be oral or intravenous depending on the situation.

■ While critical hypokalemia is treated empirically, definitive potassium replacement should be based on an estimate of the total body potassium deficit:

— As a rule of thumb, for every 1 mEq/L decrease in serum potassium, the total body deficit is 150 to 400 mEq.

— Total body potassium and estimated deficit is based on age, sex, and body size.

  ● For example, the 150 mEq estimated deficit is appropriate for an elderly woman with low muscle mass. But for a young, muscular man, an estimated deficit of 400 mEq for every 1 mEq/L decrease in serum K^+ is more appropriate.

TABLE 6. Common Causes of Hypokalemia

Decreased Intake
■ Poor dietary intake
■ Malnutrition

Gastrointestinal and Sweat Losses
■ Vomiting (including eating disorders[15])
■ Nasogastric suction
■ Diarrhea (including laxative[16] or enema[17] abuse)
■ Malabsorption syndromes
■ Enteric fistula
■ Ureterosigmoidostomy
■ Loss through sweating (heavy exercise, heatstroke, febrile illnesses)

Increased Renal Losses
■ Diuretic use
■ Renal tubular acidosis
■ Primary aldosteronism
■ Secondary aldosteronism (renal artery stenosis, CHF, cirrhosis plus ascites, excess of ACTH or glucocorticosteroids)
■ Licorice ingestion[18,19]
■ Chewing tobacco[20,21]
■ Rare causes of renal loss:
— Bartter's syndrome: Disorder of renal tubules causing high aldosterone, low potassium, and metabolic alkalosis
— Liddle's syndrome: Autosomal dominant condition of renal tubules causing increased potassium secretion

Medications
■ Aminoglycosides
■ Penicillins (eg, Carbenicillin)
■ Cisplatin, amphotericin B
■ L-Dopa
■ Lithium
■ Thallium
■ Theophylline

Redistribution: Extracellular to Intracellular Potassium Shifts
■ Redistribution with pH changes:
— Acidosis (or fall in pH) raises serum K^+
— Alkalosis (or rise in pH) lowers serum K^+
■ Treatment of diabetic ketoacidosis
■ Insulin administration
■ Hypomagnesemia
■ β_2-Adrenergic agents (eg, albuterol)
■ Hypokalemic periodic paralysis (congenital disorder causing intermittent episodes of muscle weakness due to low serum potassium)

TABLE 7. Decreasing Serum Potassium Levels and Most Frequently Associated ECG Findings

Serum Potassium Range (mEq/L)	Frequent ECG Findings
2.5 to 3	■ U waves begin, flattened T waves, low QRS voltage, prominent P waves
2 to <2.5	■ More prominent U waves, more ST-segment changes
<2	■ Widened QRS complexes, arrhythmias, PEA, asystole

— Because changes in pH affect serum potassium, another rule of thumb has evolved: Serum K$^+$ decreases by about 0.3 mEq/L for every 0.1 unit increase in pH above normal.

  ● Consequently a patient with alkalosis (pH >7.45) will have a lower serum potassium than expected on the basis of total body potassium.

  ● The astute clinician will decrease the amount of replacement potassium for an alkalotic patient with hypokalemia if the alkalosis is also corrected.

■ Base decisions about route (oral versus IV) and speed (fast versus slow) of potassium replacement on the clinical condition of the patient.

— In general, oral potassium replacement is preferable.

— Rapid correction is appropriate only for clinically unstable patients.

— IV potassium replacement can cause life-threatening hyperkalemia, so this route of replacement is usually reserved for the following conditions:

  ● The patient cannot tolerate oral K$^+$

  ● The deficit is severe (K$^+$ <2.5 mEq/L)

  ● Extenuating circumstances exist (eg, cardiac arrhythmias, low potassium in the setting of digoxin toxicity)

■ Stable patients: Limit potassium replacement dose to approximately 10 to 20 mEq/h.

— Maximum concentration: Approximately 40 mEq in 1 L of normal saline. Peripheral IV sites are preferable. Use a central line for concentrations greater than 20 mEq/L.

— Maximum rate: Approximately 40 mEq in 1 hour. A 40 mEq infusion will acutely raise the serum potassium concentration by approximately 0.50 mEq/L.

— Monitor the ECG continuously during IV potassium infusion. If potassium is infused through a central line, the tip of the catheter should not be in the right atrium. Potassium infusion into the coronary sinus is thought to contribute to life-threatening arrhythmias.

The Periarrest Hypokalemic Patient

■ Patients with severe hypokalemia will often have serious or life-threatening signs and symptoms:

— Serious: Muscle breakdown (rhabdomyolysis), paralytic ileus, bowel obstruction

— Life-threatening: Ascending paralysis, impairment of respiratory function, unstable cardiac arrhythmias

■ Treatment of malignant ventricular arrhythmias:

— Give an initial infusion of KCl, 2 mEq/min IV over 10 minutes (20 mEq total)

— Follow with 1 mEq/min over the next 10 minutes (10 mEq total)

— Document in the chart that the rapid infusion is intentional to treat life-threatening hypokalemia.

— As the patient improves and stabilizes, reduce the KCl infusion rate.

Sodium

Physiology

■ Under normal conditions the serum sodium concentration and serum osmolality are controlled through the *renin-angiotensin-aldosterone system* and with the *antidiuretic hormone* (ADH, also known as arginine vasopressin or AVP).

■ Sodium, the most abundant positive ion in the extracellular space, determines the size of the extracellular fluid (ECF) volume. Abnormalities in sodium concentration generally reflect abnormalities of total body water.

— When the body's total sodium content *increases,* ECF will increase, resulting in volume overload. Sodium retention and ECF volume overload occur frequently with congestive heart failure (CHF), congestive cirrhosis of the liver, and the nephrotic syndrome.

— When the total sodium content *decreases,* ECF volume also decreases (volume depletion), producing signs of poor skin turgor, tachycardia, and orthostatic hypotension.

— Remember these general rules:

1. High serum sodium concentration generally indicates free water depletion; low serum sodium concentration indicates free water overload.

2. Abnormally high or low serum sodium concentration usually indicates volume-related problems.

3. Clinical problems related to inappropriate intravascular volume (eg, CHF, edema, orthostatic syncope) often reflect problems in sodium concentration.

■ Sodium is an extracellular ion. It is present in relatively small concentrations intracellularly and relatively large concentrations extracellularly (in the interstitial space).

— Rapid or large changes in serum sodium concentration can lead to free water shifts that can produce severe cardiovascular, respiratory, and neurologic complications.

— An acute change in serum sodium produces acute movement of free water between the vascular space and the interstitial space. This movement continues until osmotic equilibrium is achieved between the interstitial and vascular spaces.

 • An *acute fall* in serum sodium can cause an acute fall in serum osmolality, creating a temporary gradient between intravascular and interstitial osmolality. Free water will move from an area of low osmolality (the vascular space) to an area of higher osmolality (the interstitial space) until osmotic equilibrium is restored. This acute shift of free water from the vascular to the interstitial space can produce cerebral edema.[22,23]

 • Conversely, an *acute rise* in serum sodium concentration (eg, rapid correction of hyponatremia) will produce a temporary gradient between interstitial and intravascular osmolality, and free water will shift from the area of lower osmolality (the interstitial space) to an area of higher osmolality (the vascular space). A rapid or substantial intravascular free water shift can produce a variety of complications, including rhabdomyolysis,[24,25] pontine myelinolysis,[26-28] and cerebral bleeding.

— Monitor neurologic function closely during evaluation and treatment of either hypernatremia or hyponatremia. Whenever possible correct serum sodium slowly, over 48 hours, and avoid overcorrection.[29,30]

— Free water can also shift into and out of the cells when needed to maintain equilibrium between the intracellular and the extracellular spaces. However, protective mechanisms within brain cells can influence the magnitude of these shifts and prevent acute fluid losses from these cells unless or until changes in sodium are significant.

Hypernatremia

Normal sodium range: 135 to 145 mEq/L

Causes

■ Hypernatremia, defined as a serum sodium concentration above 145 to 150 mEq/L, is generally caused by 1 of 3 mechanisms:

1. Insufficient water intake, resulting most often in *normovolemic hypernatremia*

2. Loss of water and sodium (but water loss in excess of sodium loss), resulting most often in *hypovolemic hypernatremia*

3. Gain of water and sodium (but sodium gain exceeds water gain), resulting most often in *hypervolemic hypernatremia*

■ Table 8 lists the most common causes of hypernatremia according to these 3 mechanisms. This method of classification helps identify the cause of the hypernatremia and provides guidance for therapy.

— The most frequent clinical scenario is loss of both water and sodium, but more water relative to sodium (hypovolemic hypernatremia). Most hypernatremic patients in periarrest status are hypovolemic.

— Somewhat counterintuitively, patients with hypernatremia usually have an absolute reduction in *total* body sodium. As serum sodium is lowered to a safe level, these patients will require administration of normal saline to replenish total body stores.

Diagnosis

■ Hypernatremia causes water to shift from the interstitial space into the vascular space. Significant hypernatremia can cause a shift of free water from the cellular space, causing intracellular dehydration. The severity of symptoms depends on the acuteness and severity of the rise in serum sodium. If the sodium concentration rises quickly or substantially, the signs and symptoms will be more severe.

— **Neurologic symptoms:** An acute free water shift from the interstitial to the vascular space can cause nausea and vomiting, lack of appetite, irritability, and fatigue.

— **Neurologic signs:** Physical signs include confusion, stupor, and coma; seizures; altered mental status; muscle weakness, twitching, or spasticity; tremor or ataxia; or focal neurologic signs such as paresis or abnormal plantar reflexes.

■ Patients with hypernatremia caused by decreased water intake or excessive water loss in relation to sodium loss (hypovolemic hypernatremia) will have signs and symptoms of dehydration and hypovolemia.

— These patients will usually report excessive thirst, fatigue, and orthostatic symptoms such as dizziness and lightheadedness.

Treatment

- It is important to remember that sodium abnormalities indicate primarily water problems. The major therapeutic approach is *not* to remove excess sodium but to replace the lost water.

  — Most hypernatremic patients are hypovolemic. They have a deficit of free water and sodium, but the free water deficit is more significant than the sodium deficit. Treatment requires careful replacement of both volume and sodium while avoiding a rapid fall in serum sodium and osmolality.[22]

  — Too rapid a fall in serum sodium will cause dangerous fluid shifts (from the interstitial to the vascular space) and risk of cerebral bleeding or other physiologic derangements.

- **Calculation of water deficit:** Correct the water deficit (usually with normal saline) and stop ongoing water losses by treating the underlying cause. The key step is to calculate the quantity of water needed to correct the water deficit. Use the following equation:

$$\text{Water deficit (in L)} = \frac{([Na^+]_{measured} - 140) \times TBW}{140}$$

$$TBW_{in\ L} = (0.6_{men}\ or\ 0.5_{women}) \times weight_{in\ kg}$$

- Total body water is approximately 60% of lean body weight in men and 50% in women.

- **Rate of replacement:** Fluid is administered to decrease the serum sodium slowly, generally no faster than 0.5 to 1 mEq/L per hour.

  — In the first 24 hours the decrease in serum sodium should be limited to a maximum of approximately 12 mEq/L (eg, a decrease from 160 to 148 mEq/L in the case example).

TABLE 8. Common Causes of Hypernatremia
Reduced Intake of Free Water: Normovolemic or Hypovolemic Hypernatremia
■ Mild free water loss, such as increased insensible water losses
■ Conditions that lead to inability to obtain free water:
— Infancy
— Coma, dementia
— Bed confinement, intubation
— Injuries
— Environmental emergencies (wilderness travel, castaways)
Significant Loss of Free Water (With Moderate Loss of Sodium): Hypovolemic Hypernatremia
■ Gastrointestinal losses: vomiting, diarrhea, nasogastric suctioning, fistulas
■ Renal losses:
— Osmotic diuresis such as mannitol administration
— Diabetes insipidus with loss of concentrating ability: central (no vasopressin from pituitary gland) or nephrogenic (no renal response to vasopressin)
— Postobstructive state
■ Dermal losses: sweating, burns
Significant Gain of Sodium (With Moderate Gain of Free Water): Hypervolemic Hypernatremia
■ Excessive sodium bicarbonate administration
■ Hypertonic saline administration, salt tablets, errors in formula preparation
■ Seawater ingestion
■ Excess mineralocorticoid (primary aldosteronism)
■ Excess glucocorticoid (Cushing's disease, exogenous, ectopic ACTH syndromes)

Correction of Hypovolemic Hypernatremia
■ Case example: If a 70-kg man has a serum Na^+ concentration of 160 mEq/L, calculate his estimated free water deficit:
$$\text{Water deficit} = \frac{160 - 140\ mEq/L}{140\ mEq/L} \times (70\ kg \times 0.6\ L/kg) = 6\ L$$
■ Calculate the rate of free water replacement. The goal of therapy will be to administer 6 L of free water, usually as 0.9% sodium chloride (normal saline) or 0.45% sodium chloride (half-normal saline), while reducing the serum sodium concentration by 20 mEq/L (from 160 to 140 mEq/L). Avoid D_5W because it produces decreases in serum sodium that are too rapid.

— Proper total correction should take at least 48 hours (from 148 to 140 mEq/L over the next 24 hours in the case example).

■ You must monitor the patient and check the serum sodium concentration frequently to avoid rapid correction and complications.

■ Select the route of replacement of free water based on the patient's clinical status:

— Stable, asymptomatic: Give fluids by mouth or through a nasogastric tube.

— Symptomatic but not significantly hypovolemic: Typically use 0.45% sodium chloride (half-normal saline) IV.

— Symptomatic, significantly hypovolemic: Use 0.9% sodium chloride (normal saline) IV to correct the hypovolemia; then correct the free water deficit with 0.45% sodium chloride (half-normal saline).

The Periarrest Hypernatremic Patient

■ These hypernatremic patients will be severely hypovolemic and markedly dehydrated with shock.

■ The key for the periarrest hypernatremic patient is rapid volume replacement with normal saline:

— Give normal saline 500 mL "wide open" as a *medical bolus,* and evaluate clinical response. Repeat every 20 to 30 minutes until the patient is hemodynamically stable.

— Alternatively, give 10 to 20 mL/kg over 20 minutes (700 to 1400 mL for a 70-kg person), and evaluate hemodynamic response.

■ Calculate and correct the free water deficit as outlined above when the patient is hemodynamically stable.

Hyponatremia

Normal sodium range: 135 to 145 mEq/L

Causes

■ Hyponatremia reflects an excess of free water relative to sodium.[31-33]

— Most patients with hyponatremia have reduced renal free water excretion despite normal water intake.

— Retention of excess free water may develop in association with a variety of conditions (see Table 9).

■ Most patients with hyponatremia have low serum osmolality (so-called *hypo-osmolar hyponatremia*).

— An important exception to this association of hyponatremia with a hypo-osmolar state is severe hyperglycemia. Significant hyperglycemia can lead to a hyperosmolar state even if serum sodium is below normal *(hyperosmolar hyponatremia).*

■ Table 9 presents the most common causes of hyponatremia grouped in relation to loss or gain of sodium and volume, similar to the causes of hypernatremia (Table 8).

TABLE 9.   **Common Causes of Hyponatremia**

Increased Retention of Free Water (Inadequate Free Water Excretion): Normovolemic Hyponatremia
■ Syndrome of inappropriate antidiuretic hormone secretion (SIADH)
■ Hypoadrenalism (ie, adrenal insufficiency)
■ Hypothyroidism
■ Renal failure
■ Polydipsia (psychogenic)
Significant Retention of Free Water (With Moderate Retention of Sodium): Hypervolemic Hyponatremia
■ Edematous states:
— Congestive heart failure
— Hepatic cirrhosis
— Nephrotic syndrome (renal failure)
Significant Loss of Sodium (With Moderate Loss of Free Water): Hypovolemic Hyponatremia
■ Gastrointestinal losses: vomiting, diarrhea, nasogastric suctioning, fistulas
■ Renal losses
■ Third space losses
■ Excessive sweating
■ Addison's disease
Miscellaneous Causes
■ Sampling error
■ Pseudohyponatremia: hyperlipemia, hyperproteinemia
■ Redistributive hyponatremia: hyperglycemia, mannitol

■ The most frequent cause of potentially life-threatening hyponatremia is the *syndrome of inappropriate antidiuretic hormone secretion* (SIADH).[31,32,34]

— SIADH can occur in a wide variety of clinical situations common to ACLS patients (see Table 10). An acronym, "CONDM," can be used to recall the major causes of SIADH:

- **C:** Central nervous system disease or injury

- **O:** Other (pain, post-op, hypothyroidism)

- **N:** Nonmalignant pulmonary disease (COPD, pneumonia)

- **D:** Drugs

- **M:** Malignancy

— SIADH is caused by the nonphysiologic release of vasopressin (antidiuretic hormone, or ADH; also known as arginine vasopressin, or AVP) from either the posterior pituitary or an ectopic source, such as a malignant tumor.

— ADH stimulates renal retention of free water with continued excretion of sodium. This results in multiple abnormalities: normovolemia, combined with low sodium and low osmolality in serum; and high sodium, and high osmolality (>100 mOsm/kg) in urine.

— The hallmark finding of SIADH is a highly concentrated urine, with a urine osmolality that is higher than the serum osmolality. This hallmark finding confirms SIADH as the cause of the hyponatremia. Hyponatremia caused by nonrenal sodium losses would be associated with a low urine osmolality (renal sodium retention and thus minimal excretion of sodium in the urine).

— Untreated SIADH can be fatal or can result in significant neurologic complications. SIADH should be ruled out when significant hyponatremia develops.

Diagnosis

■ Hyponatremia is usually asymptomatic unless it develops rapidly or is severe (<125 mEq/L).

— An abrupt fall in sodium produces an acute extravascular fluid shift that causes neurologic symptoms such as nausea, vomiting, headache, irritability, and lethargy.

— At serum sodium concentrations <120 mEq/L, cerebral edema, seizures, coma, or even death can occur.

■ If the hyponatremia is associated with marked hypovolemia, the major symptoms may include hypotension and even shock.

Treatment

■ First, assess intravascular volume. Determine if the patient is hypervolemic (edematous states), hypovolemic, or normovolemic.

— Signs of hypervolemia with volume overload: CHF, peripheral edema, elevated jugular veins, rales, weight gain, S_3 heart sound.

— Signs of hypovolemia with volume depletion: Tachycardia, resting and orthostatic hypotension, dry mucous membranes, poor peripheral perfusion, poor skin turgor.

■ Second, plan treatment based on the severity of symptoms and volume status.[32]

— Volume depletion: Replace volume with normal saline.

— Volume overload: Restrict water and initiate diuresis with furosemide. *Note:* Some researchers have reported superior outcomes with IV normal saline or 3% saline administration instead of fluid restriction.[30,35,36]

TABLE 10. Common Causes of the Syndrome of Inappropriate Antidiuretic Hormone Secretion (SIADH)

CNS Disease or Injury
■ Stroke
■ Brain injury, infarction, tumor, abscess
■ Meningitis
■ Encephalitis
Other
■ Pain
■ Postoperative complications
■ Hypothyroidism
Nonmalignant Pulmonary Disease
■ Acute respiratory distress syndrome
■ Pneumonia
■ Tuberculosis
■ Lung abscess
■ Cystic fibrosis
■ Asthma
Drugs
■ Vasopressin (exogenous)
■ Diuretics
■ Chlorpropamide
■ Vincristine
■ Cyclophosphamide
■ Thioridazine
Malignancies
■ Lung cancer
■ Pancreatic cancer
■ Duodenal cancer
■ Oat cell carcinoma
■ Lymphoma
■ Hodgkin's disease

— Normal or near-normal ECF volume (eg, with SIADH, hypothyroidism, adrenal insufficiency): Restrict fluid intake to one half to one third maintenance fluid requirements and treat underlying cause.

— Asymptomatic: Aim for gradual restoration of serum sodium, limiting the increase in Na^+ to no more than 0.5 mEq/L per hour (maximum increase of 12 mEq/L in the first 24 hours).

— *Note:* Rapid increases in Na^+ can lead to a higher plasma osmolality that can dehydrate and injure the brain. This life-threatening condition, called *osmotic demyelination syndrome* or *central pontine myelinolysis,* is caused by rapid fluid shifts in the brain.[24,26,27]

The Periarrest Hyponatremic Patient

■ Hyponatremic patients will often present with alarming neurologic symptoms, such as seizures or coma, with increased intracranial pressure that can lead to cardiac arrest. Rapid deterioration is more likely with rapid development of hyponatremia.

■ These patients require aggressive treatment of their hyponatremia to prevent irreversible brain damage or cardiac arrest:

— To contol neurologic symptoms: Give 3% saline IV. Aim to correct the serum sodium concentration at a rate of 1 mEq/L per hour until the neurologic symptoms are controlled.

— After neurologic symptoms controlled: Correct serum sodium at a rate of 0.5 mEq/L per hour.

— Gradual correction is particularly important for treatment of chronic hyponatremia.

■ Use 3% saline with great caution. Overly aggressive treatment with hypertonic saline can be lethal. Do not use hypertonic saline to *normalize* Na^+; use it only to raise the serum sodium sufficiently to control neurologic symptoms.

■ Recommended steps for using 3% saline (see "Clinical Case: Using 3% Saline for Life-Threatening Hyponatremia"):

— Step 1: Calculate the sodium deficit with the following formula[22]:

$$Na^+ \text{ deficit} = ([Na^+]_{desired} - [Na^+]_{measured}) \times \text{total body water}$$
$$= ([Na^+]_{desired} - [Na^+]_{measured}) \times 0.6^* \times \text{body weight (kg)}$$

(*use a body weight coefficient of 0.6 for men, 0.5 for women)

— Step 2: Calculate the volume of 3% saline (513 mEq Na^+/L) required to reduce the deficit a total of 4 mEq/L in 4 hours (4 mEq/L × TBW = mEq Na^+).

— Step 3: Administer the required volume of 3% saline over 4 hours at a rate that will increase sodium by 1 mEq/L per hour.

— *Note:* Some experts recommend more aggressive correction if the patient is obtunded or comatose (2 mEq/L per hour) or demonstrating seizures (2 to 4 mEq/L per hour).[23] This would require administration of the amount of 3% saline calculated above over 1 to 2 hours instead of over 4 hours.

Clinical Case: Using 3% Saline for Treatment of Life-Threatening Hyponatremia

A 78-year-old woman weighing 70 kg presents with seizures and a serum sodium concentration of 108 mEq/L. To control these neurologic symptoms it will be necessary to give 3% saline.

Note: Aim to raise the sodium concentration at a rate of **1 mEq/L per hour for the next 4 hours, or a total of 4 mEq/L** (desired sodium = 108 + 4 = 112 mEq/L).

Step 1: Calculate the sodium deficit:

Na^+ deficit $= ([Na^+]_{desired} - [Na^+]_{measured}) \times$ **total body water**

Na^+ deficit $= (112 \text{ mEq/L}_{desired\ Na} - 108 \text{ mEq/L}_{measured\ Na}) \times 0.5_{wt\ coefficient} \times 70 \text{ kg}_{body\ wt}$

$= (112 - 108 \text{ mEq}) \qquad \times (0.5 \qquad \times 70)$

$= 4 \text{ mEq} \qquad\qquad\qquad \times 35$

$= 140 \text{ mEq}$

Step 2: Calculate the volume of 3% saline required to replace this 140 mEq deficit:

Volume = Na^+ deficit ÷ Na^+ concentration of 3% saline

Volume = 140 $\text{mEq}_{deficit}$/513 $\text{mEq}_{per\ L\ of\ 3\%\ saline}$ = 0.27 L (270 mL) of 3% saline

Step 3: Administer 3% saline at a rate that will increase sodium by 1 mEq/L per hour or 4 mEq/L over 4 hours:

Volume = 270 mL of 3% saline over 4 hours = 270/4 = rate of 67 mL/h

Monitor neurologic status closely. Check serum Na^+ frequently.

■ *Note:* Some experts recommend administering 3% saline to correct hyponatremia at a rate of **2 to 4 mEq/L per hour** when a patient has ongoing seizures. In the calculations above, you determined the amount of 3% saline to raise the serum sodium 1 mEq/L per hour over 4 hours. If you administer this volume (270 mL) in 1 to 2 hours, it should correct the sodium at a rate of 2 to 4 mEq/L per hour. Begin at the rate of 270 mL/h until seizures stop; then decrease the rate to 67 to 135 mL/h (to raise the sodium at a rate of 1 to 2 mEq/L per hour).[23]

Calcium

- Calcium, the most abundant mineral in the body, mediates myriad intracellular enzymatic reactions. Many processes depend on intracellular calcium, such as receptor activation, muscle contraction, cardiac contractility, and platelet aggregation.

  — Calcium is essential for bone strength and neuromuscular function.

  — Alterations in serum calcium concentration have direct effects on the strength and rate at which muscle (including the myocardium) contracts.

- Only 1% of total body calcium is extracellular. Of this amount, only 50% is in the biologically active, ionized form; the other half binds to albumin.

  — Ionized calcium concentration is inversely related to the serum pH. Alkalosis (or a rise in serum pH) reduces ionized calcium because it increases the binding of calcium to albumin. Acidosis (or a fall in serum pH) increases ionized calcium. Total calcium is unchanged by pH.

  — Total serum calcium concentration is directly related to the albumin concentration. One gram of serum protein (predominantly albumin) binds to 0.8 mg of calcium. For this reason a 1 g decrease in albumin leads to a 0.8 mg/dL decrease in total calcium with no change in the level of ionized calcium. Proportionately more of the total calcium is ionized at lower albumin concentrations, so the serum ionized calcium (the functional portion of the calcium) is unchanged when the total calcium falls with a fall in serum albumin.

  — Often the widely used "metabolic panels" that present findings of multiple laboratory tests report total serum calcium but not ionized calcium. A very low total calcium level may be reported for a patient with hypoalbuminemia. To calculate the true total calcium adjusted for the hypoalbuminemia, use the following formula:

  True calcium$_{total}$ = measured calcium$_{total}$ + [(0.8) × (protein$_{normal}$ − protein$_{measured}$)]

  — If the patient is unstable or if symptoms of hypocalcemia are present, request a specific measurement of ionized calcium. The more comprehensive metabolic panels include both total and ionized calcium.

- Calcium is primarily an extracellular ion. Calcium and sodium are actively pumped out of cells. Because calcium antagonizes the effects of both potassium and magnesium at the cell membrane, it is the agent of choice for treating both severe hyperkalemia and hypermagnesemia.

- Because of the critical role of calcium, the serum calcium concentration is controlled within a narrow range. This control is chiefly exerted by secretion of parathyroid hormone (PTH) from the parathyroid gland in response to low ionized calcium levels.

  — PTH has direct effects on gastrointestinal (GI) and renal calcium resorption, on the activity of calcitonin on bone osteoclasts, and on the level of the active vitamin D metabolite, calciferol.

  — The Figure, below, depicts schematically the body's typical response to a low level of ionized serum calcium. The opposite response occurs with elevated calcium.

FIGURE. Regulation of serum calcium concentration. This figure illustrates the body's response to an abnormally low level of calcium. Low ionized serum calcium results in increased release of parathyroid hormone (PTH). PTH in turn has 3 major effects: (1) PTH decreases calcitonin. Because calcitonin inhibits the activity of bone osteoclasts, a decrease in calcitonin allows more bone turnover, resulting in an increase in serum calcium. (2) PTH increases calcium resorption in the kidneys, resulting in a rapid rise in serum calcium. (3) PTH activates vitamin D to the more active metabolite, calciferol, which causes increased gastrointestinal (GI) absorption of calcium. PTH also has a direct effect on calcium absorption in the GI tract.

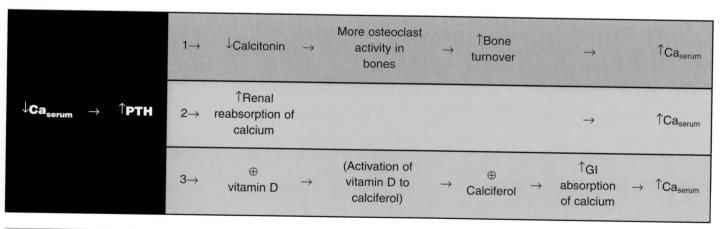

Hypercalcemia

Normal total calcium range: 8.5 to 10.5 mg/dL

Normal ionized calcium range: 4.2 to 4.8 mg/dL

Causes

- More than 90% of reported cases of hypercalcemia are caused by malignancy or hyperparathyroidism.[37]

  — Some malignancies secrete a parathormone-like substance, causing increased calcium release from the bone.

  — Primary hyperparathyroidism causes increased gut resorption of calcium.

- In the presence of decreased renal clearance, many conditions associated with increased calcium release from the bone or increased calcium absorption from the gut produce hypercalcemia.

- Table 11 presents the common causes of hypercalcemia.

- The overall incidence of hypercalcemia in the general population is 0.3% to 6%, making it much more common than hypocalcemia.

Diagnosis

- Total calcium ≥10.5 mg/dL or ionized calcium >4.8 mg/dL defines hypercalcemia. Patients are generally asymptomatic until total calcium is >12 mg/dL.

- Total calcium concentration = 12 to <15 mg/dL: Symptoms of hypercalcemia begin to appear.

  — Most common are neurologic symptoms of depression, weakness, fatigue, and confusion.

  — Cardiac contractility can actually increase until the calcium level is >15 mg/dL.

- Total calcium concentration = 15 to <20 mg/dL: Patients are usually weak, lethargic, and confused. They often exhibit hallucinations, disorientation, hypotonicity, and coma.

TABLE 11.	Common Causes of Hypercalcemia

Primary Hyperparathyroidism and Malignancy (>90% of Cases)
■ Cancers causing osteolytic bone metastases: Lung, breast, kidney, myeloma, leukemia
■ Paraneoplastic tumors: Parathyroid hormone–related proteins, bone-resorbing substances, ectopic production of calciferol
Pulmonary and Granulomatous Diseases
■ Berylliosis
■ Adult respiratory distress syndrome
■ Histoplasmosis
■ Coccidioidomycosis
■ Tuberculosis
■ Sarcoidosis
Drugs
■ Lithium
■ Thiazide diuretics
■ Hormonal therapy for breast cancer (estrogens)
■ Hypervitaminosis A and D
■ Calcium ingestion
Endocrine Disorders (Nonparathyroid)
■ Hyperthyroidism
■ Adrenal insufficiency
■ Pheochromocytoma
■ Acromegaly
■ Vasoactive polypeptide-producing tumors (intestinal)
Miscellaneous Causes
■ Immobilization
■ Paget's disease of bone
■ Milk-alkali syndrome
■ Acute renal failure, recovery phase

  — At these levels myocardial depression begins to occur with decreased automaticity and shortened ventricular systole.

  — A shortened refractory period leads to arrhythmias.

  — Many patients with hypercalcemia also develop hypokalemia, another risk factor for cardiac arrhythmias.

  — Digitalis toxicity is worsened.

  — Hypertension is common.

- ECG changes of hypercalcemia:

  — Shortened QT interval (usually when serum calcium is >13 mg/dL)

  — Prolonged PR and QRS intervals

  — Increased QRS voltage

  — T wave flattening and widening

  — Notching of QRS

  — AV block (often progressing to complete heart block and even cardiac arrest when serum calcium is >15 to 20 mg/dL)

- GI signs of hypercalcemia: Dysphagia, constipation, peptic ulcers, and pancreatitis.

- Renal signs of hypercalcemia: Diminished ability to concentrate urine; polyuria or diuresis results in loss of sodium, potassium, magnesium, and phosphate; renal lithiasis.

  — Loss of these electrolytes produces a negative cycle of calcium reabsorption that further worsens the hypercalcemia.

- Classic *memory aid* for frequent signs and symptoms of hypercalcemia: *Stones, bones, moans and groans, and psychologic overtones:*

  — Stones: Renal lithiasis

  — Bones: Osteolysis releasing calcium (metastatic disease)

  — Moans and groans: Abdominal pain in general, plus pancreatitis, peptic ulcers

  — Psychologic overtones: Apathy, depression, stupor and coma, irritability, hallucinations

Treatment

- If the hypercalcemia is due to malignancy, carefully consider the patient's prognosis and wishes before starting treatment. A patient dying of cancer may need no treatment. In all other cases aggressive treatment is needed.

- Total calcium concentration = 12 to <15 mg/dL: Begin the treatment outlined below for symptomatic patients.

- Total calcium concentration = >15 mg/dL: Begin treatment whether the patient is symptomatic or not. There are 4 components to hypercalcemia therapy. ACLS providers will seldom be responsible for more than the first two: volume restoration and starting calcium elimination through the kidneys.

- **First, restore volume:**

  — Establish vascular access with a large-bore IV.

  — Infuse normal saline (0.9% sodium chloride) at 300 to 500 mL/h until fluid deficits are replaced. Volume replacement promotes increased excretion of calcium by the kidneys.

  — Decrease infusion rate to 100 to 200 mL/h once you establish adequate rehydration.

- **Second, increase renal calcium elimination:**

  — The saline diuresis induced by volume restoration will usually decrease the serum calcium concentration by 1.5 to 2.5 mg/dL.

  — Consider furosemide 1 mg/kg, especially for patients in heart failure. But do *not* administer loop diuretics until you have restored intravascular volume. *Note:* Use of furosemide in hypercalcemia is controversial because it can foster reuptake of calcium ions, worsening the hypercalcemia.

  — Some experts recommend empirically adding magnesium (15 mg/h) and potassium (up to 10 mEq/h) during volume restoration because they are excreted during saline diuresis.

- **Third, reduce calcium release from bones** by administering drugs that inhibit osteoclast activity. These drugs do not work immediately (onset of action and peak effect may take several hours).

  — Calcitonin inhibits osteoclast activity and promotes calcium deposition in bone, but it produces only modest reductions in serum calcium concentration.

  — Pamidronate (Aredia) and etidronate (Didronel) are 2 currently approved inhibitors of osteoclastic activity.

  — Glucocorticoids, indomethacin, gallium nitrate, and oral phosphates are other options.

- **Fourth, treat the primary disorder** causing the hypercalcemia. For example, discontinue any causative medications; perform parathyroidectomy for hyperparathyroidism; and provide specific treatment for paraneoplastic syndromes, nonparathyroid endocrine disorders, or granulomatous diseases.

The Periarrest Hypercalcemic Patient

- These hypercalcemic patients will present with severe neurologic symptoms such as profound lethargy, confusion, hallucinations, and even coma; with cardiac arrhythmias such as complete heart block; with extreme hypovolemia; or with cardiac arrest.

- Urgent treatment:

  — Rapid fluid resuscitation with normal saline infusion: 500 mL "wide open" as a *medical bolus.* Evaluate clinical response. Repeat every 20 to 30 minutes until patient is hemodynamically stable.

  — In severe cases give 10 to 20 mL/kg of normal saline over 20 minutes (700 to 1400 mL for a 70-kg person), and assess hemodynamic response.

  — Consider furosemide 1 mg/kg (see above).

- Patients with heart failure or renal insufficiency:

  — Begin hemodialysis rapidly to decrease serum calcium concentration.

Hypocalcemia

Normal total calcium range: 8.5 to 10.5 mg/dL

Normal ionized calcium range: 4.2 to 4.8 mg/dL

Causes

- The incidence of hypocalcemia in the general population is 0.6%.

- Calcium exchange is dependent on adequate serum concentrations of potassium and magnesium. Effective treatment of hypocalcemia often requires administration of all 3 electrolytes. The most important and frequent causes of hypocalcemia are acute pancreatitis, lack of parathyroid hormone, lack of vitamin D, and medications (see Table 12).

TABLE 12. Common Causes of Hypocalcemia

Insufficient Parathyroid Hormone
■ Post-parathyroidectomy for hyperparathyroidism
■ Neck surgery (eg, thyroidectomy)
■ Post–neck irradiation
■ Destruction of parathyroid glands by metastatic carcinoma, infiltrative diseases
Insufficient Vitamin D
■ Malnutrition, dietary abnormalities
■ Malabsorption
■ Congenital rickets
■ Chronic liver disease
■ Chronic renal disease
■ Sunlight deficiency
■ Hypo- or hypermagnesemia
■ Advanced bone disease
Medications
■ Cimetidine (most frequent cause of drug-induced hypocalcemia)
■ Phosphates (from enemas, laxatives)
■ Dilantin, phenobarbital
■ Gentamicin, tobramycin, actinomycin
■ Calcitonin, mithramycin
■ EDTA (citrate from blood administration)
■ Heparin, protamine
■ Theophylline
■ Glucagon
■ Norepinephrine
■ Loop diuretics
■ Nitroprusside
Miscellaneous Causes
■ Pancreatitis
■ Shock or sepsis
■ Burns
■ Toxic shock syndrome
■ Magnesium deficiency

Diagnosis

- Signs and symptoms of hypocalcemia usually occur when the level of ionized calcium falls below 2.5 mg/dL:

  — Acute signs and symptoms: Paresthesias of the extremities and face, fatigue, muscle cramps, carpopedal spasm, stridor, tetany and seizures, confusion, impaired memory

  — Acute physical findings: Hyper-reflexia, positive Chvostek's sign (tap over facial nerve in front of ear produces twitch of eyelid or corner of mouth) or positive Trousseau's sign (carpal spasm of hand and fingers after BP cuff has been inflated above systolic pressure for 3 minutes; the BP cuff inflation induces ischemia of the ulnar nerve)

  — Acute cardiac symptoms: Decreased contractility, low blood pressure, heart failure

  — ECG changes of hypocalcemia:

    - QT-interval prolongation
    - Terminal T-wave inversion
    - Bradycardias, heart blocks
    - VT or torsades de pointes

Treatment

- Treatment of hypocalcemia involves calcium administration. When calcium is administered intravenously, monitor the infusion site closely because inadvertent tissue infiltration can cause skin necrosis, and some calcium preparations can cause sclerosis of veins.

- *Calcium gluconate* tends to be less irritating to tissues than calcium chloride. Because patients with hypocalcemia may require continuous IV infusions, many clinicians prefer calcium gluconate to calcium chloride in this situation.

  — Calcium gluconate for symptomatic hypocalcemia: Administer 10% calcium gluconate (9.3 mg/mL or 93 mg/10 mL of elemental calcium). Give 10 to 20 mL (93 to 186 mg) over 10 minutes.

— Follow calcium gluconate with an IV infusion of 540 to 720 mg elemental calcium (58 to 77 mL of 10% calcium gluconate) in 500 to 1000 mL D_5W. Infuse at a rate of 0.5 to 2 mg/kg per hour (10 to 15 mg/kg).

■ Alternatively *calcium chloride* may be used in doses that provide the same amount of elemental calcium. Prolonged infusion with this agent, however, is not recommended.

— Calcium chloride: Administer 10% solution (27.3 mg/mL, or 273 mg/10 mL of elemental calcium). Give 5 mL (136.5 mg of elemental calcium) over 10 minutes. Follow in the next 6 to 12 hours with up to 1 g (36.6 mL of 10% calcium chloride) by IV infusion.

■ Treatment details:

— Evaluate serum calcium every 4 to 6 hours. Aim to maintain the total serum calcium concentration between 7 and 9 mg/dL.

— Correct abnormalities in magnesium, potassium, and pH simultaneously.

— *Note:* Untreated hypomagnesemia will often make hypocalcemia refractory to therapy. Therefore, evaluate serum magnesium when hypocalcemia is present and particularly if hypocalcemia is refractory to initial calcium therapy.

The Periarrest Hypocalcemic Patient

■ These hypocalcemic patients will present with seizures, tetany, laryngospasm, hypotension or shock, profound bradycardias from heart block, acute congestive failure, or coma.

■ For the cardiac arrest patient:

— Establish IV access with a large-bore catheter and administer normal saline bolus.

— Calcium gluconate: Administer 10% calcium gluconate (9.3 mg/mL or 93 mg/10 mL of elemental calcium). Give 30 mL (279 mg) of a 10% solution over 1 to 3 minutes.

— Calcium chloride: Administer 10% solution (27.3 mg/mL or 273 mg/10 mL of elemental calcium). Give 10 mL (273 mg) over 1 to 3 minutes.

Magnesium

Physiology

■ Magnesium is the second most abundant intracellular cation (after potassium). Located predominantly inside cells, magnesium is the fourth most common mineral in the human body. Serum magnesium levels are unreliable predictors of total body magnesium stores because

— 50% of total body magnesium is found in bone

— 33% of extracellular magnesium is bound to serum albumin

■ Many critical physiologic processes depend on magnesium:

— Magnesium is essential for the movement of sodium, potassium, and calcium into and out of cells.

— In prospective studies low potassium in combination with low magnesium is a risk factor for multiple arrhythmias, including VF.[12] Correction of hypokalemia, however, may be impossible unless hypomagnesemia is also corrected.

— Magnesium plays an important role in stabilizing excitable membranes. Magnesium infusion is an important therapy for treating atrial and ventricular arrhythmias in patients with low serum levels or total body deficits.

Hypermagnesemia

Normal magnesium range: 1.35 to 2.2 mEq/L

Causes

■ Emergency providers will rarely encounter hypermagnesemia. When hypermagnesemia does occur, it is almost always associated with significant renal failure since normally functioning kidneys easily excrete large amounts of magnesium.

■ The major causes of hypermagnesemia are increased magnesium load, impaired elimination from the GI tract, and increased renal absorption.

— Excess intake of magnesium-containing drugs, particularly laxatives and antacids such as Maalox, is an important cause in the elderly and in patients with renal insufficiency.

— The most common causes of hypermagnesemia are listed in Table 13.

Diagnosis

■ Hypermagnesemia causes neurologic symptoms of muscular weakness, paralysis, ataxia, drowsiness, and confusion. Nausea and vomiting are common GI symptoms. Other symptoms include flushing, transient tachycardia followed by bradycardia, hypoventilation, and cardiorespiratory arrest.[12]

■ ECG changes of hypermagnesemia:

— Increased PR and QT intervals

— Increased QRS duration

— Decrease in P-wave voltage

— Variable degree of T-wave peaking

— Complete AV block

— Asystole

Treatment

■ General treatment for hypermagnesemia:

— Stop any oral or parenteral sources of magnesium.

— Support the ABCDs of ACLS.

— Dilute serum magnesium concentration with administration of IV fluids.

TABLE 13. Most Common Causes of Significant Hypermagnesemia

Renal Failure (Acute or Chronic) or Increased Magnesium Load
■ Laxatives, antacids, or enemas containing magnesium
■ Treatment of pre-eclampsia or eclampsia (may affect both mother and neonate)
■ Rhabdomyolysis
■ Tumor lysis syndrome
Impaired Elimination of Magnesium From GI Tract
■ Anticholinergics
■ Narcotics
■ Chronic constipation
■ Bowel obstruction
■ Gastric dilatation
Increased Magnesium Absorption by Kidneys
■ Hyperparathyroidism
■ Hypothyroidism
■ Adrenal insufficiency
■ Mineralocorticoid deficiency
■ Lithium therapy

— Antagonize the cellular effects of elevated magnesium with calcium gluconate or calcium chloride.

— Remove excess magnesium from the body.

■ Antagonize the effects of hypermagnesemia:

— Administer *either* calcium gluconate 10 mL IV of a 10% solution or calcium chloride 5 to 10 mL IV of a 10% solution over 5 to 10 minutes.

■ Remove excess magnesium from the body:

— Induce diuresis with normal saline IV at 500 mL/h plus furosemide 1 mg/kg if renal function is normal. Saline diuresis will hasten magnesium excretion by the kidneys.

— *Note:* Saline diuresis may increase calcium excretion, making signs and symptoms of hypermagnesemia worse. Be prepared also to administer calcium chloride 10% solution IV.

The Periarrest Hypermagnesemic Patient

■ The severity of symptoms will increase as the serum magnesium rises:

— 3 to <4 mEq/L: Neuromuscular irritability, somnolence, and loss of deep tendon reflexes

— 4 to <5 mEq/L: Increasing muscle weakness

— 5 to <8 mEq/L: Onset of severe vasodilation and hypotension

— ≥8 mEq/L: Onset of cardiac conduction abnormalities, neuromuscular paralysis, hypotension, ventilation failure, and cardiac arrest

■ In urgent situations immediately antagonize the effects of hypermagnesemia at the neuromuscular cellular level:

— Administer calcium gluconate 10 mL IV of a 10% solution given as a slow bolus.

— An alternative is to give calcium chloride 5 to 10 mL IV of a 10% solution slow bolus.

— Repeat calcium administration every 5 to 10 minutes until patient stabilizes.

■ As the patient stabilizes, begin removal of magnesium with saline diuresis and a diuretic (if renal function is normal):

— Normal saline 500 mL/h IV

— Furosemide 1 mg/kg IV bolus

■ As treatment continues the patient may require cardiorespiratory support. Provide this support immediately because once the serum magnesium level decreases, the patient should be fine. Dialysis is ultimately the treatment of choice, but ready availability is a problem in some clinical settings.

Hypomagnesemia

Normal magnesium range: 1.3 to 2.2 mEq/L

Causes

■ Hypomagnesemia occurs in 11% of all hospitalized patients and in up to 65% of severely ill patients.[38]

■ Hypomagnesemia usually results from either decreased magnesium intake or increased magnesium loss, from either the kidneys or the gut (see Table 14). Alterations in parathyroid hormone, certain medications (eg, pentamidine and diuretics), and alcoholism also can induce hypomagnesemia.

— Multiple neurohumoral mechanisms become activated in patients with decompensated congestive heart failure, leading to hypomagnesemia and other acid-base and electrolyte

TABLE 14. Common Causes of Hypomagnesemia

Decreased Intake
■ Alcoholism
■ Malnutrition
■ Starvation
Increased Loss
■ Gastrointestinal loss: Bowel resection, pancreatitis, diarrhea
■ Burns
■ Lactation
■ Renal disease
Miscellaneous Causes
■ Drugs: Diuretics, pentamidine, gentamicin, digoxin
■ Parathyroid abnormalities
■ Hypothermia
■ Hypercalcemia
■ Diabetic ketoacidosis
■ Hyper- or hypothyroidism
■ Phosphate deficiency

disturbances.[38] These patients face a high risk of deleterious arrhythmias.

Diagnosis

- Most patients with hypomagnesemia are asymptomatic.

- Patients with symptomatic hypomagnesemia most commonly present with one or more of the following symptoms: muscular tremors, fasciculations, vertigo, ataxia, altered mentation, Chvostek's or Trousseau's sign, and various paresthesias. Many of the symptoms indicate the presence of hypocalcemia.

- Other possible symptoms are ocular nystagmus, tetany, dysphagia, and seizures.

- Hypomagnesemia is often associated with hypokalemia or hypocalcemia. Providers should always check the levels of potassium and calcium in patients with low serum magnesium.

- ECG changes of hypomagnesemia:
  - Prolonged QT and PR intervals
  - ST depression
  - T-wave inversion
  - Flattening or inversion of precordial P waves
  - Widening of the QRS interval
  - Torsades de pointes
  - Treatment-resistant VF (and other arrhythmias)
  - Worsening of digitalis toxicity

Treatment

- Treatment of hypomagnesemia depends on its severity and the clinical status of the patient. In patients with renal insufficiency, replace magnesium cautiously; there is a significant risk of life-threatening hypermagnesemia.[39]

- Mild or chronic hypomagnesemia:
  - Oral replacement is the preferred route for mild hypomagnesemia. (Parenteral magnesium administration is indicated if symptoms are present even if hypomagnesemia is mild.)
  - Give magnesium sulfate ($MgSO_4$) 400 mg PO once or twice a day.
  - Several weeks of therapy may be required to replenish total body magnesium stores.

- Moderate hypomagnesemia:
  - Give $MgSO_4$ IV at a rate of 1 to 2 g over 15 minutes, then 6 g in IV fluid per 24 hours. This problem may require 3 to 7 days for correction.
  - Monitor magnesium level and deep tendon reflexes.

- Significant symptomatic hypomagnesemia:
  - Start with $MgSO_4$ 1 to 2 g IV over 15 minutes.
  - Add 6 g magnesium to the daily IV fluids for the next 3 to 7 days.
  - Check the patient's magnesium levels and reflexes daily.

- Acute seizures:
  - Give $MgSO_4$ 2 g IV over 10 minutes.
  - Add calcium chloride 5 to 10 mL of a 10% solution because most patients with hypomagnesemia are also hypocalcemic.

- Torsades de pointes associated with hypomagnesemia:
  - Give up to 2 g of $MgSO_4$ over 1 to 2 minutes (over 5 to 60 minutes if pulse is present).

The Periarrest Hypomagnesemic Patient

- These patients will present with either seizures or unstable ventricular arrhythmias, most often torsades de pointes.

- Administer $MgSO_4$ 2 g IV (generally administer over 10 minutes; give over 1 to 2 minutes for the most urgent cases).
  - You may repeat the dose in 10 to 15 minutes if the patient remains unstable.

- Administer calcium gluconate 10 mL of a 10% solution or calcium chloride 5 to 10 mL of a 10% solution because most patients with hypomagnesemia are also hypocalcemic.

Life-Threatening Acid-Base Abnormalities
Physiology

- The healthy human body closely regulates serum pH between 7.35 and 7.45.
  - When pH falls below 7.35, *acidosis* is present.
  - When pH rises above 7.45, *alkalosis* is present.

- There are 4 main types of acid-base imbalances:
  - Metabolic acidosis
  - Metabolic alkalosis
  - Respiratory acidosis
  - Respiratory alkalosis

- There are mixed acid-base disturbances as well. Whenever acid-base imbalances occur, the body attempts to correct the abnormality and bring the pH back toward the normal range.

Diagnostic Approaches to Acid-Base Abnormalities

Using the ABG: pH, Pco_2, Bicarbonate

- To assess a patient's acid-base status, obtain an arterial blood gas (ABG) analysis. The ABG is critical for identifying acid-base abnormalities and the degree of any compensation. In addition to Po_2 and O_2 saturation, the following variables appear on a typical ABG report (normal range follows variable):
  - pH: 7.35 to 7.45
  - Pco_2 (partial pressure of carbon dioxide): 35 to 45 mm Hg

— Bicarbonate (HCO_3^-): 22 to 32 mEq/L

— Base deficit or base excess: −2 to +2

■ An average P_{CO_2} value of 40 mm Hg is used in calculations to compare the *predicted pH* with the *measured pH*. The magnitude and direction of any difference between predicted and measured pH provide a rough estimate of whether a metabolic or respiratory acidosis or alkalosis is present.

■ **Comparing predicted pH with measured pH:** When interpreting the ABG, you must evaluate both the P_{CO_2} and the pH to identify any acid-base disorder and metabolic and respiratory components. You make this assessment by first predicting the pH from the P_{CO_2}:

— Step 1: Determine if the pH is acidotic (<7.35), alkalotic (>7.45) or normal (7.35 to 7.45), and note if the patient is hypercarbic (P_{CO_2} >45) or hypocarbic (P_{CO_2} <35). Hypocarbia indicates a respiratory alkalosis, and hypercarbia indicates a respiratory acidosis. Now to identify the primary problem and any compensation, you need to determine the contribution of the P_{CO_2} to any acidosis or alkalosis.

— Step 2: Subtract the patient's measured P_{CO_2} from 40 (estimated normal P_{CO_2}). The result will be either positive (if the patient's P_{CO_2} is low) or negative (if P_{CO_2} is high).

— Step 3: Multiply the result of step 2 by 0.008. Note that the product may be a positive or negative number because Step 2 may result in a positive or a negative number.

— Step 4: Add the positive or negative product obtained in Step 3 to 7.4. This will result in either the addition of a number to 7.4 or subtraction of a number from 7.4. The resulting number is the pH predicted from the P_{CO_2}. Every 1 mm Hg

uncompensated rise in P_{CO_2} above 40 mm Hg (more hypercarbic) is predicted to make the pH fall by 0.008 (more acidotic).

— Overall, $(40 - P_{CO_2}) \times 0.008 = \pm\Delta$ in pH from 7.4.

■ If the patient's measured pH is higher than the calculated pH, *metabolic alkalosis* must be associated with the hypocarbia or hypercarbia. If the measured pH is lower than the calculated pH, *metabolic acidosis* must be associated with the hypocarbia or hypercarbia.

Example: ABG: pH 7.30, P_{CO_2} 30 mm Hg

■ Perform the calculation steps noted above:

— Step 1: The pH is acidotic (<7.35). You also note that the P_{CO_2} of 30 mm Hg is hypocarbic, so the patient has a respiratory alkalosis.

— Step 2: Subtract the measured P_{CO_2} (30) from 40. The difference is +10.

— Step 3: Multiply the +10 difference from Step 2 by 0.008. The product is + 0.08.

— Step 4: Add the product of step 3 (0.08) to 7.4. This represents the change in pH predicted from the P_{CO_2} alone. Adding + 0.08 to 7.4 yields a predicted pH of 7.48.

■ **Interpretation:** On the basis of the P_{CO_2} level of 30, this patient's predicted pH is 7.48. But this patient's measured pH is 7.30, which is quite acidotic. The conclusion is that the much lower measured pH is due to the presence of a *primary metabolic acidosis*. The respiratory alkalosis represents partial compensation (the pH is still acidotic), so your conclusion is primary metabolic acidosis with partial respiratory compensation.

■ **Compensation in acid-base disturbances:** Why is the patient's P_{CO_2} in the example above less than the normal range of 35 to 45 mm Hg?

— The patient is attempting to compensate for the metabolic acidosis by increased ventilation, or "blowing off CO_2."

— As the CO_2 is "blown off" and the P_{CO_2} falls, the pH rises—what is called a *compensatory respiratory alkalosis*. Provided the patient is alert and has no compromise of the airway, respiratory compensation will be almost immediate.

— If the acidosis were respiratory, the kidneys would attempt to compensate by retaining bicarbonate (a base). Unlike respiratory compensation, which is immediate, metabolic compensation for underlying respiratory acid-base problems takes 8 to 48 hours to occur.

— Note that a compensatory mechanism is terminated when the pH approaches normal. A compensatory mechanism will not "overcorrect" the pH (see "The Overcompensation Rule," below).

■ **Primary respiratory acidosis with compensatory metabolic alkalosis:** A common example of a primary respiratory acid-base disturbance occurs in chronic obstructive pulmonary disease with CO_2 retention (see Case Scenario).

— As the P_{CO_2} rises, the pH falls, leading to a *primary respiratory acidosis*.

— Over time the kidneys will retain extra bicarbonate (HCO_3^-) to neutralize the acid created by the retained CO_2 in an attempt to restore the pH to near-normal.

— This response is called a *compensatory metabolic alkalosis,* or *metabolic compensation.*

■ **Using the measured base deficit or base excess:** Another factor to use in interpreting the acid-base balance from the ABG is the base deficit or base excess. It is normally between −2 and +2.

Case Scenario

Mr B is a 74-year-old, 40-pack-year smoker with advanced chronic obstructive pulmonary disease. He is a known "CO_2 retainer." He presents to the ED with another in a long series of acute exacerbations. He is tachypneic, cyanotic, and obviously struggling to breathe. He becomes more obtunded as he is being examined. A STAT ABG reveals the following results (patient is on 2 L O_2):

pH 7.30, PCO_2 80, PO_2 58, HCO_3^- 38, base excess +12, oxygen saturation 89%

Perform your analysis of the ABG:

- Step 1: First note that the pH is below the normal range, so *acidosis* is present.

Next look at the PCO_2. At 80 it is elevated to twice normal, indicating that respiratory acidosis is present. You know that as PCO_2 rises, the pH falls unless there is metabolic compensation. Now you should determine if there is any compensation.

- Step 2: Subtract the patient's PCO_2 (80 mm Hg) from 40. This yields –40.

- Step 3: Multiply the result of Step 2 (– 40) by 0.008. This yields a product of – 0.32.

- Step 4: Add the result of Step 3 (–0.32) to 7.4. The pH predicted from the PCO_2 of 80 would be 7.08. Because the pH is 7.3 there must be some metabolic compensation for the respiratory acidosis. This metabolic alkalotic compensation is confirmed by the base excess of +12.

- Then note the HCO_3^-. It is elevated to 38 mEq/L (normal: 22 to 32 mEq/L). This finding shows that the patient's kidneys have resorbed excess bicarbonate to compensate for his respiratory acidosis. The sustained resorption of bicarbonate by the kidneys accounts for the base excess of +12. As noted above, this base excess indicates a *metabolic alkalosis*.

- **Interpretation:** The analysis of Mr B's arterial blood gas, then, is *primary respiratory acidosis with compensatory metabolic alkalosis (or primary respiratory acidosis with partial metabolic compensation).*

— If the base deficit is more negative than –2, a *metabolic acidosis* is present (base deficit less than –2 indicates metabolic acidosis).

— If a base excess is more positive than +2, *metabolic alkalosis* is present.

- **The Overcompensation Rule:** An additional useful rule to keep in mind with acid-base disturbances is that *compensatory mechanisms are unlikely to **overcompensate** in acid-base abnormalities.*

— As the pH approaches normal, the compensatory mechanisms "shut off."

— By this rule Mr B's primary problem cannot be a metabolic alkalosis because his pH remained acidotic. His body would not have overcompensated with CO_2 retention to the point of causing an acidosis just to fix a metabolic alkalosis.

— If a patient with chronic respiratory failure presents with an *alkalotic* pH, this does not represent metabolic compensation because a compensatory mechanism for respiratory acidosis will not overcorrect the pH to the alkalotic range. You should look for a condition responsible for a metabolic alkalosis. For example, hypochloremic or hypokalemic metabolic alkalosis can develop in patients with chronic respiratory failure. This can occur during diuretic (eg, furosemide) therapy if the patient does not receive adequate potassium chloride supplementation).

— Keeping this rule in mind, the ACLS provider can determine which is the primary acid-base disturbance and which is the compensatory mechanism.

Anion Gap

- The *anion gap* is another calculated value that can help identify the underlying cause of an acid-base disturbance.

— The number of positive ions in the body (eg, sodium and potassium) should be approximately equal to the number of negative ions (chloride and bicarbonate). But this balance never occurs because there is always a difference (the gap) caused by unmeasured negative ions such as ketones and lactic acid.

— This anion gap quantifies the difference between the serum sodium concentration and the serum chloride plus bicarbonate concentrations:

$$\text{Anion gap} = [Na^+] - ([Cl^-] + [HCO_3^-])$$

Normal anion gap: 10 to 15 mEq/L

- **Interpretation:** With an anion gap in the normal range (12 to 15), any existing acidosis will be due to the negative ions in the equation, chloride and bicarbonate.

— A *normal anion gap acidosis* occurs with diarrhea because a fall in serum bicarbonate is balanced by a rise in serum chloride (hyperchloremic metabolic acidosis).

— With an anion gap that is abnormally high (>15 mEq/L), any existing acidosis is caused by an accumulation of unmeasured negative ions, such as ketones or lactic acid, or a fall in serum bicarbonate that is not balanced by a rise in serum chloride.

— The classic example of a high anion gap acidosis is diabetic ketoacidosis.

Diabetic Ketoacidosis

Pathophysiology

- Diabetic ketoacidosis (DKA) is the most frequent life-threatening acid-base abnormality that ACLS providers will encounter. A relative insulin deficiency is the primary cause of DKA.

- It is important to understand the major abnormalities in the pathophysiology of DKA because these problems define the therapeutic approach:

  — **Hyperglycemia:** Without sufficient insulin, glucose cannot enter the cells, so it reaches higher and higher concentrations in the blood (hyperglycemia). The blood glucose is further elevated by the effects of the hormone *glucagon,* which is released by the liver during insulin deficiency, and catecholamines, which stimulate gluconeogenesis (glucose is made).

  — **Dehydration:** The hyperglycemia causes an osmotic diuresis (polyuria), with excretion of glucose-containing urine (glucosuria). Significant volume can be lost during this osmotic diuresis. This volume loss leads to severe dehydration, worsening acidosis, and hypotension.

  — **Ketoacidosis:** Without intracellular glucose the body begins to metabolize existing lipids (fat stores). These lipids are partially oxidized into free fatty acids and acetoacetic acids. The free fatty acids accumulate and the acetoacetic acid is converted into ketones. These processes result in the development of ketoacidosis. These ketones and free fatty acids account for the high-anion-gap metabolic acidosis invariably present in DKA.

  — **Hypokalemia:** Total body potassium stores decrease during the osmotic diuresis and dehydrating volume loss of DKA. The serum potassium, however, may be normal or even slightly elevated when the patient presents with DKA. *The ketoacidosis (low pH) results in an acute shift of potassium from the intracellular to the extracellular (including the vascular) space. This explains how the serum potassium may be normal or even elevated despite the total body loss of potassium.* During treatment of DKA and correction of the acidosis, the potassium returns to the intracellular space (from the vascular space). This can result in severe hypokalemia if the ACLS provider fails to anticipate the shift and initiate potassium replacement.

Causes of DKA

- Although DKA can develop in patients with insulin-dependent diabetes, it can be the presenting sign of diabetes. If the patient has no history of insulin-dependent diabetes, clinicians can lose valuable time under the mistaken assumption that DKA is a diagnostic impossibility.

  — DKA can be the initial presentation of a person with undiagnosed diabetes. In one study from the 1980s, 20% of all patients admitted for DKA had newly diagnosed diabetes.[40]

  — Furthermore, patients with non–insulin-dependent diabetes may develop insulin dependency that is not recognized until they experience an episode of DKA.[40]

- DKA frequently results when a patient with insulin-dependent diabetes stops or reduces insulin therapy. About 15% of patients with DKA are not taking insulin at the time of emergency presentation.

- The clinical history of many insulin-dependent diabetics qualifies them as "brittle diabetics." The reason for frequent episodes of DKA is unclear: the DKA may develop despite uninterrupted insulin therapy.

- The risk factors for DKA are well known for most patients with insulin-dependent diabetes. One commonly used memory aid for the more common precipitants of DKA is the so-called *6 I's: infection, infarction, ignorance, ischemia, intoxication, and implantation.*

  — *Infection:* Pneumonia and urinary tract infections are the infections that most commonly precipitate an episode of DKA.

  — *Ignorance* (poor understanding of diabetes): Noncompliance with insulin regimens or dietary restrictions, and errors of commission and omission in insulin therapy.

  — *Infarction* (brain): Stroke syndromes, especially those leading to coma, are often associated with rapid deterioration in insulin-dependent diabetics.

  — *Ischemia:* Acute myocardial infarction, with its associated stress and hyperadrenaline state, will often induce DKA.

  — *Intoxication:* Excessive alcohol consumption is a common offender.

  — *Implantation:* This "I" refers to the many complications that diabetic women can experience during pregnancy.

- Signs and symptoms of DKA:

  — The clinical presentation of DKA is highly variable and often non-specific. All healthcare professionals must maintain the stereotypical "high index of suspicion" in emergency settings, especially when an insulin-dependent diabetic presents with virtually any complaint.

  — The most common symptoms associated with DKA are nausea, vomiting, and vague abdominal pain. The widely repeated clinical axiom that *"any GI complaint in an insulin-dependent diabetic is DKA until proven otherwise"* merits both compliance and repetition.

Treatment of DKA

- DKA is a life-threatening condition. The ACLS provider must be able to recognize it and treat it effectively.

- Begin general assessment and therapy following the 5 Quadrads Approach of ACLS:

  - **Airway patency and breathing effectiveness:** If the obtunded patient demonstrates hypoventilation, intubation may be necessary for airway maintenance and protection and for oxygenation and ventilation.

  - **Circulation:** Dehydration and hypovolemia are virtually always present.

  - **Diagnosis:** Initially order a 12-lead ECG, serum electrolytes, ABG, and urinalysis.

  - **Assess vital signs:** Evaluate temperature, blood pressure, heart rate and rhythm, respirations (rate and pattern), and oxygen saturation (on room air and in response to low-flow oxygen).

  - **Oxygen-IV-monitor-fluids:** Provide oxygen, start an IV, attach a cardiac monitor, and initiate fluids.

- The 4 major pathophysiologic abnormalities in DKA provide a helpful way to organize therapy. Providers should address the abnormalities in this order of priority:

  1. Correct dehydration
  2. Correct hypokalemia
  3. Correct hyperglycemia
  4. Correct ketoacidosis

■ Correct Dehydration

1. Administer normal saline (0.9% sodium chloride) IV: Establish IV access with a large-bore catheter and infuse 1 L rapidly; follow with 1 to 2 L over the first and second hours.

2. When volume status is stable, give half-normal saline (0.45% sodium chloride) IV at 150 to 300 mL/h.

3. When serum glucose falls to less than 300 mg/dL, provide dextrose 5% with half-normal saline at 150 to 300 mL/h. This switch to glucose-containing solutions will help prevent the patient from developing hypoglycemia from the IV insulin.

4. Determine the effectiveness of fluid resuscitation by close observation of hourly urine output. Most patients with DKA will require insertion of a urinary catheter.

   - Ideally urine output should be at least 1 mL/kg per hour after the initial fluid resuscitation.

   - If urine output fails to reach this level by the second hour, more aggressive fluid therapy will be needed, provided the patient has normal renal function. Rather than change to half-normal saline, continue with normal saline at higher rates.

■ Correct Hypokalemia

1. Add KCl to the above IV fluids at a rate of 10 to 20 mEq/L. Exceptions will be patients with initial hyperkalemia (>6 mEq/L or with ECG signs of high potassium), patients with renal failure, or patients who are not producing urine as confirmed by hourly urine output.

2. For patients with documented hypokalemia on presentation, add KCl at a rate of 40 mEq per hour (not per liter!).

3. The clinical goal is to maintain potassium levels in the normal range while recognizing 2 major caveats:

   - First, DKA patients have severe depletion of total body potassium stores. Because these patients are severely acidotic, they often initially have a false "normal" potassium (as pH falls, potassium moves from intracellular to extracellular space). A normal serum potassium of 3.6 mEq/L in a patient with DKA is likely to represent severe depletion of total body potassium stores.

   - Second, as therapy corrects the acidosis, the serum potassium will fall because the potassium returns to the intracellular spaces (from the extracellular spaces, including from the vascular space). This shift can lead to life-threatening hypokalemia. ACLS providers should anticipate this shift and start IV potassium therapy early.

   - A historical side note illustrates the importance of these caveats (see "Relevant Research"). Medical historians speculate that literally decades of unnecessary deaths occurred after the discovery of insulin in 1922.[41,42] Until the early 1950s clinicians failed to recognize both that correction of the acidosis in DKA could produce life-threatening hypokalemia and that intravenous therapy with potassium could be life-saving.[42]

■ Treat Hyperglycemia

1. Insulin is needed to help glucose enter the cells. Start with regular insulin 10 U IV push. Then infuse 5 to 10 U/h IV (0.1 U/kg per hour).

2. In terms of treatment priorities, insulin follows initial fluid resuscitation and potassium replacement. The serum potassium should be high enough to prevent hypokalemia (K^+ >3.7 mEq/L) before you initiate the insulin infusion.

3. It is important to reduce the serum glucose concentration gradually. Aim for a gradual reduction of 10% per hour and no faster than 50 to 100 mg/dL per hour.

- If the serum glucose concentration is reduced faster than 100 mg/dL per hour, the fall in serum osmolality may be associated with a shift of free water from the vascular to the interstitial space, with the risk of cerebral edema.

- Remember that severe hyperglycemia increases the serum osmolality and dilutes the serum sodium. As the serum glucose falls, the serum sodium should rise. The risk of cerebral edema is thought to be high if the serum sodium does not rise as the serum glucose concentration falls. For every 100 mg/dL fall in serum glucose, the serum sodium should rise 1.6 mEq/L (see "Cerebral edema," below).

4. Once glucose drops to <300 mg/dL, change fluids to D_5/0.45% sodium chloride. This switch to glucose-containing solutions will help prevent hypoglycemia from the IV insulin.

5. Once insulin therapy begins, further ketone formation should cease, the anion gap should lessen, and bicarbonate should increase. IV insulin infusion should continue until bicarbonate is >15 mEq/L, there is no anion gap, the patient can tolerate oral food and liquids, *and* for about 1 hour after the first dose of subcutaneous insulin.

■ **Correct Ketoacidosis**

1. Bicarbonate administration is *not* routine therapy for DKA. The increase in pH from bicarbonate can be severely deleterious, shifting potassium into cells and producing life-threatening hypokalemia[43,44] and cerebral edema, especially in children.[45,46] In addition, the sodium bicarbonate will increase serum osmolality that is already high from the hyperglycemia.

2. The generally accepted indications for bicarbonate administration in DKA are

   — Hyperkalemia producing ECG changes

   — Severe acidosis: pH <7.1 (some experts recommend no bicarbonate until pH is <7.0)

   — Severe depletion of buffering reserve: bicarbonate <5 mEq/L

   — Shock or coma

   — Acidosis-induced cardiac or pulmonary dysfunction

3. If indicated, administer sodium bicarbonate by adding 50 to 100 mEq to 1 L of 0.45% sodium chloride and infusing the 1 L over 30 to 60 minutes. To avoid hypokalemia, some experts recommend the addition of 10 mEq potassium to the 1 L of 0.45% sodium chloride.

4. If bicarbonate therapy is initiated, do not try to normalize pH. Just raise the pH enough to *get the patient out of trouble.*

The Periarrest Patient With DKA

■ Be particularly alert for the following life-threatening problems in patients with DKA:

   — **Life-threatening cardiac arrhythmias from hypokalemia:** To repeat: *Beware of the false "normal" potassium level in DKA patients as therapy begins.* Volume replacement with normal saline and insulin infusion will begin a rapid shift of potassium into the cells. You should expect that the serum potassium will fall as the serum pH rises.

   — **Life-threatening cardiac arrhythmias from hyperkalemia:** With profound acidosis, potassium can shift outside the cells to such a degree that life-threatening arrhythmias from hyperkalemia may develop before the DKA is treated. In such an event follow the treatment

---

Relevant Research: Recognition of the Importance of Potassium in DKA[42]

The introduction of insulin into clinical medicine made a "dramatic" difference in the mortality resulting from diabetic coma. This is true in the sense that before 1922 DKA was almost uniformly fatal, and even in the 1950s the mortality in many large hospitals was as high as 30% to 50%. Often the autopsy did not establish a cause of death. Many deaths may have been a result of hypokalemia, a complication that was not recognized until 1946. In that year in the *Journal of the American Medical Association,* Jacob Holler described a patient who developed respiratory paralysis 12 hours into treatment. After several hours in an iron lung, the patient was cured by potassium infusion.[41] In the 5 years after Holler's paper there were many reports of deaths resulting from hypokalemia as well as several "near misses," but clinicians were extremely cautious about early replacement, probably because "the frightening effects of IV injections of potassium made clinicians reluctant to believe in a lack of potassium as a cause of trouble, except in very rare conditions such as familial periodic paralysis." It had been known since 1923 that insulin lowered serum potassium, but this was not of great interest because the symptoms of hypokalemia were not known. Also, potassium was not an electrolyte with which clinicians were familiar. Until the introduction of flame photometry in 1950, it was measured only in research studies because chemical methods took several hours to complete.

—*Condensed abstract from Reference[42]*

sequence outlined in Table 5 for hyperkalemia. Generally the patient will require only urgent addition of calcium chloride or calcium gluconate plus sodium bicarbonate since IV insulin and high levels of glucose are already in place.

— **Shock and lactic acidosis** from prolonged dehydration and volume depletion, hypotension, and tissue hypoxia: Suspect these problems in DKA patients who have a persistent anion gap and metabolic acidosis despite appropriate initial therapy. These patients need aggressive fluid resuscitation and, as noted above, some may receive sodium bicarbonate administration.

— **Cerebral edema (osmotic encephalopathy):** The precise mechanism of this complication is not known, but it has been theorized to include rapid correction of hyperglycemia (>100 mg/dL per hour) and a fall in serum osmolality.

- Suspect the development of cerebral edema in patients with DKA who show signs of increasing intracranial pressure, such as headache, altered mental status, or pupil dilation.

- Hyponatremia provides an important clue to imminent overhydration and pending cerebral edema. DKA patients will initially have a low serum sodium concentration, which may be normal in the presence of hyperglycemia.

  ♦ For every increase in serum glucose of 100 mg/dL above 180 mg/dL, the serum sodium concentration will be reduced by 1.6 mEq/L below 135 mEq/L.

  ♦ For this reason you should watch for a matching rise in serum sodium (ie, 1.6 mEq/L rise for every 100 mg/dL fall in serum glucose) as hyperglycemia is corrected.

  ♦ Failure of serum sodium to rise appropriately as the glucose falls, or an actual fall, is a red flag for cerebral edema.

- Urgent CT scanning can establish this diagnosis, which should be treated urgently with IV mannitol.

Nonketotic Hyperosmolar Syndrome

Pathophysiology

- The nonketotic hyperosmolar syndrome (NKHS) is a life-threatening acid-base abnormality that occurs in diabetic patients.[47]

  — DKA occurs predominantly in insulin-dependent (type 1) diabetes mellitus; NKHS occurs almost exclusively in non–insulin-dependent (type 2) diabetes mellitus.

  — NKHS is nonketotic because residual insulin secretion, although insufficient to prevent hyperglycemia, effectively inhibits the breakdown of lipids and the production of free fatty acids and ketones *(ketogenesis)*.

- Other than ketoacidosis, all the pathophysiologic abnormalities of DKA occur with NKHS: hyperglycemia with osmotic diuresis develops, leading to dehydration and volume loss, and depletion of potassium through increased renal output.

Causes

- Most of the same processes that initiate DKA also precipitate NKHS. Patients with NKHS often omit or are unable to take their regular oral antidiabetic agents.

- Other precipitating factors include infection, infarction (stroke), and indiscretions with medications or diet. NKHS often develops in patients who are manifestly ill and debilitated with near-obtundation.

Diagnosis

- Providers should suspect NKHS in any patient who appears to be ill and is known to have type 2 diabetes. Patients

will frequently be severely dehydrated and may be obtunded. The syndrome has often been called "nonketotic hyperosmolar coma" because so many of these patients are unconscious and unresponsive on presentation.

- The laboratory findings are classic and diagnostic:

  — Hyperglycemia, often with blood sugar >600 mg/dL

  — Hyperosmolality, with plasma osmolality >320 mOsm/L

  — Absence of acidosis

  — Absence of ketones in the urine and blood

Treatment

- For the ACLS provider the initial treatment approach for NKHS is the same as the approach for DKA:

  — Volume replacement with normal saline

  — Potassium replacement

  — Treatment of hyperglycemia with insulin

  — Close monitoring of electrolytes and pH (usually lactic acidosis in NKHS rather than ketoacidosis), and response to therapy

The Periarrest Patient With NKHS

- Life-threatening NKHS is most likely to occur in elderly patients with known type 2 diabetes. On presentation these patients are often comatose with severe hypotension or overt shock. The mainstay of treatment for the unstable patient with NKHS is rapid volume replacement and consideration of pressor agents for shock.

- By definition NKHS patients rarely have the ketoacidosis of DKA with the associated intracellular to extracellular shift of potassium, so the patients are not as likely to develop the intracellular potassium shift (and fall in serum potassium) during therapy.[47] For this reason these patients are less prone to the life-threatening cardiac arrhythmias that may develop in patients with DKA.

- The same recommendations noted above for periarrest patients with DKA apply to these NKHS patients. Although cerebral edema can occur in NKHS, it seems to be diagnosed less often. Children with NKHS, like children with DKA, are much more likely than adults to develop cerebral edema during resuscitation.[48,49]

Summary: Electrolyte and Life-Threatening Acid-Base Abnormalities

Electrolyte abnormalities can cause severe physiologic and metabolic derangements, including cardiac arrhythmias and other types of cardiovascular decompensation.

Table 15 provides a quick summary of the associated ECG changes and the treatments recommended in this chapter.

Clinicians should maintain a high index of suspicion for possible electrolyte disturbances. Prompt diagnosis and aggressive treatment can often prevent life-threatening complications.

TABLE 15. Life-Threatening Electrolyte Abnormalities With Associated ECG Findings and Recommended Treatment Approaches

Electrolyte Problem and Normal Range	Associated ECG Findings	Recommended Treatment Approach
Hyperkalemia 3.5 to 5 mEq/L	■ 5.5 to <6: Tall, peaked T waves ■ 6 to <6.5: Prolonged PR interval (first-degree heart block), increase in QT interval ■ 6.5 to <7: Flattened P waves, depressed ST segment ■ 7 to <7.5: Widened QRS complexes ■ 7.5 to <8: Deepening S waves, merging of S and T waves ■ 8 to <10: Sine wave–shaped complexes, idioventricular complexes and rhythms ■ ≥10: PEA (sine wave look), VT/VF, asystole	*Sequence begins with recommendations for the most urgent (arrest) hyperkalemic patient.* **Antagonize effects at cellular level:** ■ *Calcium chloride* 5 to 10 mL IV 10% solution (500 to 1000 mg) **Shift potassium into cells:** ■ *Sodium bicarbonate* 50 mEq (1 ampule) IV bolus or 1 mEq/kg; repeat in 15 min; then 2 ampules (100 mEq) in 1 L D_5W ■ *Regular insulin plus glucose:* 10 U regular insulin IV plus 50 mL D_{50} (25 g) glucose; then 10 to 20 U regular insulin with 500 mL $D_{10}W$ IV over 1 hour PRN ■ *Albuterol* (nebulized) 10 to 20 mg over 15 min; may repeat PRN **Remove potassium from body:** ■ *Furosemide* 40 to 80 mg IV bolus ■ *Kayexalate* 15 to 50 g PO or 50 g PR with sorbitol ■ *Peritoneal dialysis* or *hemodialysis*
Hypokalemia 3.5 to 5 mEq/L	■ 2.5 to 3: Prominent U waves, flattened T waves, low QRS voltage, prominent P waves ■ 2 to <2.5: More prominent U waves, more ST-segment changes ■ <2: QT interval more prolonged, QRS complex widens, wide-complex tachyarrhythmias, VT, VF	**Rough estimates of total body deficits based on serum K:** ■ $[K^+]$ = 3 to <3.5 mEq/L Deficit = 100 to 200 mEq ■ $[K^+]$ = 2.5 to <3 mEq/L Deficit = 200 to 300 mEq ■ $[K^+]$ = 2 to <2.5 mEq/L Deficit = 300 to 400 mEq **Maximum peripheral IV concentration:** KCl approximately 40 mEq in 1 L NS **Maximum rate:** KCl approximately 40 mEq total in 1 h **Cardiac arrest (maximum limit):** ■ Infuse KCl IV at 2 mEq/min for 10 min (20 mEq) ■ Follow with KCl at 1 mEq/min for 10 min (10 mEq)

Electrolyte Problem and Normal Range	Associated ECG Findings	Recommended Treatment Approach
Hypernatremia 135 to 145 mEq/L	■ Expect sinus tachycardia in these volume-depleted patients ■ Otherwise hypernatremia produces no diagnostic ECG findings	**Estimate total body water deficit:** ■ Water deficit (in L) $$= \frac{([Na^+]_{measured} - 140)}{140} \times (0.6_{men} \text{ or } 0.5_{women}) \times weight_{in\ kg}$$ ■ Replace water deficit with 0.9% or 0.45% sodium chloride (normal or half-normal saline) at a rate that reduces $[Na^+]$ no faster than 0.5 to 1 mEq/L per hour and no more than approximately 12 mEq/L in first 24 h **Cardiac arrest:** ■ Rapid fluid replacement: NS 500 mL "wide open"; evaluate response; repeat every 20 to 30 min until stable
Hyponatremia 135 to 145 mEq/L	May have sinus tachycardia if volume depleted. Otherwise hyponatremia produces no diagnostic ECG findings. **Steps for use of 3% saline:** 1. Calculate total Na deficit (in mEq): $([Na^+]_{desired} - [Na^+]_{measured}) \times TBW_{in\ L}$ $TBW_{in\ L} = (0.6_{men} \text{ or } 0.5_{women}) \times Weight_{in\ kg}$ 2. Calculate volume of 3% saline needed to reduce Na deficit by 4 mEq/L over 4 hours (3% saline = 513 mEq/L) 3. Give calculated volume at rate to increase Na by 1 to 4 mEq/L per hour (correction at rate of 2-4 mEq/L per hour is reserved for patients with severe neurologic symptoms or ongoing seizures)	**If hypervolemic or with SIADH:** ■ Restrict water ■ Consider furosemide diuresis **If normovolemic:** ■ Restrict water ■ Identify and treat underlying abnormality **If hypovolemic:** ■ Replace volume with NS **Limit Na correction rate (unless symptomatic):** ■ To approximately 0.5 mEq/L per hour ■ To maximum of approximately 12 mEq/L in first 24 h **Cardiac arrest (seizures, coma, arrest):** ■ Use 3% saline IV (see steps for use of 3% saline)

(Continued on next page)

TABLE 15. Continued

Electrolyte Problem and Normal Range	Associated ECG Findings	Recommended Treatment Approach
Hypercalcemia Total calcium: 8.5 to 10.5 mg/dL Ionized calcium: 4.2 to 4.8 mg/dL	■ Key: Markedly shortened QT intervals ■ Prolonged PR and QRS intervals ■ Decreased automaticity ■ Shortened and depressed ST segments ■ Flattening and widening of T waves ■ Bundle branch blocks may occur ■ AV block; may progress to complete heart block and cardiac arrest (usually with levels >15-20 mg/dL)	*Total calcium 12 to <15 mg/dL:* Treat if symptomatic *Total calcium >15 mg/dL:* Treat whether symptomatic or not **Restore volume:** ■ Infuse NS at 300 to 500 mL/h until fluid deficit is replaced ■ Decrease rate to 100 to 200 mL/h with restoration **Increase renal calcium excretion:** ■ Induce diuresis (see above) ■ Consider furosemide 1 mg/kg IV every 2 to 4 h ■ Consider empiric Mg (up to 15 mg/h) administration ■ Consider empiric K (up to 10 mEq/h) administration **Cardiac arrest:** ■ Rapid fluid replacement: NS 500 mL "wide open"; evaluate response; repeat every 20 to 30 min until patient is hemodynamically stable ■ Magnesium sulfate 1 to 2 g IV push ■ Consider KCl 1 to 2 mEq/min (may be administered empirically in patients with hypercalcemia and cardiac arrest) ■ Diuretics
Hypocalcemia Total calcium: 8.5 to 10.5 mg/dL Ionized calcium: 4.2 to 4.8 mg/dL	■ Prolonged QT interval due to prolonged ST segment ■ Terminal T-wave inversion ■ May experience VT or torsades de pointes ■ Bradycardias, heart block	**Urgent treatment (symptomatic hypocalcemia):** ■ Calcium gluconate 10 to 30 mL of 10% solution IV over 10 min or ■ Calcium chloride 5 to 10 mL of 10% solution IV over 10 min **Cardiac arrest:** ■ Calcium gluconate 10 to 20 mL of 10% solution over 1 to 3 min (may give up to 30 mL in periarrest) or ■ Calcium chloride 10 mL of 10% solution over 1 to 3 min
Hypermagnesemia 1.3 to 2.2 mEq/L	■ Increased PR and QT intervals ■ Increased QRS duration ■ Decrease in P-wave voltage ■ Some degree of T-wave peaking ■ Complete AV block ■ Asystole	*Sequence begins with recommendations for the most urgent (arrest) hypermagnesemic patient:* **Antagonize effects at cellular level:** ■ Calcium gluconate 10 mL of 10% solution IV over 1 to 3 min or ■ Calcium chloride 5 to 10 mL of 10% solution IV over 1 to 3 min ■ Repeat calcium every 5 to 10 min until stable **Remove magnesium from body:** ■ Induce saline diuresis: NS 500 mL/h IV ■ Furosemide 1 mg/kg IV bolus
Hypomagnesemia 1.3 to 2.2 mEq/L	■ Prolonged PR and QT intervals ■ Wide QRS complexes ■ ST depression ■ Broad, flat T waves with precordial T-wave inversion ■ Torsades de pointes	**Noncardiac arrest:** ■ Magnesium sulfate 1 to 2 g IV over 5 to 10 min ■ Follow initial 1 to 2 g with 6 g in next 24 h **Cardiac arrest:** ■ Magnesium sulfate up to 2 g IV push over 1 to 2 min

References

1. Jackson MA, Lodwick R, Hutchinson SG. Hyperkalaemic cardiac arrest successfully treated with peritoneal dialysis. *BMJ*. 1996; 312:1289-1290.

2. Voelckel W, Kroesen G. Unexpected return of cardiac action after termination of cardiopulmonary resuscitation. *Resuscitation*. 1996;32: 27-29.

3. Niemann JT, Cairns CB. Hyperkalemia and ionized hypocalcemia during cardiac arrest and resuscitation: possible culprits for post-countershock arrhythmias? *Ann Emerg Med*. 1999;34:1-7.

4. Allon M. Hyperkalemia in end-stage renal disease: mechanisms and management. *J Am Soc Nephrol*. 1995;6:1134-1142.

5. Lin JL, Lim PS, Leu ML, Huang CC. Outcomes of severe hyperkalemia in cardiopulmonary resuscitation with concomitant hemodialysis. *Intensive Care Med*. 1994;20:287-290.

6. Allon M, Shanklin N. Effect of bicarbonate administration on plasma potassium in dialysis patients: interactions with insulin and albuterol. *Am J Kidney Dis*. 1996;28:508-514.

7. Wang P, Clausen T. Treatment of attacks in hyperkalaemic familial periodic paralysis by inhalation of salbutamol. *Lancet*. 1976;1: 221-223.

8. Allon M, Dunlay R, Copkney C. Nebulized albuterol for acute hyperkalemia in patients on hemodialysis. *Ann Intern Med*. 1989;110: 426-429.

9. Mandelberg A, Krupnik Z, Houri S, Smetana S, Gilad E, Matas Z, Priel IE. Salbutamol metered-dose inhaler with spacer for hyperkalemia: how fast? How safe? *Chest*. 1999; 115:617-622.

10. Montoliu J, Lens XM, Revert L. Potassium-lowering effect of albuterol for hyperkalemia in renal failure. *Arch Intern Med*. 1987;147: 713-717.

11. Paltiel O, Salakhov E, Ronen I, Berg D, Israeli A. Management of severe hypokalemia in hospitalized patients: a study of quality of care based on computerized databases. *Arch Intern Med*. 2001;161:1089-1095.

12. Higham PD, Adams PC, Murray A, Campbell RW. Plasma potassium, serum magnesium and ventricular fibrillation: a prospective study. *Q J Med*. 1993;86:609-617.

13. Gennari FJ. Hypokalemia. *N Engl J Med*. 1998;339:451-458.

14. Schulman M, Narins RG. Hypokalemia and cardiovascular disease. *Am J Cardiol*. 1990; 65:4E-9E.

15. Mehler PS. Eating disorders. *N Engl J Med*. 1999;341:614-615.

16. Chin RL. Laxative-induced hypokalemia. *Ann Emerg Med*. 1998;32:517-518.

17. Eisele JW, Reay DT. Deaths related to coffee enemas. *JAMA*. 1980;244:1608-1609.

18. Brayley J, Jones J. Life-threatening hypokalemia associated with excessive licorice ingestion. *Am J Psychiatry*. 1994;151:617-618.

19. Famularo G, Corsi FM, Giacanelli M. Iatrogenic worsening of hypokalemia and neuromuscular paralysis associated with the use of glucose solutions for potassium replacement in a young woman with licorice intoxication and furosemide abuse. *Acad Emerg Med*. 1999;6:960-964.

20. Blachley JD, Knochel JP. Tobacco chewer's hypokalemia: licorice revisited. *N Engl J Med*. 1980;302:784-785.

21. Conn JW, Rovner DR, Cohen EL. Licorice-induced pseudoaldosteronism: hypertension, hypokalemia, aldosteronopenia, and suppressed plasma renin activity. *JAMA*. 1968;205:492-496.

22. Adrogue HJ, Madias NE. Aiding fluid prescription for the dysnatremias. *Intensive Care Med*. 1997;23:309-316.

23. Fraser CL, Arieff AI. Epidemiology, pathophysiology, and management of hyponatremic encephalopathy. *Am J Med*. 1997;102:67-77.

24. Gross P, Reimann D, Henschkowski J, Damian M. Treatment of severe hyponatremia: conventional and novel aspects. *J Am Soc Nephrol*. 2001;12(suppl 17):S10-S14.

25. Menashe G, Borer A, Gilad J, Horowitz J. Rhabdomyolysis after correction of severe hyponatremia. *Am J Emerg Med*. 2000;18: 229-230.

26. Soupart A, Decaux G. Therapeutic recommendations for management of severe hyponatremia: current concepts on pathogenesis and prevention of neurologic complications. *Clin Nephrol*. 1996;46:149-169.

27. Laureno R, Karp BI. Myelinolysis after correction of hyponatremia. *Ann Intern Med*. 1997;126:57-62.

28. Gross P, Reimann D, Neidel J, Doke C, Prospert F, Decaux G, Verbalis J, Schrier RW. The treatment of severe hyponatremia. *Kidney Int Suppl*. 1998;64:S6-S11.

29. Brunner JE, Redmond JM, Haggar AM, Kruger DF, Elias SB. Central pontine myelinolysis and pontine lesions after rapid correction of hyponatremia: a prospective magnetic resonance imaging study. *Ann Neurol*. 1990;27: 61-66.

30. Ayus JC, Krothapalli RK, Arieff AI. Treatment of symptomatic hyponatremia and its relation to brain damage: a prospective study. *N Engl J Med*. 1987;317:1190-1195.

31. Anderson RJ, Chung HM, Kluge R, Schrier RW. Hyponatremia: a prospective analysis of its epidemiology and the pathogenetic role of vasopressin. *Ann Intern Med*. 1985;102: 164-168.

32. Schrier RW. Treatment of hyponatremia. *N Engl J Med*. 1985;312:1121-1123.

33. Adrogue HJ, Madias NE. Hyponatremia. *N Engl J Med*. 2000;342:1581-1589.

34. Miller M. Syndromes of excess antidiuretic hormone release. *Crit Care Clin*. 2001;17: 11-23, v.

35. Ayus JC, Arieff AI. Chronic hyponatremic encephalopathy in postmenopausal women: association of therapies with morbidity and mortality. *JAMA*. 1999;281:2299-2304.

36. Knochel JP. Hypoxia is the cause of brain damage in hyponatremia. *JAMA*. 1999;281: 2342-2343.

37. Barri YM, Knochel JP. Hypercalcemia and electrolyte disturbances in malignancy. *Hematol Oncol Clin North Am*. 1996;10: 775-790.

38. Milionis HJ, Alexandrides GE, Liberopoulos EN, Bairaktari ET, Goudevenos J, Elisaf MS. Hypomagnesemia and concurrent acid-base and electrolyte abnormalities in patients with congestive heart failure. *Eur J Heart Fail*. 2002;4:167-173.

39. Navarro-Gonzalez JF. Magnesium in dialysis patients: serum levels and clinical implications. *Clin Nephrol*. 1998;49:373-378.

40. Faich GA, Fishbein HA, Ellis SE. The epidemiology of diabetic acidosis: a population-based study. *Am J Epidemiol*. 1983;117: 551-558.

41. Holler JW. Potassium deficiency occurring during the treatment of diabetic acidosis. *JAMA*. 1946;131:1186-1189.

42. Tattersall RB. A paper which changed clinical practice (slowly): Jacob Holler on potassium deficiency in diabetic acidosis (1946). *Diabet Med*. 1999;16:978-984.

43. Viallon A, Zeni F, Lafond P, Venet C, Tardy B, Page Y, Bertrand JC. Does bicarbonate therapy improve the management of severe diabetic ketoacidosis? *Crit Care Med*. 1999; 27:2690-2693.

44. Kannan CR. Bicarbonate therapy in the management of severe diabetic ketoacidosis. *Crit Care Med*. 1999;27:2833-2834.

45. Glaser N, Barnett P, McCaslin I, Nelson D, Trainor J, Louie J, Kaufman F, Quayle K, Roback M, Malley R, Kuppermann N. Risk factors for cerebral edema in children with diabetic ketoacidosis. The Pediatric Emergency Medicine Collaborative Research Committee of the American Academy of Pediatrics. *N Engl J Med*. 2001;344:264-269.

46. Dunger DB, Edge JA. Predicting cerebral edema during diabetic ketoacidosis. *N Engl J Med*. 2001;344:302-303.

47. Magee MF, Bhatt BA. Management of decompensated diabetes: diabetic ketoacidosis and hyperglycemic hyperosmolar syndrome. *Crit Care Clin*. 2001;17:75-106.

48. Gottschalk ME, Ros SP, Zeller WP. The emergency management of hyperglycemic-hyperosmolar nonketotic coma in the pediatric patient. *Pediatr Emerg Care*. 1996;12:48-51.

49. Ellis EN. Concepts of fluid therapy in diabetic ketoacidosis and hyperosmolar hyperglycemic nonketotic coma. *Pediatr Clin North Am*. 1990;37:313-321.